The LAF Surveys

What we learned about the causes and treatment of lone atrial fibrillation

BY

HANS R. LARSEN MSc ChE

FOREWORD BY:

Dr. Patrick Chambers MD

PUBLISHED BY:

INTERNATIONAL HEALTH NEWS

www.yourhealthbase.com

The LAF Surveys
Published by:

International Health News
1320 Point Street
Victoria BC
Canada V8S 1A5
(250) 384-2524
E-mail: editor@yourhealthbase.com
www.yourhealthbase.com

Also by Hans Larsen

Lone Atrial Fibrillation: Towards a Cure [2015]
Thrombosis and Stroke Prevention {2018]

The LAF Surveys
Contents

This book is dedicated to my wife Judi without whose help and encouragement it would never have been completed.

I would also like to extend my heartfelt [in normal sinus rhythm] thanks to the hundreds of afibbers whose participation in the LAF surveys made the book possible.

Foreword

Atrial fibrillation has long been viewed as emblematic of an aging heart. In most professional circles it is ALWAYS the sequelae of some form of heart disease. Anything that backs up the plumbing and puts stress on the left atrium, such as congestive heart failure, heart attack, hypertension, mitral valve disease, ..., often results in atrial fibrillation. In other words it is ALWAYS pathologic.

However, in recent years an entity called lone atrial fibrillation (LAF) has struggled to gain acceptance. Even now many cardiologists refer to it as "so-called LAF", denigrating its legitimacy. Many still treat it with digitalis even though this has been shown to exacerbate LAF episodes. Others refuse to accept the demonstrated differences in age, body type, autonomic tone, stroke risk, ... in those afflicted with LAF vs pathologic AF.

Mainstream medicine is quite slow to adapt to our changing environment. Professional American medical societies (AMA, American College of Cardiology, ...) are the last to embrace/endorse new, rational, and successful approaches to the treatment of disease. Part of this is due to a conservative Hippocratic approach ("First do no harm") but a growing part is due to Big Pharma. No company is going to make the big bucks if MDs are recommending increased magnesium/potassium intake and exercise when statins and weight loss drugs are so readily available. Patients have slowly been programmed to believe that technology is the ultimate solution. We have become lazy and entitled.

Everything must be "evidence based" and that means a prospective, randomized double-blind, placebo-controlled study, which is very expensive. Common sense and simple observation are irrelevant. Instead MDs are duped by studies that tout relative benefit and ignore absolute benefit or studies that compare a favored drug over the competition at a suboptimal dose. As Mark Twain so eloquently stated "There are three kinds of lies: lies, damned lies, and statistics."

And even if a study comparing a non-pharmaceutical approach were to be done, it would be suppressed. For example, all local practitioners recommend a flu vaccine every year for the elderly. Yet the number needed to treat or NNT to avoid one case of the flu is 40 for the vaccine but only 33 for Vitamin D supplementation.

The practice of medicine has become more high powered and expensive. But we have lost something in the transition. For LAF this book contains that something. It is for those both willing to step off the conveyer belt of traditional medicine and sufficiently curious to explore alternative approaches to LAF, the unwelcome visitor. I know because I was on that conveyor belt until the unwelcome visitor made an unexpected appearance. While this book promotes the alternative approach, it also discusses the pros and cons of pharmaceutical drug therapy and

1

recognizes and appropriately recommends ablation in specific and comprehensive detail.

Here you will find the distilled summary of accumulated knowledge from an extensive data base. Several peer-reviewed articles based on the surveys have appeared in the medical literature. You will not find such an exhaustive compilation in a single source.

The surveys clearly demonstrate that LAF is by no means an "old age" disease. The average age at diagnosis is 48 years. LAF strikes its victims at the most productive time of their lives and can wreak havoc with work, relationships, and leisure activities. On the positive side – it would appear that lone afibbers are substantially less likely to have diabetes or hypertension.

Among the more intriguing findings uncovered in the surveys is evidence that LAF may be inherited and that having undergone tonsillectomy in adolescence may be associated with a substantial increase in the risk of developing LAF later in life.

Perhaps the most important contribution of Hans' book is the descriptions of protocols used by more than 100 lone afibbers to eliminate their afib episodes without ablation or surgery.

Hans Larsen is a Professional Engineer and holds a Master's degree in Chemical Engineering from the Technical University of Denmark. He developed a lifelong interest in biochemistry and nutrition through his early studies with Professor Henrik Dam, the Nobel Prize-winning discoverer of vitamin K.

Hans has devoted much of his life to expanding our practical knowledge of the causes and treatment of lone atrial fibrillation. He has written no less than eight books, six of which address LAF. He has advised eternally grateful celebrities.

Although I am no celebrity, I am also eternally grateful for his help in overcoming this persistent malady.

Patrick Chambers, MD
Laboratory Director, Torrance Memorial Medical Center, retired

P.S. Although there are lots of tables and charts, the writing style is very straightforward and analyses are easily digested.

Patrick Chambers received his baccalaureate degree from Princeton University in Mathematics in 1971 followed shortly thereafter by completion of medical studies at the University of California at Davis. He completed his specialty training in pathology at the Los Angeles County/University of Southern California Medical Center. After more than 25 years as a practicing pathologist and laboratory director at Torrance Memorial Medical Center he retired to Kailua, Hawaii.

Introduction

I was diagnosed with **lone** atrial fibrillation [LAF] in December 1989. During the first 5 years of my afib journey I experienced only a couple of episodes a year but during 1998 I experienced 23 episodes lasting an average of 11 hours each. It was then that I started to do some serious research into my condition and in late 2000 I decided to share my research with the readers of my monthly newsletter "International Health News" in a separate newsletter named "The Afib Report". The first issue was published on my new website [afibbers.org] in January 2001.

I began my search for a cure or at least a viable treatment option for lone atrial fibrillation by reading all the literature I could find on the subject. As it turned out, medical science did not have a lot to say about it. Essentially, LAF was treated with drugs that had not been specifically designed for LAF and therefore often had a very poor benefit: risk ratio. The options of catheter ablation and maze surgery had just appeared on the horizon, but were yet too new to be seriously considered.

Having been involved in major scientific research projects during most of my career I decided that the first step on the "road to victory" would have to be to determine the "nature of the beast" and find the answers to questions like:

- Why do some people get LAF while others don't?
- Why do some afibbers have frequent and severe episodes while others get off pretty lightly?
- Are there afibbers who have overcome their condition without drugs or surgery and, if so, how did they do it?

In order to find answers to these questions 18 surveys [LAF Surveys} were carried out between 2001 and 1013. Please note that I have not attempted to consolidate the responses from the surveys, but rather have discussed the most important of them in chronological order so as to maintain the excitement involved in gradually "building up the case".

Although much of the information in the book may appear "dated" there is no reason to believe that triggers for afib, natural protocols for preventing afib, or the general characteristics of afibbers have changed; however, it is clear that great improvements have been made in the fields of catheter ablation and cardiothoracic surgery since the last survey in 2013.

The surveys clearly reveal that LAF is by no means an "old age" disease (average age at diagnosis is 48 years) and that 80% of its victims are male. The surveys establish which drugs are optimal and which drugs should be shunned by LAF patients. The importance of supplements, particularly magnesium, is thoroughly investigated and protocols used by over 100 LAF patients who have managed to eliminate their afib episodes without ablation or surgery are described. The latest survey presents data for over 1000 catheter ablations and maze procedures and draws clear conclusions regarding the factors affecting success and failure of these procedures.

I coined and use throughout the book the terms "afib" and "afibbers" in order to provide less doom-laden terms to describe **lone** atrial fibrillation and patients with lone atrial fibrillation. Although LAF can be extremely debilitating it is, on its own, not life-threatening and does not increase the risk of suffering an ischemic stroke. Thus it is quite a different condition from the much more common atrial fibrillation associated with heart disease and a substantially increased risk of stroke.

The original definition of LAF was:

Lone atrial fibrillation (LAF) – atrial fibrillation in the absence of structural heart disease (aortic or mitral valve defects, atrial septal defect, and other cardiac structural defects).

It was well recognized that LAF as such did not confer an increased risk of ischemic stroke and anticoagulation was not recommended unless the patient had at least two risk factors [age above 75 years, hypertension, diabetes, congestive heart failure] or had suffered a previous stroke or TIA.

Over the years the definition of afib [lone atrial fibrillation] has been gradually tightened to exclude most atrial fibrillation patients from the **lone** category by requiring the absence of conditions that previously were considered **risk factors** for LAF-related stroke:

Lone atrial fibrillation (2014) – Age less than 60 years and absence of clinical and echocardiographic evidence of cardiopulmonary disease, including hypertension and diabetes [1].

The *2014 AHA/ACC/HRS Guideline* recommends against using the term **lone** atrial fibrillation altogether. It also recommends that all atrial fibrillation patients with a CHA$_2$DS$_2$-VASc stroke risk score of 2 or greater should be anticoagulated. This means that all atrial fibrillation patients 75 years old or older should be prescribed anticoagulants and that all AF patients 65 years or older should be prescribed anticoagulants if they have just one risk factor such as hypertension or diabetes. [1]

This distinction is important in that the information contained in this book is based on the original definition of lone atrial fibrillation and the associated less stringent requirement for anticoagulation.

1. January CT, et al. 2014 ACC/AHA/HRS Guideline for the Management of Patients with Atrial Fibrillation. Journal of the American College of Cardiology, Vol. 64, No. 21, 2014.

Hans R. Larsen MSc ChE
Victoria, BC, Canada, April 2020

What is Atrial Fibrillation?

Atrial fibrillation involves a chaotic movement of electrical impulses across the atria and leads to a loss of synchrony between the atria and the ventricles. Once an episode has begun the atria may quiver or fibrillate at a rate as high as 300 to 600 times per minute. This causes a very inefficient filling and emptying of the atria; the chaos is transferred to the ventricles causing them to lose their regular rhythm and begin to contract fast and in a totally irregular manner. This is what gives rise to the fast and irregular pulse rate felt during an AF episode (90-160 beats/minute).

Atrial fibrillation in itself is not a disease, but rather a symptom of some other disorder of the body. Coronary heart disease, heart attack, heart surgery, valvular heart disease, hypoglycemia, electrolyte imbalances, hyperthyroidism, pheochromocytoma, strenuous exercise, binge drinking, consumption of tyramine-containing foods, and exposure to emotional or physical stress can all trigger atrial fibrillation. Recent research has found that an inflammation of the heart lining (myocardium) is often involved in atrial fibrillation.

Most cases of atrial fibrillation involve heart disease or an abnormality of the heart. However, between 12 and 30% of all cases do not involve an underlying heart problem. These cases are classified as *lone atrial fibrillation* (LAF). It should be kept in mind that the validity of the diagnosis is highly dependent on the quality and quantity of the tests done to rule out underlying heart problems. Just recently researchers at the Cleveland Clinic confirmed that inflammation, presumably of the heart lining, is frequently present in patients who have been diagnosed as having LAF [1].

Lone atrial fibrillation (LAF) is characterized by the absence of detectable structural heart abnormalities and heart disease. This means that LAF is not life-threatening and is less likely to precipitate a stroke than is atrial fibrillation involving heart problems.

It is likely that LAF only develops when three conditions are met:

1. The autonomic nervous system is dysfunctional
2. The heart tissue is abnormally sensitive and capable of being triggered into and sustaining an afib episode
3. A trigger or precipitating cause capable of initiating an afib episode is present.

An abnormally sensitive heart tissue, if triggered, becomes a source of premature atrial complexes (PACs) that, if frequent enough, may run together to create atrial fibrillation. Individual heart cells are capable of "beating" on their own outside the control of the autonomic system. Sometimes agglomerations of very active cells form and create a focus for so-called ectopic or premature beats (beats originating outside the sino-atrial node). The junctions between the left atrium and the pulmonary veins are particularly popular spots for these "rogue" cell agglomerations and some arrhythmias can be successfully treated by removing or isolating them through ablation or the maze procedure.

German researchers have confirmed that most atrial fibrillation episodes are preceded by a series of premature atrial beats (PACs). They analyzed 297 AF episodes in 33 patients and found that the PACs originated in the left atrium in 77.5% of the episodes. The frequency of PACs increased from an average of 0.8 PACs per minute to 4.1 per minute in the two minutes preceding the onset of an episode [2].

Lone atrial fibrillation is a chronic disorder like diabetes or arthritis rather than an acute disorder like the flu or a bout of pneumonia. It comes in three "flavours" – *paroxysmal, persistent*, and *permanent*. Paroxysmal AF converts to normal sinus rhythm on its own and episodes last less than 7 days (most less than 24 hours); persistent AF episodes last more than 7 days, but cardioversion is effective in conversion to normal sinus rhythm; permanent LAF is permanent and does not respond to cardioversion.

It is possible, but probably rare, to have just one episode of LAF. Far more common is the paroxysmal (intermittent) form of LAF. The frequency and duration of episodes vary greatly, but generally increase with age and the number of years the disorder has been present. In some cases LAF becomes permanent, that is, the irregular, rapid heartbeat becomes a constant companion.

Violent palpitations, breathlessness, dizziness and frequent urination are common features of LAF episodes. Many LAF patients suffer greatly during their episodes while others have no symptoms at all and are diagnosed only by chance through a routine electrocardiogram.

Dr. Philippe Coumel of the Lariboisiere Hospital in Paris discovered in 1982 that a dysfunction of the autonomic nervous system plays a major role in LAF. He found that there are two varieties of paroxysmal LAF, an *adrenergic* form and a *vagal* form [3, 4].

Adrenergic type LAF is intimately connected with an over-active sympathetic (adrenergic) nervous system and is primarily found in older people. Episodes occur almost exclusively during daytime and are often preceded by exercise or emotional stress. This type of LAF can also be a symptom of hyperthyroidism or pheochromocytoma. Some cardiologists feel that adrenergic type LAF may involve some sort of unrecognized heart abnormality.

Vagal type LAF is associated with an overactive parasympathetic (vagal) nervous system and is often observed in athletes and people with digestive problems. It is most common among men aged 40 to 50 years. The commonest feature is that of weekly episodes, lasting from a few minutes to several hours. The essential feature is the occurrence of episodes at night, often ending in the morning. Rest, digestive periods (particularly after dinner), and alcohol consumption are also predisposing factors. Exercise or emotional stress does not trigger the arrhythmia. On the contrary, on feeling the sensation of an oncoming episode (repeated atrial premature beats), many patients have observed that they can prevent an episode by exercising, but the relaxation period that follows an effort or an emotional stress frequently coincides with the onset of vagal LAF. There is no indication that vagal LAF involves any heart abnormality and vagal LAF rarely if ever develops into a permanent condition.

Some LAF patients experience both vagal and adrenergic episodes and are classified as having a mixed variety of LAF.

Frequent urination (every 20 minutes or so) often occurs during the early phase of an episode and is due to the release of atrial natriuretic peptide from the fibrillating atria.

1. Chung, Mina K., et al. C-reactive protein elevation in patients with atrial arrhythmias: inflammatory mechanisms and persistence of atrial fibrillation. Circulation, Vol. 104, December 11, 2001, pp. 2886-91
2. Kolb, C., et al. Modes of initiation of paroxysmal atrial fibrillation from analysis of spontaneously occurring episodes using a 12-lead Holter monitoring system. American Journal of Cardiology, Vol. 88, No. 8, October 15, 2001, pp. 853-57
3. Coumel, Philippe. Paroxysmal atrial fibrillation: a disorder of autonomic tone? European Heart Journal, Vol. 15, suppl A, April 1994, pp. 9-16
4. Coumel, Philippe. The role of the autonomic nervous system in atrial flutter and fibrillation, chapter 6. In Atrial Flutter and Fibrillation: From Basic to Clinical Applications, edited by N. Saoudi, et al. Armonk, NY, Future Publishing, 1998

Definition of Terms

- Paroxysmal – Episodes occurring intermittently and tending to terminate spontaneously - usually within 48 hours.
- Persistent – Episodes lasting longer than 7 days and not terminating spontaneously, but can be terminated with chemical or electrical cardioversion.
- Permanent – Constant (chronic, 24/7) afib not amenable to effective termination by cardioversion.
- Adrenergic – Episodes occurring almost exclusively during daytime, often in connection with exercise or emotional or work-related stress.
- Vagal – Episodes tending to occur during rest, at night or after a meal. Alcohol and cold drinks are common triggers.
- Mixed (random) – Episodes occur anytime and do not consistently fit the adrenergic or vagal pattern.

Catheter Ablation and Maze Procedures

- Focal ablation – The original radiofrequency (RF) ablation procedure in which specific active foci of aberrant impulses are located and ablated.
- Pulmonary vein ablation (PVA) – An ablation procedure in which a ring of scar tissue is placed just inside the pulmonary veins where they enter the left atrium. The original PVA carries a high risk of pulmonary vein stenosis, so it is rarely used in this form anymore. Thus, the term PVA is now associated with ablation around the pulmonary veins when a more specific description (SPVI, CAPVI or PVAI) is not provided by the EP or the exact type of PVA is not known by the respondent.
- Pulmonary vein isolation (PVI) – An ablation procedure, also known as ostial ablation, in which a ring of lesions is placed on the left atrium wall such as to encircle each pulmonary vein. This procedure reduces the risk of stenosis since the scar tissue is created in the atrium wall rather than inside the pulmonary veins themselves
- Segmental pulmonary vein isolation (SPVI or Haissaguerre procedure) – In this procedure electrophysiological mapping (using a multipolar Lasso catheter) is used to locate the pathways taken by aberrant impulses from the pulmonary veins and these pathways are then eliminated by ablation around the veins approximately 5 to 10 mm from the ostium of the veins.
- Pulmonary vein antrum isolation (PVAI or Natale procedure) – This procedure is a variant of the SPVI procedure. It involves locating aberrant pathways through electrophysiological mapping (using a multipolar Lasso catheter) and ablating these pathways guided by an ultrasound (ICE) catheter. The ablation is performed as close as possible to the outside edge (antrum) of the junction between the pulmonary veins and the atrial wall. All four pulmonary veins as well

as the superior vena cava (if indicated) are isolated during the procedure.

- Circumferential anatomical pulmonary vein isolation (CAPVI or Pappone procedure) – In this procedure anatomical mapping (CARTO) is used to establish the exact location of the pulmonary veins. Two rings of lesions are then created in the left atrium - one completely encircling the left pulmonary veins and another completely encircling the right pulmonary veins; the two rings are usually joined by a linear lesion.

- All three variants of the PVI procedure may be followed by focal ablations involving other areas of the atrium wall or creation of linear lesions in order to eliminate sources of afib located outside the pulmonary veins.

- Right atrial flutter ablation – This procedure involves the application of radiofrequency energy to create a block of the cavotricuspid isthmus in the right atrium so as to interrupt the flutter circuit. A right atrial flutter ablation is usually successful in eliminating the flutter, but rarely helps eliminate atrial fibrillation and may even, in some cases, initiate the development of atrial fibrillation.

- Left atrial flutter ablation – Left atrial flutter is a common complication of ablation for atrial fibrillation. It most often resolves on its own, but if not it may be necessary to re-enter the left atrium, locate the offending circuit, and block it via radiofrequency catheter ablation.

- Cryoablation – In this procedure a nitrogen-cooled or argon-cooled, rather than electrically-heated, catheter is used to create the ablation lesions.

- Maze procedure – The original surgical procedure, the full maze or Cox procedure, used a cut-and-sew protocol for creating lesions forming a "maze" that conducts the electrical impulse from the SA to the AV node, while at the same time interrupting any "rogue" circuits. The cut-and-sew method has now largely been replaced by the use of RF-powered devices, but cryosurgery, microwave application, and high-intensity focused ultrasound (HIFU) have all been tried as well and are preferred by some surgeons. Creating the full set of maze lesions usually requires open-heart surgery and the use of a heart/lung machine.

- Mini-maze procedure – The so-called mini-maze procedure also involves lesions on the outside of the heart wall, but access to the heart is through incisions between the ribs rather than via open-heart surgery. The mini-maze may involve the creation of the full maze set of lesions, but usually focuses on pulmonary vein isolation. The procedure does not involve the use of a heart/lung machine and lesions are usually created by the application of RF energy or cryoenergy.

- AV node ablation – This ablation approach aims at eliminating the effects of fibrillation in the atria on ventricular performance by isolating the AV node [the ventricular beat controller] from any extraneous impulses and feed it its "marching orders" from an implanted pacemaker.

Statistical Terms

- N – The number of respondents in a sample.
- Mean – The average value for a group of data, i.e. the sum of the values of all data points divided by the number of data points.
- Median – The value in the middle of a group of data, i.e. the value above which half of all individual values can be found and below which the remaining 50% can be found.
- Statistical significance – In this study average values are considered different if the probability of the difference arising by chance is less than 5 in 100 using the two-tailed t-test. This is expressed as "p" [probability] being equal to 0.5 or less. Lower values of p are indicative of a greater certainty that observed differences are truly significant..

Definition of Success

- Complete success – No afib episodes, no antiarrhythmics, consistent sinus rhythm (success score=10)
- Partial success – No afib episodes, but on antiarrhythmics to maintain consistent sinus rhythm (success score=5)
- Failure – Afib episodes still occurring with or without the use of antiarrhythmics (success score=0)
- Blanking period – The first 6 months following the final procedure
- Index period – The last 6 months of the 12-month period following the final procedure for the purpose of curing afib
- Initially successful – No afib episodes and no antiarrhythmics during the index period.
- Uncertain – Cases where insufficient data is available or where less than 3 months has gone by since the procedure and afib episodes are still occurring.

Catheter Ablation and Surgery

The procedures used to cure atrial fibrillation can be divided into two groups: – catheterization procedures and surgical procedures. Both types involve the creation of lesions on the heart wall (right and/or left atrium) in order to stop the propagation of impulses not involved in conducting the heart beat "signal" directly from the sino-atrial (SA) node to the atrio-ventricular (AV) node.

Catheterization procedures create the lesions from the inside via an ablation catheter threaded through the femoral vein and are performed by electrophysiologists (EPs). Surgical procedures create the lesions from the outside and access is either through incisions between the ribs or may involve open-heart surgery and the use of a heart/lung machine. Surgical procedures are carried out by cardiothoracic surgeons.

The overwhelming majority of catheterization procedures use radiofrequency (RF) energy to create the lesions, but some EPs prefer the use of nitrogen-cooled catheters (cryoablation) rather than RF-powered ones due to their reduced risk of creating pulmonary vein stenosis.

The original surgical procedure, the full maze or Cox procedure, used a cut-and-sew protocol for creating lesions forming a "maze" that conducted the electrical impulse from the SA to the AV node, while at the same time interrupting any "rogue" circuits. The cut and sew method has now largely been replaced by the use of RF-powered devices, but cryosurgery, microwave application, and high-intensity focused ultrasound (HIFU) have all been tried as well and are preferred by some surgeons.

The so-called mini-maze procedure also involves lesions on the outside of the heart wall, but access to the heart is through incisions between the ribs rather than via open-heart surgery. The mini-maze may involve the creation of the full maze set of lesions, but usually focuses on pulmonary vein isolation. The procedure does not involve the use of a heart/lung machine.

Most of the rogue electrical impulses that create afib originate in the area where the pulmonary veins join the left atrium. Thus, all catheterization procedures aimed at curing afib involve electrical isolation of the pulmonary veins from the left atrium wall. Depending on the origin of the afib, catheterization procedures may also involve ablations of the superior vena cava and coronary sinus (thoracic veins), linear ablation of the left atrial roof, and a standard cavotricuspid isthmus (right flutter) ablation.

2001 General Survey

By Hans R. Larsen [2001]

Demographics and General Background

A total of 50 afibbers completed the initial parts of this our first LAF survey. Of these 40 were men over the age of 30 years, 3 were men younger than 30 years, and 7 were women. The average age of the whole group was 54 years (range 18-82 years). The average age of the older men was 54 years with 83% of this group being between the ages of 45 and 65 years. The average age of the younger men was 25 years, and the average age of the women was 64 years. Overall 62% of all respondents were between the ages of 45 and 65 years.

The members of our afib group tended to be tall with an average height of 6 feet (183 cm) for the older men, 6 ft. 2 in. (187 cm) for the younger men, and 5 ft. 6 in. (168 cm) for the women. Weight tended to be within normal ranges with an average weight among men of 185 lbs (84 kg) and among women of 150 lbs (69 kg). The average weight for women decreased to 138 lbs (63 kg) when one overweight woman was excluded.

Body mass index (BMI) averaged out at 25 (25 for older men and 24 for both women and younger men). However, there were still a significant number of overweight men in the over 40-age group. Fifty per cent had a body mass index over 25 and 3 or 7.5% had a BMI over 30 thus being classified as obese. In comparison, a recent survey of over 17,000 US army personnel concluded that 54% of these young (75% under the age of 35) supposedly fit people were overweight and 6.2% were obese [1].

The average pulse rate among respondents was 61 bpm (range 45-92), the resting systolic pressure 132 mm Hg (range 98-146), and the resting diastolic pressure 76 mm Hg (range 62-89). Only 7% of respondents were taking medications for hypertension.

The survey respondents are a highly educated group and include 3 MDs, 3 PhDs, 12 people with master's degrees, 13 with bachelor's degrees, and 13 with a college degree or at least some college education. In other words, 88% has at least a college education.

The largest percentage (28%) of respondents is retired. This group is closely followed by engineers/scientists at 24%, people involved in business at 22%, lawyers at 8% and MDs at 4%. Perhaps the most interesting conclusion is that 98% of all respondents are, or before retirement were, involved in brainwork.

Interesting observations, but not really conclusive. These demographic data may characterize a group prone to afib, but then again, they may also characterize a group with ready access to the Internet who is motivated to find a solution to their health problems.

The question about "dominant personality" is an interesting one. It is obvious that a fair amount of soul-searching took place before answering it – and even so, the spouse's opinion often carried the day! About 74% of all respondents described themselves as aggressive (tense, up-tight) or ambitious (competitive, tenacious). About 28% (33% among the men over 40) described themselves as being easily upset (sensitive) and 32% as being laid-back (easy-going, calm). Another 14% saw themselves as workaholics (driven, hardworking) and 12% were energetic (enthusiastic, restless). Twelve per cent felt one of their main characteristics was that they were friendly, caring, people persons.

So it is certainly not obvious that afibbers are characterized by one particular personality trait. While 74% say they are aggressive or ambitious, 60% are laid-back and easily upset. Please note that many respondents listed more than one trait so the percentages do not add up to 100. Assigning respondents to personality types indicate that 41% are type A (aggressive, ambitious), 22% are type B (calm, laid-back) with the remaining 37% being a mixture of the two types.

Over 50% (54%) of all respondents had never smoked; 34% were former smokers and 12% were occasional smokers at this time. So LAF cannot be blamed on the weed!

Most respondents, 74% to be exact, had received a diagnosis of paroxysmal (intermittent) lone atrial fibrillation [LAF]. Ten per cent had permanent LAF and the remaining 16% had been diagnosed with LAF, but had some additional risk factors, most commonly high blood pressure.

A full 44% reported digestive problems and many felt that there was a correlation between these problems (bloating, belching, reflux, etc.) and their LAF episodes.

In general respondents were healthy with only 36% reporting other disorders than LAF. Anxiety, asthma, and high cholesterol were most prevalent. Only 17% were taking pharmaceutical drugs for disorders other than LAF.

The average number of years that respondents had suffered from LAF was 8. However, the range was wide. Among older men the range was 1 to 40 years, among younger men 1 to 14 years, and among women 2 to 64 years. Leaving out one woman who had had LAF from childhood (64 years) the range for women changes to 2 to 13 years and the average to 5 years. I guess this data shows that one can live a long time with LAF and, unless we come up with a viable solution, we just may have to!

Triggers and Episode Characteristics

Triggers

Most survey participants have a vivid memory of their first LAF episode. The most common trigger of that first one was emotional or work-related stress (26%) closely followed by physical overexertion at 24%. Caffeine, alcohol, and ice-cold drinks were next at 10%, 6% and 8% respectively. Other less common triggers were severe illness or a viral infection (experienced by 6% of respondents), dehydration (4%), and rest (4%). Digestive periods, coughing and burping, pharmaceutical drugs, surgery, electromagnetic radiation, and toxic chemicals round off the list of initial triggers with 2% (1 respondent) each.

The triggers of subsequent episodes follow in the footsteps of the first one. The overwhelming favorite for the title of most important trigger is emotional or work-related stress. A full 50% of all respondents listed stress as a trigger. Physical overexertion was next at 24% closely followed by alcohol (including wine) and rest at 22% each. The digestive period following a heavy meal was a trigger for 18%, caffeine was mentioned by 16%, and an ice-cold drink by 12%. Ten per cent reported that MSG (monosodium glutamate) was a trigger for them and 6% said that lying on the left side would set off an episode. Aspartame (NutraSweet) was mentioned as a trigger by two respondents (4%) as was chocolate, coughing and burping, and flying (at high altitudes). Three men over 30 years of age (6%) felt that their episodes were cyclical in nature and not related to any specific trigger. Other triggers mentioned were aged cheese, sugar, food additives, acid indigestion, a hot bath, NyQuil (a cold remedy), electromagnetic radiation, toxic chemicals, hypoglycemia, high blood pressure, and changes in weather patterns. Please note that the percentages do not add up to 100 because many respondents listed more than one trigger.

The triggers uncovered in the LAF survey are similar to those found by James Driscoll in his on-line survey (www.dialsolutions.com/af/database/stats.html). In James' survey based on 105 entries stress again was the clear "winner" followed by alcohol, caffeine, exercises, fatigue, and rest and resting after exercise. Cold drinks, MSG, chocolate, bending over or lying on the left side were other important triggers.

It is clear that the triggers for LAF are many and varied and highly specific to each individual except for excessive emotional and physical stress which is pretty well universal.

Amalgam fillings

Seventy-four per cent of all respondents had amalgam fillings in their teeth – an average of 10 fillings each. A preliminary look at the data shows that afibbers without amalgam fillings tended to have significantly fewer episodes than afibbers with amalgams (2 episodes versus 18 episodes over the past 6 months). This is indeed an intriguing clue and will be investigated further.

Most respondents (70%) had not had their amalgams replaced; 10% had done so and 6% were in the process of doing so. The remaining 14% did not have any to replace. Of the 5 who had had their amalgams replaced 3 followed up with a proper detoxification program. Here are their answers to the question: "Have you noticed any difference in the frequency of episodes?"

- Yes, four to one improvement.
- I would guess the frequency was reduced by about a third. So even though I know I am sensitive to mercury it was not the whole answer for me.
- No, my real relief came with the removal of large varicose veins from my left leg that were affecting my circulation because of blood pooling in the leg.

Forty-six per cent of respondents had dissimilar metals in their mouth and 46% did not. The remaining 8% did not know whether they had or not. It is interesting that 4 out of the 5 respondents with permanent afib did have dissimilar metals in their mouth. There was no significant difference in episode frequency between respondents with dissimilar metals and those without.

Hypoglycemia
A quarter of all respondents have hypoglycemia (low blood sugar) and another 24% have symptoms of hypoglycemia. About half the ones having diagnosed hypoglycemia felt that there was a definite correlation between a hypoglycemia episode and a LAF episode. This, in a way, is good news as it is fairly simple to quickly abort a hypoglycemic episode.

Common symptoms of hypoglycemia are:

- craving for sweets;
- irritability or weakness if meal is missed;
- dizziness when standing up suddenly;
- heart palpitations;
- afternoon fatigue; tiredness an hour or so after eating;
- depression and mood swings.

Hypoglycemia is formally diagnosed through a 3-hour or, better yet, a 6-hour glucose tolerance test. Basically if your fasting glucose level is below 50 mg/dL or if your glucose level 4 to 6 hours after a meal falls below the fasting value you have hypoglycemia. However, the actual blood glucose level that causes hypoglycemic reactions can vary considerably between individuals.

Hypoglycemia has been implicated in such diverse conditions as criminal behaviour, premenstrual syndrome, migraine headaches, atherosclerosis, and atrial fibrillation.

Hypoglycemia is best controlled by religiously avoiding foods with a high glycemic index (sugar, white and whole grain bread, bananas, raisins, potatoes, rice, and wheat cereal) and by eating frequent small meals throughout the day. Alcohol should also be avoided and the intake of dietary fiber increased. A daily multivitamin (and minerals) capsule is very important and a minimum intake of 200-400 micrograms/day of chromium is essential.

A hypoglycemia-induced LAF episode can often be aborted by quickly consuming a "power bar" or a high glycemic index food like bananas or raisins. It is best to follow up with a snack of low glycemic index food (apple, orange, raw carrot or some nuts) in order to avoid a "yo-yo" effect. Hypoglycemia is relatively easy to keep in check and doing so may significantly reduce the number of LAF episodes.

Episode characteristics
Most (56%) could feel an episode coming on. This again is good news as they may have enough time to abort the event by getting up and exercising (vagal) or taking a beta-blocker (adrenergic). Almost 90% experience ectopic (premature) heart beats from time to time and 70% of those felt there is a correlation between ectopic beats and a LAF event.

The most common side effect of a LAF episode is fatigue which is felt by 63% of all respondents. This is followed by dizziness (33%), anxiety or fear (17%), shortness of breath (11%), increased urination frequency (11%), nausea (9%), and tightness across the chest (9%). Seventeen per cent reported no side effects at all. Please note that the percentages do not add up to 100 as many respondents reported more than one symptom.

The maximum pulse rate during an episode ranged from 60 to 260 bpm with an average of 145. The minimum rate was between 35 and 100 bpm with an average of 72.

Most people with intermittent (paroxysmal) LAF did not go to the hospital or emergency clinic when experiencing an episode. The remaining 13% did go to the hospital with about half of them receiving cardioversion. Interestingly, only two of the six respondents who did go to the hospital felt that this helped to convert to sinus rhythm quicker.

The frequency and duration of individual episodes varied considerably among survey participants. The average number of episodes over the past 12 months was 27 (30 for men over 30 years, 6 for men under 30, and 21 for women). The range was 0 to 200 episodes and 5 out of the 50 respondents had permanent LAF.

The average number of episodes for the past 6 months was 16 (18 for men over 30 years, 2 for men under 30, and 11 for women) with a range of 0 to 125. The episodes lasted an average of 30 hours (35 hours for men over 30, 14 hours for men under 30, and 13 hours for women) with a range of a couple of minutes to over 500 hours.

The average total time spent in fibrillation over the past 6 months [**afib burden**] worked out to 172 hours (203 hours for men over 30, 29 hours for men under 30, and 71 hours for women). The average length of the longest episode was 387 hours (455 hours for men over 30, 16 hours for men under 30, and 187 hours for women). All told the average time spent in fibrillation over the past 180 days (ignoring permanent LAF) worked out to about 4% or about 1 day (24 hours) per month. The range varied widely from 0 to 17%.

The most "popular" time for an episode to start was between 6 PM and midnight (38% of all episodes) followed by the period between midnight and 8 AM (32%). Episodes were rarest in the morning (8 AM to noon) at 13% and a little more common between noon and 6 PM at 17%. This would indicate that about 32% of all episodes are of a purely vagal nature, 13% are probably purely adrenergic, and the remaining 55% could be either adrenergic or vagal. They are most likely vagal if they occur after lying down or during a digestive period.

Afib effect on quality of life
The time to recover fully from an episode varied from a few minutes to two weeks with an average time of 32 hours. About 13% of all respondents did not feel that having LAF had affected their quality of life. Forty-two per cent felt they had been moderately affected and 17% felt their life had been severely affected if not devastated. Here are some of the more poignant comments from the survey:

- "Basically it has, over the last 30 years, changed my life. While I look at it as a life lesson(s) - HA! I really do not have any other option. It concerns me to the extent that you never know when an episode will occur – while it is not that frequent – I still know that it could happen anytime or anywhere. It has and will have input on travelling, activities etc. It is just a limitation on my system – and one that I have to understand – or it will remind ME!!! I guess it's like having a 30-year electrical short in your car and not being able to find it!! It does influence where you take it and where you park it. I have always looked on life as a glass half full – so in all honesty, while afib is my albatross, it has taught me a lot about myself that I never would have learned. So, for that reason, I am very thankful. You learn to play with the cards that the dealer gives you!!"
- "I'm nervous travelling, I drink much less, I have completely changed my eating patterns, I get depressed easily, I have quit my job - apart from that, not much!! On the other hand, I've had to re-evaluate what matters in life, slow down, and learn to accept the unfairness and try to reach a state of calm."
- "It has wrecked my love of racquetball because I'm afraid I am going to have an attack while I play since the meds don't feel like they hold any more like they used to. I am leery of travel now until I find out what stage I am at."
- "LAF has had an enormous effect on my life. I am anxious about travelling and making any kind of arrangement in advance."
- "I was once a very active long distance runner and bicyclist. I have had to curtail those activities. I have been far less active physically in the past 2 years – inhibited mainly by LAF."

> - "Causes restrictions in planning too far ahead, increases food cravings during episodes (because of stomach "butterflies", etc.). I am prematurely retired and feel constrained from taking on any work commitments. When the attacks occur, I strongly feel the symptoms and the irregular beats and this generates depression and negative outlooks for the future."
> - "Very badly affected. I used to play a lot of sports and be very active physically, but I can't even swing a golf club for 30 minutes now without going into AF. I don't eat out much now and my social life and travel have been dramatically reduced."

Prevention and Treatment

Preventing and terminating episodes

Fifty percent of survey respondents did not know how to abort an episode. Others have had some limited success in stopping an episode before it takes hold, but there certainly does not seem to be any one sure-fire way of aborting one. Following are some of the comments received on this subject:

- Sometimes deep breathing appears to avoid onset.
- On two occasions I may have shortened the episode by drinking a teaspoon of Epsom salt in a glass of water.
- I think maybe taking atenolol may be helping abort episodes.
- I try to calm down and very carefully clear my throat and get the tickling feeling out of my throat and I seem to recover. I also drink water and take a small Ativan (tranquillizer).
- Valsalva and I/V magnesium infusion following by vigorous exercise.
- Walking, changing position in bed to the right side has worked sometimes.
- I lie down and listen to calming music. I have a special CD that works, but only after my heart beats crazy for a few hours. It doesn't work right away after an episode begins.
- Sometimes with ectopic beats I do a Valsalva type maneuver and the odd beats go away.
- Sometimes getting up and moving works if I have been lying down and feel premature beats coming.
- I am not on a regular administration of any anti-arrhythmic drugs, but I sometimes take sotalol (40-80 mg) when I feel an episode coming on. Since my pulmonary vein ablation on 12/1/00 I have been increasingly fibrillation-free. I have had no episodes for 40 days at this writing.
- No reliable way, but sometimes it helps to take 12.5 or 25 mg of atenolol (Tenormin).
- Celery juice (thanks to a posting on your site) seems to stave episodes sometimes, but not every time.

- I can sometimes delay the onset if I raise my heart beat (by running up a flight of stairs when I have the first ectopic beats) but I'll be in AF within an hour or so.
- Once the episode starts I have found that exercise 24 hrs later ends it; this does not work if the attack was precipitated by exercise.
- I used to be able to stop an episode with extra CoQ10, L-carnitine and Mg.
- During the day, standing up immediately and moving around. Sometimes in doing this, I will burp, which relieves pressure, which aborts the episode.
- Yes, stopped it with verapamil.
- Rapid beats stopped by using the Valsalva maneuver.
- I take a quick bite out of a 10 mg propranolol tablet that is always in my pocket, and let it dissolve under my tongue. It seems very effective, almost always works.
- I was a permanent afibber and the only thing that helped me was to take a Xanax because I used to get anxiety and panic attacks along with the afib that didn't help the afib.
- Rest and breathe slowly and deliberately.
- Yes, I do some deep breathing (yoga) exercises focusing particularly on the exhaling, really squeezing the midriff.
- Burping and compressing have worked quite often for me.
- Sit down, loosen clothing, start deep breathing/biofeedback, take an aspirin and I usually convert in 15- 20 minutes.

Prevention with supplements

Most respondents (78%) used supplements. Almost 18% thought they definitely helped, but the majority (63%) was not sure whether they helped or not. The most popular supplements were:

Supplement	Users – Percentage of Total Respondents	Percentage of Users Reporting Benefits
Magnesium	70%	86%
Multivitamins	60%	57%
Vitamin C	53%	57%
Vitamin E	50%	71%
Coenzyme Q10	43%	43%
Fish oil	40%	100%
Calcium	25%	-
Potassium	23%	-
B-complex	20%	43%
Selenium	18%	43%
Hawthorn	13%	-
L-carnitine	13%	-
Vitamin B12	13%	-

Overall 39% supplemented with fish oil (tissue oil) and 4% with cod liver oil. This is encouraging as fish oil has been found to help prevent arrhythmias, heart attacks, angina, and sudden cardiac death. There is also evidence that eating fish or supplementing with fish oils (eicosapentaenoic acid and docosahexaenoic acid) help prevent breast and prostate cancer. For more information on the benefits of fish oil see www.oilofpisces.com.

Only 10% of respondents had had their intracellular magnesium level measured. All (100%) were found to have levels below the normal range. Seven respondents (14%) had had magnesium infusions. Three had felt a definite benefit, 3 some improvement, and only 1 reported no improvement; however, this person did not know if his magnesium level was low to begin with.

Prevention with pharmaceutical drugs
Sixty-four per cent (of paroxysmal afibbers) took one or more pharmaceutical drugs to prevent future LAF episodes. The most widely used drugs were:

Drug	Percentage Use
Atenolol [Tenormin]	21%
Other Beta-blockers	25%
Flecainide [Tambocor]	18%
Sotalol [Betapace]	14%
Propafenone [Rythmol]	11%
Verapamil	7%
Digoxin [Lanoxin]	7%

About half of the drug users had side effects with the most common symptoms being fatigue (25%) and dizziness (11%).

A preliminary comparison of the number of episodes experienced by afibbers on preventive drugs and afibbers who took no drugs showed that drug users tended to have more episodes (23 versus 19 average over 6 months) than did non-drug users. The episodes were similar in duration. At first glance this seems rather improbable; that preventive drugs would actually make things worse. However, taking a closer look at the prescription pattern it becomes clear why this could indeed be the case. Over 70% of afibbers with the vagal variety were prescribed drugs that are known to worsen their condition (digoxin and beta-blockers).

The most popular drug used to speed conversion to sinus rhythm was flecainide (Tambocor) which was used by 12% (either at home or in hospital). However, most people (53%) just rested or otherwise waited out the episode. Seven per cent found light exercise to be beneficial and 5% found sexual intercourse to shorten a long episode. One respondent was able to terminate a hypoglycemia-related episode within 5 minutes by eating a "power bar".

Atenolol (Tenormin) was used by 22% to slow down the heart rate during an episode followed by verapamil at 13%, propafenone (Rythmol) at 9%, and sotalol (Betapace) at 7%. Forty-eight per cent of all respondents did not use any drugs for slowing down the rate.

Stroke prevention
Most (39%) took a daily aspirin to help prevent a stroke. Another 20% took Coumadin (warfarin) on a regular basis. Twelve per cent used fish oil or cod liver oil specifically for stroke prevention, 4% used ginkgo biloba while 8% took an aspirin only at the beginning of an episode. Actually as blood clots are more likely to be released after an episode ends and particularly if it lasts more than 24 hours it is advisable to continue with the aspirin for a week or two after a long episode. The remaining 17% took no specific precautions against stroke.

The original recommendations for anti-thrombotic therapy for people with lone atrial fibrillation and no risk factors were [2001 ACC/AHA/ESC Guidelines for the Management of Patients with Atrial Fibrillation]:

- age under 60 and no heart disease – no therapy or aspirin if desired;
- age between 60 and 75 and no risk factors – daily aspirin;
- age over 75 years – warfarin (Coumadin) if no contraindication.

Afibbers with risk factors such as rheumatic heart disease, prior stroke, heart failure, echo systolic dysfunction, diabetes or hypertension are advised to use warfarin at all ages. Warfarin is also prescribed for 3 weeks before and 3 weeks after attempted cardioversion.

Ninety per cent of respondents reported no adverse effects from their stroke prevention regimen and some had been on it for 10 years or more.

Catheter ablation and maze surgery
Six out of 53 respondents (11%) had had either RF ablation or maze surgery to eliminate LAF. One maze procedure was deemed entirely successful with no further episodes for two years. Two RF ablations were deemed successful with no episodes for 2 and 16 months respectively after surgery. One RF ablation prevented episodes for 8-10 months and was then followed by maze surgery, but it is too early to say if this was successful. One RF procedure was definitely not successful and one was done very recently so it is too early to tell. So at this point it really is not clear whether ablation or surgery is worthwhile. The success rate is probably highly dependent on the skill of the surgeon and the location of the misfiring cells. However, new techniques, especially for ablation, are constantly developing so hopefully the picture will become clearer within the next year or so.

Thirty per cent of the remaining respondents had considered ablation or surgery, but not proceeded with this option. Four had had an electrophysiology study (EPS) with the results that there was nothing to ablate. Only three of all respondents had considered implantation of a defibrillator and none had proceeded with this option.

Relaxation and exercise

Twelve out of 50 respondents (24%) reported that they were doing yoga or other relaxation exercises. Ten (83%) felt a definite benefit while 2 were not sure if they benefited. Thirteen reported praying or meditating on a regular basis and 77% found it helpful while 15% found it somewhat helpful. Seven (14%) of respondents had tried Traditional Chinese Medicine and 5 had found it helpful or somewhat promising.

Thirty-six per cent of respondents jogged or ran daily, 31% walked daily, and 14% had a daily workout or engaged in swimming or golf on a regular basis. Only 7% did not exercise at all and 12% did very strenuous exercise on a regular basis. There was not a great deal of difference in the exercise pattern before and after the first LAF episode except that the proportion of strenuous exercisers dropped from 31% to 12%. Most (45%) considered themselves strongly athletic, 19% thought they were athletic, and 31% somewhat athletic. Only 5% considered themselves to be sedentary.

The Exercise Connection

Long-term endurance training (vigorous regular exercise) profoundly affects the body's physiology. Among other things it significantly lowers the heart rate and testosterone levels [2, 3]. It is also known that, while exercise in the short term increases adrenergic tone (activates sympathetic nervous system), its long-term effect is an increase in vagal tone (predominant parasympathetic system) [4, 5].

Most vagal type afibbers are heavy exercisers. This raises the tantalizing possibility that they might actually be able to reduce their number of episodes by cutting back on exercise. A recent study carried out in Spain found that "detraining", i.e. cessation or reduction in exercise resulted in profound changes. Blood volume decreased, heart rate increased, and adrenergic tone increased after 2 to 4 weeks without training [6].

One of the members of our group has actually observed that giving up on exercise one week out of every four significantly reduced his frequency of episodes.

Of course, abruptly stopping all exercise carries with it a whole new set of problems so a gradual approach is definitely in order. Might be worth experimenting with if you are a vagal afibber!

Respondents' approach to reducing episode frequency

Adrenergic afibbers

- Haven't really found a way, except avoid known triggers.
- Avoiding emotional stress, late nights and strenuous physical activity, and of course, alcohol, coffee, chocolate, and sweets.

Mixed afibbers

- Reducing stressful situations.
- I mainly rely on medications (flecainide and atenolol) to limit the frequency of attacks as well as controlling the stress levels as much as possible. Food intake is another factor.
- If I work out only 3 out of every four weeks of the month it seemed to go away for 6 months. Prior to that it went away for a year.
- For me the key thing was having surgical removal of large varicose veins in my left leg. Only one episode since last July when I had the surgery, and it came when I over-exercised, stood too long, and ate too much - all in the same afternoon.

Vagal afibbers

- Maintain a background of flecainide - it has completely eliminated my attacks.
- Try to keep in touch with my emotions. Understand the flow of "energy" (overwork, getting too intense, diet, not eating when nervous, limiting my exposure to crowds, etc.) that I know occurs in my external and internal worlds that causes this thing.
- I mostly live my life as usual, merely avoiding hard alcohol and keeping up my supplements.
- Eat carefully, avoid constipation and practice relaxation.
- Meditation/diet/exercise/positive outlook.
- Removing amalgams under strictest protocol.
- Eat smaller meals, calm down and avoid caffeine and aspartame.
- Learn your triggers and avoid them.
- Not to drink alcohol and get overtired. Don't eat big meals and nothing after 5 pm.
- I take a beta-blocker (metropolol) before a known stressful event. I believe magnesium helps.
- Taking digestive enzymes.
- Taking verapamil and generally relaxing more.
- Stay calm, eat every 2-3 hours, and don't get overtired.
- Deep breathing exercises and getting off digoxin.
- Trying to eliminate the production of gas in my chest.

Respondents' approach to regaining normal sinus rhythm

- Lie down and try and relax.
- 200 mg of flecainide
- The most successful has been indulging in sex. This has worked almost every time except if I have just gone into an episode. Then, it seems nothing will work, but on the average sex will work 7 times out of 10. (Editor's note: Indulging in sex has also been found effective in terminating permanent hiccups).
- I only have one – wait it out!
- Prior to maze, taking atenolol every few hours until I converted.

- Most recently – shock!! I would prefer to find a different approach that would work. The shock returns normal rhythm, but since I have a very sensitive nervous system I am concerned about the overall effect.
- Exercising to my tolerance seems to help. Otherwise waiting it out.
- Taking things easy (exercise hasn't helped me), taking an extra verapamil (doctor said OK), taking Epsom salt in water.
- I converted when I totally relaxed, gave up worrying about it - plus I think my body took over.
- I rely on medications (flecainide and atenolol) to regain normal sinus rhythm.
- Atenolol
- Gentle exercise
- Staying on low-carbohydrate diet to minimize insulin resistance and adrenaline surge.
- Cardioversion is certainly the quickest, I prefer spontaneous but apparently can't always count on it.
- Go about with mundane tasks and put it out of your mind as much as you can.
- Trying to relax - stay in bed - the less active I am when in AF in general the shorter the episode will be.
- Exercise or Rythmol
- Shower, bowel movement, or just time. I have a good friend who is an E&P tech for a major medical institution and he is convinced that these are chaotic events. He believes in the "chaos" theory.
- I take a Xanax (anti-anxiety medication) and go to sleep.
- Possibly the deep breathing exercises.

Respondents' advice to fellow afibbers

- I know this is hard but learn to live with it. Try not to become too apprehensive during episodes. You know they will eventually pass.
- Yes, the answer will come from OUR PRESSURE. I would URGE everyone who has regular, predictable sessions accompanied with the BIG PEE SYNDROME, to try their utmost to get their doctors to cooperate in a testing program through the cycle. Testing changing levels of electrolytes in blood and effluent, changes in ECGs, etc., as one GOES THROUGH THE CYCLE FROM THE BEGINNING OF AF TO WHERE SINUS IS RESTORED. Something is happening. The answer is to be found in the changes that are taking place. But the stumbling block is the total unwillingness of the medical people to listen to patients. They trust their pharmaceutical approach, and nothing else is to be even considered.
- Try flecainide, 50 mg twice a day...nothing else.
- Although quite frightening sometimes I believe it to be not too serious a condition.
- Read everything you can, avoid known triggers, consider the maze surgery if medications are failing (none of them do any good to the rest of your system).

- Remember it is not life threatening; keep notes and try to identify triggers; keep up the electrolyte supplements – magnesium, calcium, potassium.
- Find the most experienced electrophysiologist familiar with LAF and if your heart is otherwise structurally normal get it done (ablation).
- Presently, I do not know any – but if I did, it would be to first relax; it is not (at least in my case) a life- threatening disease and there are hundreds, if not thousands, of worse problems a person could have. Every time I have to go to the emergency room I thank God that I have only afib! Next, try to get to understand your system(s) and what circumstances initiate your own afib episodes. Try to understand its pattern(s) and what is happening inside your body to cause these changes. I like to use the following metaphor: for some reason my nervous system is wired with #14 wire and the breaker fuse is 15 amps. While this meets code and can withstand "normal" day-to-day loads it will break when more load is put on this circuit. My "breaker" surfaces in the sinus node where it is diagnosed as afib. I believe the same type of "overloading" occurs in other people with a low tolerance wiring system, but they are diagnosed as having migraine headaches, etc. It is hard for some people to understand our low tolerance system because their system is wired with #12 wire (with a 20-amp fuse!). We all have also met individuals who have 100-amp systems – but I won't go into that!!! Learn to recognize what is plugged into your system – that raises the amperage - and learn to unplug things before adding more!!
- Knowing yourself is so very important; e.g. if you are a type A blood type your natural wiring system is already running a few amps – with nothing plugged in!!! There are so many cultural, social, external, factors, as well as some, which we may not even be consciously aware of, that can and will "load the system". The list of these factors is almost unending. I believe that each individual only has to listen to his or her system and most of these factors will be obvious.
- Last and probably the most important is how you deal with present situations. And that you really understand how each – no matter how little or big the situation – can affect your nervous system. They do (at least in my case) have an accumulative effect. I try to keep in touch with myself and to sense when my "bank" deposits are getting low – but this is recognizably very hard, especially when the individual (as I find myself) is very creative and intense and tends at times to get involved "in the process". I find the best thing I can do is to have an "automatic" investment plan – yoga, meditation, a good diet, etc.
- To me, afib is basically an internal imbalance of energy; when I exceed the edge I have afib and in my case (at least the last few times) only an equal surge of energy - cardioversion - can get it back into balance.
- Maybe there's more to this mind and body thing than we thought.... try not to get obsessive about it (I'm working hard to ignore my heartbeat!).... Keep it in perspective.... don't let it rule your life!

- Have mercury testing done. I found mine to be high. Maybe there is a connection. I am having my amalgams removed and plan to detoxify.
- Keep a positive outlook and MEDITATE - find a spiritual path.
- The antiarrhythmic medication I am taking has some potentially dangerous side effects. Given the opportunity again, I am not so sure I would rely on these dangerous medications to control the LAF.
- Get rid of mercury under the strictest of protocols. Control anxiety with yoga/Qigong. Hang in there!
- Be prepared to do whatever you have to to get rid of this terrible condition. Know your own body and respond to its demands. If you feel you need to get fixed and you can't wait and don't want to wait then thank The Lord there is the maze procedure. If you want to give the ablation a shot then go to the best in the country where they are doing dozens of them every week and they have the latest technology and mapping equipment. I will take the offensive if things get worse.
- Take antioxidants, (2) Do not eat meat but eat fish instead, (3) Eat vegetables, fruits, soy products and avoid dairy products, (4) read the following: The Antioxidant Miracle by Lester Packer, PhD (John Wiley & Sons, Inc.); The Total Guide to a Healthy Heart by Seth J Baum M.D. (Kensington Publishing Corp. 1999); Heart Healthy Magnesium by James B. Pierce, PhD (1994 Avery Publishing Group).
- Learn as much you can, learn your triggers by keeping notes, avoid triggers by changing lifestyle, do not panic and run to the emergency room at first sign (not a medical opinion), share your condition with others in the AF Forum. Seek asecond opinion from another doctor about any procedure or drugs.
- Remain calm, pray to God and do anything at all that is reasonable such as talk to friends, etc. in order to take your mind off the AF. I ONLY revert during the time my mind has been deflected from myself and the anxiety of being in AF. Remain hopeful that a non-maze cure for AF is not far away (possibly one of the new ablation procedures). By the way, I am skeptical of the evidence so far advanced that purports to show that removal of amalgams will cure AF.
- Avoid digoxin as long as condition is LONE afib and intermittent!
- Investigate the latest forms of RF ablation.
- Make a log of your episodes - the time of day, the activity, and the length. Next time you see your cardiologist hand it in - he'll be delighted. Try to stay as healthy and as fit as you can. Try to not let it rule your life.
- Provided it is "lone" AF, you probably have some greater latitude to try alternative methods of treatment and avoid reliance on drugs that seem to be the medical profession's first but not necessarily the only choice.
- Try to remain calm and relax.
- Watch the drug flecainide - while it kept my episodes to 1-4 per year, the severity of those episodes was intense - pain and discomfort, light-headedness, and complete incapacitation; always required cardio-conversion at the hospital. Since stopping this drug the episodes are

daily but I am able to function (somewhat) and do not experience any pain.

- Relax and do not worry as the more you worry the more AF episodes you will get. After 14 years of AF I finally decided to go to the hospital and my AF episode got worse!!!! I have had an afib episode in the middle of the Rockies in Canada more than 3000 meters up with just a friend and I. I lay down for 1 hour, ate as much food and drink as I could, and it went away. Then I carried on down the mountain on my bike at 40 km per hour. AF is a worrying condition, but it should not stop you from doing what you want as long as you do not have another more serious heart/medical condition.
- Personally, I believe my life is in the hands of God so I pray about my situation and the situation of others on this list. I would also say that to let this condition get you down ultimately results in cheating yourself out of many pleasures of life. Find someone you can talk to!
- If you can identify triggers, pay a lot of attention to avoiding them. If a rapid heartbeat is your trigger, consider carrying a beta-blocker with you and using it as needed.
- Take the stress out of your life, keep your weight down, do deep breathing exercises, hike, swim, ski, etc. without overdoing it, eat a good varied diet, and see if you can get off medications.

Correlation Analysis

We now have full or partial data from 75 respondents. Sixteen of these have permanent LAF, 27 have the vagal variety, 20 the adrenergic variety, and the remaining 12 have a mixture of vagal and adrenergic LAF. Although not a large sample, we are now able to draw some tentative conclusions from the data.

One thing is quite obvious. There is a very large variability in the severity of the LAF between respondents; this, unfortunately, makes it difficult to reach conclusions that are valid in strict statistical terms, but we certainly can spot trends.

We have gathered data on 3 measures of severity of the condition: the number of episodes within the last 6 months, the average duration of these episodes, and the total time spent in fibrillation over the past 6 months [afib burden].

Afib burden
Probably the most useful expression of severity is the total time spent in fibrillation over the past 6 months [afib burden]. The average for all respondents with paroxysmal (intermittent) LAF is 143 hours with a minimum of 0 hours and a maximum of 936 hours. In comparison, an afibber with permanent LAF would have spent 4320 hours in fibrillation over the 6-month period. Vagal afibbers had the easiest time with an average of 97 hours spent in afib (range: 0-576 hrs). Mixed afibbers were next with an average of 173

hours (range: 0-750 hrs) followed by the adrenergic group at 197 hours (range: 0-936 hrs).

There is a strong, statistically significant correlation between time spent in afib and the number of episodes experienced over a 6-month period (r=0.59 p=0.0001). Adrenergic afibbers had an average of 14 episodes in 6 months (range: 0-90), vagal afibbers 17 episodes (range: 0-150), and those with the mixed variety 24 episodes (range: 0-125).

The correlation between the average duration of the episodes and total time spent in fibrillation is much less pronounced. There is a slight upward trend, but it is not statistically significant. The average episode lasted 11 hours for the mixed group (range: 0-37 hrs), 15 hours for the vagal group (range: 0-168 hrs), and 20 hours for the adrenergic group (range: 0-72 hrs).

Correlation with age
There is a statistically non-significant trend (r=0.22 p=0.09) for the time spent in fibrillation to increase with age. Thus, according to the trend line, the average time spent in fibrillation was about 50 hours (over 6 months) at age 30 years and about 125 hours at age 50 years. There were no significant correlations between age and the number of episodes experienced in 6 months nor between age and the average duration of those episodes. The average age of vagal afibbers was 48 years, adrenergic 55 years, mixed 56 years, and permanent 57 years. The age difference between vagal and permanent afibbers was statistically significant (p=0.02); the difference between vagal and adrenergic was not significant (p=0.08) nor was the difference between vagal and mixed afibbers (p=0.12). Thus it would appear that the vagal variety is associated with younger age while the permanent variety is associated with older age.

Correlation with gender
There were only 10 women in our sample (65 men) so conclusions regarding the effect of gender should be treated with some caution. Nevertheless, there were some interesting observations.

Only 1 woman had the vagal variety of LAF with the remaining 9 being evenly split between adrenergic, mixed, and permanent. Women with LAF (at least those that responded to the survey) were significantly older than men with LAF. The average age for the women was 66.3 years while that of the men was 51.2 years. This difference was statistically significant (p=0.0002).

Women spent less time in fibrillation (over a 6-month period) than did men (43 hours versus 156 hours on average). They also had fewer episodes (8 versus 18) and the average duration of their episodes was less than those of men (4 hours versus 17 hours). It was not possible to establish the statistical significance of these differences due to the small size of the group of women with paroxysmal LAF. There was no significant difference in the percentage of women and men who were taking antiarrhythmics (71% versus 62%).

Correlation with years of afib

There was no correlation between the number of years a respondent had had LAF and the time spent in fibrillation (over a 6-month period). There was a slight, but statistically non-significant (r=0.20 p=0.14) increase in the number of episodes with increasing years of LAF, but no increase in the duration of episodes. The average number of years of LAF was 6 years for both vagal and adrenergic afibbers, 7 years for mixed, and 5 years for permanent. The figure for permanent] afibbers may be a bit misleading though in that many may have had the condition [without symptoms] for several years prior to being diagnosed through a routine electrocardiogram. Nevertheless, the data does not support the idea that vagal, adrenergic or mixed LAF tends to progress to the permanent version with time.

Use of pharmaceutical drugs

Data was available for 79 lone afibbers with the paroxysmal (intermittent) variety and for 20 with the permanent variety. There were 35 vagal, 24 adrenergic, and 20 mixed variety in the paroxysmal group. Overall the 29 paroxysmal afibbers not taking any drugs spent an average of 107 hours in fibrillation over the 6-month survey period. The 50 respondents taking drugs spent an average of 125 hours in fibrillation. This difference, although not statistically significant (p=0.7), does not support the contention that antiarrhythmic drugs are uniformly beneficial for LAF patients. Afibbers on drugs had more episodes (over 6 months) than afibbers not on drugs - an average of 22 versus 12. Conversely, afibbers on drugs had shorter episodes (average duration of 11 hours) than did afibbers not on drugs [average duration of 17 hours]. These differences were not statistically significant.

My explanation of this finding, not substantiated by any other evidence that I am aware of, is that some antiarrhythmic drugs are slightly proarrhythmic at normal heart rates, thus more episodes, but do become antiarrhythmic at rapid heart rates, thus shorter episodes. The facts that antiarrhythmics can convert atrial fibrillation to atrial flutter, increase the frequency and duration of paroxysmal AF, and convert paroxysmal AF to permanent AF are well-documented [7].

There were no differences between drug users and non-drug users as far as average age, gender distribution or total years of LAF. The finding that overall, afibbers who take antiarrhythmics are no better off than afibbers who do not is indeed surprising and obviously needs further scrutiny. First of all it should be kept firmly in mind that none of the drugs prescribed for LAF have been specifically developed to deal with this condition and, as a matter of fact, several of them are not even approved for the treatment of atrial fibrillation as such. So essentially whenever a LAF patient is prescribed an antiarrhythmic it is a trial and error procedure – there is no guarantee of success. This is compounded by the fact that many afibbers are clearly receiving the wrong drugs for their particular condition. This is particularly pronounced among vagal afibbers.

Drugs in vagal afib

Twenty-six of the 35 vagal afibbers (74%) were taking antiarrhythmics or other drugs to prevent further episodes. There is ample evidence that vagal afibbers should not take digoxin (Lanoxin), beta-blockers or antiarrhythmics with beta-blocking properties as these drugs will markedly worsen their condition [8, 9]. Yet of the 26 vagal afibbers on drugs 14 (54%) were on a drug contraindicated for their condition. These people spent an average of 105 hours in fibrillation (over 6 months) as compared to 40 hours for the people on the drugs best suited for vagal LAF flecainide (Tambocor) and disopyramide (Norpace, Rythmodan).

Even vagal afibbers taking no drugs at all spent less time (90 hours) in fibrillation than did the people who were on the wrong drugs. Vagal afibbers on flecainide did the best and spent only 23 hours in fibrillation and had an average of 6 episodes (average duration of 3 hours) over the 6 months. This compares to 6 episodes (average duration of 24 hours) for non-drug users and 24 episodes (average duration of 13 hours) for people on contraindicated drugs. There was no significant difference in age or time since diagnosis between the drug and non-drug groups.

It was, unfortunately, not possible to establish the statistical significance of the above-mentioned differences because the individual sub-groups were too small and quite heterogeneous. Nevertheless, it seems clear that flecainide and disopyramide may be of benefit for vagal afibbers while other antiarrhythmics are not. Flecainide or disopyramide for that matter are not for the faint of heart though. They are highly dangerous drugs that should only be used by people with an absolutely sound heart. Side effects can be serious and potentially fatal.

Drugs in adrenergic afib

Afibbers with the adrenergic variety were somewhat older on average (53 years) than vagal afibbers (49 years). Of the 24 adrenergic afibbers 13 took no drugs and 11 (46%) were primarily on beta-blockers with atenolol (Tenormin) being the most popular (used by 55%). There was no significant difference in the time spent in fibrillation in the drug group (146 hours) and the non-drug group (155 hours). The non-drug group did, however, have more episodes than the drug group (14 versus 8 for the 6-month period). There was no significant difference in age or time since diagnosis between the drug and non-drug groups.

Drugs in mixed afib

Afibbers with the mixed variety were again older than the vagal group with an average age of 54 years. The 13 respondents in the drug group (65%) spent an average of 197 hours in fibrillation over the 6-month survey period and had an average of 39 episodes lasting an average of 11 hours. In contrast, the 7 non-drug users spent only 40 hours in fibrillation with 14 episodes lasting an average of 9 hours. Thus it would appear that mixed afibbers on drugs are substantially worse off than those not on drugs. This is really not surprising as most of the drug group were taking drugs (including 3 on digoxin) that would aggravate the vagal component of their condition.

The results and conclusions for the mixed group are somewhat confounded by the fact that the average age of the non-drug group was 48 years as compared to 58 years for the drug group. Looking closer at the regression analysis results it would appear that the age difference could account for about 25 extra hours of fibrillation in the older drug group. So even taking age into account it is still clear that drug users spent about 4 times longer in fibrillation and had almost 3 times as many episodes as did non-drug users.

Drugs in permanent afib
Afibbers with permanent afib tended to be older than paroxysmal afibbers (average age of 59 years versus 51 years). Women were also somewhat over-represented in the permanent group at 30% versus 15% in the paroxysmal group. Six of the 20 respondents with permanent LAF did not take any drugs to control their heart rates. Four took diltiazem (Cardizem, Tiazac). Four took atenolol either alone or in combination with diltiazem, two took propafenone (Rythmol), and one each took sotalol (Betapace), digoxin (Lanoxin) or amiodarone (Cordarone). One permanent afibber was on a mixture of diltiazem and propafenone. Diltiazem seemed to be the most helpful of the lot as far as keeping the heart rate under control.

It is not immediately obvious why some permanent afibbers are on antiarrhythmics as there is no evidence that this will help them convert to sinus rhythm unless they are being prepared for cardioversion – none of the respondents were. Certainly being on digoxin can only make things worse and amiodarone has some very serious long-term side effects.

In conclusion, the data collected in the LAF survey does not support the assumption that treatment with antiarrhythmics is beneficial to people with lone atrial fibrillation. There are clearly cases where afibbers have been helped by these drugs, e.g. flecainide for vagal afibbers, but in general terms they do not seem to be helpful and, in many cases, are clearly detrimental. It would appear to be up to each individual, in cooperation with his or her physician, to find the right drug or to forego antiarrhythmics altogether. Remember that LAF is not life-threatening, but antiarrhythmics can be. The best and safest approach for many afibbers may well be to just take verapamil during an episode to keep the heart rate under control.

Correlation Analysis [updated]

Since publishing the original survey results we have received an additional 24 completed questionnaires giving a total sample size of 99. Twenty respondents have permanent LAF, 35 have the vagal variety, 24 the adrenergic variety, and the remaining 20 a mixture of vagal and adrenergic. The additional 24 sets of data means that we should be able to draw more valid conclusions than with

31

just the original 75 sets. So I decided to re-evaluate all variables using all available data.

Afib burden
The average for all respondents with paroxysmal [intermittent] LAF was 127 hours spent in fibrillation over the six-month survey period. The minimum was 0 hours and the maximum 900 hours. In comparison, an afibber with permanent LAF would have spent 4320 hours in fibrillation over a six-month period. Vagal afibbers had the easiest time with an average of 83 hours spent in afib [range: 0-576 hrs]. Mixed afibbers were next with an average of 142 hours [range: 0-750 hrs] followed by the adrenergic group at 151 hours (range: 0-900 hrs).

There is a strong, statistically significant correlation between time spent in afib and the number of episodes experienced over the six-month survey period [r=0.46 p=0.0001]. Adrenergic afibbers had an average of 11 episodes in six months [range: 0-90], vagal 16 episodes [range: 0-150], and those with the mixed variety 30 episodes [range: 0-180].

There is also a statistically significant correlation between total time spent in afib and the average duration of individual episodes [r=0.25 p=0.02]. The average episode lasted 10 hours for the mixed group [range: 0.1-48 hrs], 13 hours for the vagal group [range: 0.1-168 hrs], and 17 hours for the adrenergic group [range: 0.1-72 hrs].

Correlation with age
There is a statistically significant trend for the time spent in fibrillation to increase with age [r=0.26 p=0.02]. According to the trend line, the average time spent in fibrillation over the six-month survey period was about 30 hours at age 30 years, 75 hours at age 40, 110 hours at age 50, and 155 hours at age 60.

The average age of vagal afibbers was 49 years, adrenergic 53 years, mixed 54 years, and permanent 59 years. The age difference between vagal and permanent afibbers was statistically significant [p=0.003]. The age difference between vagal and adrenergic afibbers was not statistically significant nor was the difference between vagal and mixed afibbers. Thus it would appear that the vagal variety is associated with a younger age while the permanent variety is associated with an older age.

Correlation with gender
There were 19 women in our sample. Six [32%] had permanent LAF, 6 [32%] the mixed variety, 5 [26%] adrenergic, and 2 [10%] vagal. This distribution is distinctly different from that of men [18% permanent, 18% mixed, 24% adrenergic, and 40% vagal].

Women with LAF [at least those that responded to the survey] were older than men with LAF. The average age for women was 61 years while that of men was 51 years. This difference was statistically significant [p=0.001].

It is tempting to speculate that the same mechanisms [estrogen?] that protects women against heart attacks for an extra 10 years [compared to men] is at work here, but I have no evidence of such a connection. The explanation could simply be that older women seek medical information on the Internet more often than do younger women.

Women with paroxysmal LAF spent less time in fibrillation [43 hours] than men [133 hours] over the six- month survey period. There was no significant difference in the number of episodes, but episodes among women tended to be shorter in duration (4.5 hours versus 15 hours for men). There was no significant difference in the percentage of women and men who were taking drugs to prevent future episodes (69% versus 62%).

Correlation with years of afib
There was a slight trend for the time spent in fibrillation (over six months) to increase with the number of years since diagnosis of LAF. This trend was not statistically significant (p=0.14). There was also a slight increase in the number of episodes with increasing years of AF, but again not of statistical significance (p=0.11). There was no correlation between the duration of episodes and years of LAF nor was there a statistically significant association between age and afib burden (p=0.38). The average number of years of LAF was 6 years for vagal, 5 years for adrenergic, 7 years for mixed, and 8 years for permanent. The figure for permanent afibbers may be a bit misleading though in that many may have had the condition (without symptoms) for several years prior to being diagnosed through a routine electrocardiogram.

Correlation with aspirin use
About half (47%) of all respondents with paroxysmal LAF took aspirin on a daily basis (22% among permanent afibbers). There was no significant difference in episode severity between users and non-users of aspirin. Aspirin users were older than non-users (54 versus 49 years average age) and more likely to be women (22% versus 12%). Unfortunately, the limited data did not allow consideration of these potential biases. Since one would have a positive effect and the other a negative effect it is probably fair to say that aspirin usage has little or no effect on LAF episode severity.

Correlation with digoxin use
Only 16% of paroxysmal afibbers had ever been on digoxin (Lanoxin, digitalis) and there was no significant difference in afib burden between those who had been or were on digoxin and those who were not. However, there was a clear difference in digoxin use between intermittent (paroxysmal) and permanent afibbers. Fifty per cent of permanent afibbers had used digoxin as compared to only 16% of intermittent afibbers. This finding lends further support to the contention that digoxin can convert LAF to the permanent form.

There was also a statistically significant difference (p=0.04) between the proportion of women (50%) and men (18%) who had been prescribed digoxin.

This could, at least partially, explain why more women than men fell into the permanent LAF category (32% versus 18%).

Correlation with amalgam fillings
Most (76%) paroxysmal afibbers had amalgam (silver) dental fillings as did most permanent afibbers (75%). There was a clear correlation between the time spent in fibrillation and the presence of amalgam fillings. Paroxysmal afibbers without amalgam fillings spent an average of 35 hours in fibrillation over the six- month survey period while those with amalgam fillings spent 143 hours in afib. This difference was statistically significant (p=0.04).

There was also a clear linear relationship between time spent in fibrillation and the number of fillings (r=0.42 p=0.002). An afibber with 0 fillings could expect to spend 35 hours in afib while someone with 8 fillings could expect 140 hours and someone with 20 fillings could expect an average of 300 hours in afib over a six-month period. Afibbers with amalgam fillings also tended to have more episodes (20) and of longer duration (15 hours) than afibbers without (13 episodes of average duration of 9 hours). These differences were, however, not statistically significant.

The findings that afibbers with amalgams have a higher afib burden than those without support the contention that at least part of the inflammatory response underlying LAF is caused by oxidative stress or electrical instability generated by the presence of mercury in the heart tissue.

Correlation with presence of dissimilar metals in the mouth
Seventy-six per cent of permanent afibbers (100% of female permanent afibbers) had dissimilar metals (amalgam fillings, gold crowns, bridges) in their mouth as compared to only 44% of paroxysmal afibbers (54% of female paroxysmal afibbers). There was no overall significant difference in afib burden between paroxysmal afibbers with dissimilar metals and those without. It would thus appear that dissimilar metals are primarily a problem for permanent afibbers. However, this conclusion is somewhat confounded by the fact that amalgam fillings and dissimilar metals often go hand in hand.

Correlation with fish oil supplementation
Forty-two per cent of paroxysmal afibbers supplemented with fish oils (44% among permanent afibbers). Somewhat surprisingly afibbers on fish oil spent more time in fibrillation than did those not taking fish oil (149 hours versus 97 hours over the six-month period). Fish oil users also had more episodes than non- fish oil users (25 versus 13). A closer look at the overall picture reveals that the fish oil group had quite a few "disadvantages" when compared to non-fish oil group. Afibbers who supplemented with fish oil were older (55 years versus 49), less likely to be women (12% versus 20%), and more likely to have amalgam fillings (82% versus 70%). All these factors would be expected to significantly increase afib burden.

An attempt to at least partially account for this bias was made by just considering the 18 respondents who did not have any amalgam fillings. In this case, fish oil supplementation appeared to be beneficial. Fish oil users had only 8 episodes and spent only 24 hours in fibrillation while non-users had 16 episodes and spent 40 hours in fibrillation. Adjusting for age and gender should further improve the picture.

Fish oil users were also significantly more likely to be supplementing with magnesium (76% as compared to only 33% among non-users). The effect of this confounding was eliminated by just considering non-magnesium users. In this group 21% took fish oil while 79% did not. The users of fish oil (average age of 54 years) had an average of 8 episodes and spent 89 hours in fibrillation. The non-users (average age of 45 years) had an average of 16 episodes and spent 106 hours in fibrillation.

Due to the significant confounding of the data it is difficult to draw a firm conclusion as to whether or not fish oils affect the severity of LAF. Nevertheless, considering the significant stroke protection afforded by fish oils it is probably fair to say that they are overall beneficial to lone afibbers.

Correlation with magnesium supplementation
Fifty-one per cent of paroxysmal afibbers supplemented with magnesium (50% among permanent afibbers). There was no significant overall difference in afib burden between those who supplemented and those who did not. Magnesium users were quite a bit older (55 years versus 48 years for non-users) and more likely to be women (20% versus 13%). They were also much more likely to be supplementing with fish oil; 63% of magnesium users also used fish oil as compared to only 21% among non-magnesium users. The effect of this confounding was eliminated by just considering non-fish oil users. In this group 33% took magnesium while 67% did not. The users of magnesium (average age of 55 years) had an average of 6 episodes and spent 65 hours in fibrillation. The non-users (average age of 46 years) had an average of 16 episodes and spent 112 hours in fibrillation over a 6 month period. Based on this data it is probably fair to conclude, especially in view of the considerable age difference between the groups, that magnesium is indeed beneficial for afibbers.

Correlation with digestive problems
Fifty-one per cent of all paroxysmal afibbers had digestive problems (bloating, flatulence, belching) compared to only 28% of permanent afibbers. There was a slight, statistically non-significant trend for afibbers with digestive problems to spend less time in fibrillation than those without digestive problems. Why afibbers with digestive problems should have less severe LAF than those without digestive problems is certainly a mystery and one I have no explanation for at this time.

Correlation with physical fitness
There was no correlation between afib burden and the level of physical fitness.

Comparison of the Best and the Worst
A rather intriguing way of looking at the survey data is to compare those afibbers (7) who had no LAF episodes over the six-month survey period with

those (9) who spent 450 hours or more in afib during the same period. The "best" (zero hours) afib group was younger than the "worst" group (average age of 53 years versus 60 years); they had also had LAF for a shorter period (7 years versus 11 years).

The best group was more likely to have the vagal variety of LAF (57% versus 33%). The best group was more likely to take aspirin (43% versus 22%). The worst group was more likely to take fish oil (67% versus 29%) and magnesium (51% versus 43%). Whether this is because the worst group is clearly "sicker" and therefore trying everything or whether it is because fish oil and magnesium have a detrimental effect on afib burden is not clear, but it is likely to be the former.

All members (100%) of the worst group had amalgam fillings (an average of 15 fillings each) while only 43% of the best group did (an average of 2 fillings each). This again points to the crucial role of amalgam fillings as a major cause of LAF. Perhaps the most intriguing finding is that the members of the best group were almost twice as likely to have digestive problems than were the members of the worst group (79% versus 50%). I have no explanation for this, but it is consistent with the findings of the entire survey.

Effect of Diet

We received 77 responses to the diet questionnaire. Of these 19 were from afibbers who had not participated in previous surveys. This increased the database available to investigate correlations between afib burdens and such variables as age, years of LAF, and presence of amalgam fillings to 118. Not a vast number, but still enough to give additional confidence in the results.

The same, unfortunately, cannot be said for the 77 replies concerning.diet. The results are intriguing, but raise more questions than they answer. The number of replies is simply not sufficient to draw valid, statistically significant conclusions, especially when it comes to looking for diet-related differences between vagal, adrenergic, mixed and permanent afibbers.

The total sample of 118 consisted of 47 vagal afibbers, 23 adrenergic, 29 mixed, and 19 permanent. There were a total of 26 afibbers with blood type A, 28 with type O, 3 with type B, and 5 with type AB. Blood type A was most common among vagal afibbers (63%) while type O was most common among adrenergic (50%), mixed (58%) and permanent (71%).

Non-dietary correlations
There was a strong overall correlation between time spent in fibrillation over the 6-month survey period and the number of episodes (p=0.0001) and average duration of episodes (p=0.02). The time spent in fibrillation for vagal afibbers was highly dependent on episode duration (p=0.01) while time spent in fibrillation for adrenergic afibbers was highly dependent on the number of

episodes (p=0.0001). The previously observed increase in afib burden with advancing age also held true with the larger sample (p=0.03).

The correlation between the presence of amalgam (silver) dental fillings and afib burden was confirmed in the larger sample. Afibbers without amalgams spent an average of 40 hours in fibrillation over the 6-month survey period while those with amalgam fillings spent 203 hours in afib. This difference was statistically significant (p=0.02).

There was no indication that supplementing with magnesium or fish oil affected afib burden. This is somewhat surprising as magnesium and fish oils have both been found effective in preventing other types of cardiac arrhythmias, especially ventricular arrhythmias. Perhaps is just goes to underscore that LAF truly is different from arrhythmias involving a diseased heart. Our findings, of course, do not detract from the other health benefits of magnesium and fish oil supplementation nor do they invalidate anecdotal evidence of their benefits. Nevertheless, magnesium and fish oils are clearly not "magic bullets" when it comes to preventing LAF episodes.

Effect of diet on episode frequency
Vagal afibbers seemed to have fewer episodes if they avoided pork and omega-6 oils and emphasized fish and shellfish in their diet. Adrenergic afibbers had fewer episodes if they emphasized poultry and olive oil. Mixed afibbers had more episodes on a carbohydrate-rich diet, particularly one rich in whole wheat products, fruits and vegetables.

Afibbers with blood type A tended to have more episodes if they emphasized whole wheat products, fruits and vegetables, and in general, ate a high carbohydrate diet. Poultry consumption seemed to decrease the number of episodes. There were no obvious dietary triggers for blood type O.

Effect of diet on episode duration
Vagal afibbers who consumed a lot of vegetables appeared to have longer episodes while adrenergic afibbers who ate a lot of legumes had shorter episodes.

Diet did not seem to affect episode duration for blood type A, but afibbers with type O tended to have shorter episodes with an increased intake of omega-6 oils.

Effect of diet on afib burden
There was a trend for adrenergic afibbers who emphasized poultry to spend less time in fibrillation while those emphasizing fruits and vegetables spend more. There were no clear dietary effects on time spent in fibrillation for vagal and mixed afibbers.

Diet did not seem to affect afib burden for blood type A, but afibbers with type O spent slightly longer in afib if they also had digestive problems.

Effect of diet on digestion

There were no clear correlations between diet and digestive problems among vagal afibbers. A high intake of butter appeared to worsen digestion in adrenergic afibbers while a diet rich in omega-6 oils and arachidonic acid improved it. A high fat intake, particularly of the monounsaturated fats found in meat products, equated to digestive problems among mixed afibbers whereas a high carbohydrate intake was associated with improved digestion. There was no correlation between blood type and digestive problems.

Summary of diet survey

It is difficult to give an overall interpretation of the diet survey results. All the correlations mentioned above had a statistical probability of less than 0.05, that is, the outcome has a less than a 5% probability of being due to chance – so presumably they should be significant. Nevertheless, I am extremely hesitant to draw any firm conclusions from the survey. There simply were not enough responses and the questionnaire itself, in retrospect, also left a lot to be desired (standardized serving sizes, more categories, etc.).

It does seem though that pork, poultry, fish, vegetables, fruits and overall carbohydrate consumption could be important factors. It is conceivable that hormones in poultry could affect the autonomic nervous system, as could carbohydrates through the insulin spike caused by high glycemic index foods in particular. This, however, is pure speculation on my part and can only be confirmed or rejected via a much larger, better designed and professionally interpreted study.

REFERENCES

1. Lindquist, Christine H. and Bray, Robert M. Trends in overweight and physical activity among US military personnel, 1995-1998. Preventive Medicine, Vol. 32, January 2001, pp. 57-65
2. Steinacker, J.M., et al. Training of junior rowers before world championships: effects on performance, mood state and selected hormonal and metabolic responses. Journal of Sports Medicine and Physical Fitness, Vol. 40, December 2000, pp. 327-35
3. Hackney, A.C. Endurance exercise training and reproductive endocrine dysfunction in men: alterations in the hypothalamic-pituitary-testicular axis. Curr Pharm Des, Vol. 7, March 2001, pp. 261-73
4. Matsuo, S., et al. Cardiac sympathetic dysfunction in an athlete's heart detected by 123I- metaiodobenzylguanidine scintigraphy. Japanese Circ J, Vol. 65, May 2001, pp. 371-4
5. Hautala, A., et al. Changes in cardiac autonomic regulation after prolonged maximal exercise. Clin Physiol, Vol. 21, March 2001, pp. 238-45
6. Mujika, I. And Padilla, S. Cardiorespiratory and metabolic characteristics of detraining in humans. Medicine & Science in Sports & Exercise, Vol. 33, March 2001, pp. 413-21

7. Atrial Fibrillation: Mechanisms and Management, 2nd ed., edited by R.H. Falk and P.J. Podrid. Lippincott-Raven Publishers, Philadelphia, 1997, p. 371
8. Coumel, Philippe. Paroxysmal atrial fibrillation: a disorder of autonomic tone? European Heart Journal, Vol. 15, Suppl A, April 1994, pp. 9-16
9. Prystowsky, Eric N. Management of patients with atrial fibrillation: a statement for healthcare professionals from the subcommittee on electrocardiography and electrophysiology, American Heart Association. Circulation, Vol. 93, March 15, 1996, pp. 1262-7

2002 General Survey

By Hans R. Larsen [2002]

We received 83 new completed questionnaires in our second lone atrial fibrillation survey (LAFS 2). This brings our total database to 203 afibbers, enough to enable us to draw statistically valid conclusions.

The majority (43%) of the survey participants have the vagal variety of LAF, 29% the mixed form, and 12% the adrenergic. The remaining 16% have permanent LAF. The average (mean) age of respondents with paroxysmal LAF is 53 years (median 54 years) while that of permanent afibbers is 58 years (median 57 years). The average age at diagnosis for paroxysmal (intermittent) afibbers was 46 years (median 48 years) with a range of 14 to 74 years. The majority of respondents (51%) were between 40 and 55 years of age when first diagnosed. A significant 24% of respondents were in their 20s and 30s and only 5% were over 65 when diagnosed. This finding refutes the generally held belief that atrial fibrillation is an "old age" disease – it clearly is not.

The average age at diagnosis for permanent afibbers was 49 years (median 51 years) with a range of 8 to 72 years. The majority of respondents (52%) were between 40 and 55 years of age when first diagnosed. A significant 32% were over 55 when diagnosed and only 16% were below the age of 40 when first diagnosed. Permanent afibbers are thus somewhat older than paroxysmal afibbers, but even permanent LAF is by no means an "old age" disease.

The majority (81%) of respondents are male. Whether this reflects the distribution of LAF in the general population or is an indication of the relative use of the Internet among men and women is not clear.

Severity of episodes
The number and duration of afib episodes and the total time spent in fibrillation over a 6- or 1- month period [afib burden] are our "gold standard" measures of the severity of paroxysmal LAF. It is an essential component in evaluating the effectiveness of drugs, supplements and other interventions. It is, unfortunately, very difficult to calculate a meaningful average of these values for a group of afibbers. The problem is that most respondents have fairly low values, but a small minority has greatly elevated values, which essentially makes a normal average (mean) quite meaningless in describing the overall severity for a particular group. For example, the calculated average time spent in afib per month for paroxysmal afibbers is 15 hours despite the fact the 81% of them spend less than 15 hours in afib. The average is skewed because a small group spends between 50 and 120 hours in fibrillation per month. I have, therefore, decided to use **median** rather than **mean** (average) values in describing group averages. The **median** is the value in the middle, i.e. the value above which half of all individual values can be found and below which the remaining 50% can be found. Using the median eliminates the bias introduced by a small group of "heavy hitters".

The median number of episodes over a 6-month period was 3 (mean: 13 episodes) for all paroxysmal afibbers. The median duration was 4 hours (mean: 10 hrs) and the median total time spent in fibrillation over a 6-month period was 22 hours (mean: 90 hrs). The median time spent in fibrillation per month was 3.7 hours (range: 0-120 hrs). In comparison the time spent in fibrillation by permanent afibbers is 720 hours/month.

Other findings
77% of paroxysmal afibbers have amalgam dental fillings, 52% have digestive problems, 51% take aspirin on a regular basis, 11% take warfarin and 38% take no anti-platelet or anti-coagulation medications. 78% of permanent afibbers have dental amalgams, 32% have digestive problems, 35% take aspirin regularly, 52% take warfarin and 13% take no anti-platelet or anti-coagulation medications.

Fifteen respondents have undergone ablation therapy; two have had the maze surgery. One hundred and twenty-three afibbers (61%) are taking drugs to prevent or ease episodes whilst 39% are not. A total of 81 afibbers (40%) are taking supplements, 13 have had their amalgam (silver) fillings removed, and 8 have taken other measures to prevent future episodes. In upcoming issues of The AFIB Report we will discuss the effectiveness of these interventions. In the remaining part of this issue we will briefly cover the "statistics" for the four different forms of LAF – vagal, adrenergic, mixed and permanent.

Vagal LAF
Eighty-eight respondents have the vagal form of LAF. Their median age is 53 years, age at diagnosis is 47 years, and 90% of them are men. The median number of episodes over a 6- month period was 3 with a range of 0 to 78. Median duration was 5 hours with a range of 0 to 65 hours. The median number of hours spent in fibrillation per month was 4 with a range of 0 to 120. 56% have digestive problems, 57% take a daily aspirin, 11% are on warfarin (Coumadin) and 32% take no anti-coagulation medication.

Adrenergic LAF
Twenty-four respondents have the adrenergic form of LAF. Their median age is 52 years, age at diagnosis is 47 years, and 79% of them are men. The median number of episodes over a 6- month period was 2 with a range of 0 to 20. Median duration was 7 hours with a range of 0 to 72 hours. The median number of hours spent in fibrillation per month was 4 with a range of 0 to 45. Fifty percent have digestive problems, 35% take a daily aspirin, 10% are on warfarin and the remaining 55% take no anti-coagulation medication on a regular basis.

Mixed LAF
Fifty-nine respondents have the mixed form of LAF. Their median age is 58 years, age at diagnosis is 50 years, and 68% of them are men. The median number of episodes over a 6- month period was 4 with a range of 0-90. Median duration was 2 hours with a range of 0 to 36 hours. The median number of hours spent in fibrillation per month was 4 with a range of 0 to 120. 46% have digestive problems, 48% take a daily aspirin, 12% are on warfarin and the remaining 40% take no anti-coagulation medication on a regular basis.

Permanent LAF

Thirty-two respondents have permanent LAF. Their median age is 57 years, age at diagnosis is 51 years, and 81% of them are men. 32% have digestive problems, 35% take aspirin daily, 52% are on warfarin and the remaining 13% take no regular anti-coagulation medication.

Conclusion

There is a slight trend for mixed and permanent afibbers to be older. The most common form of LAF for women is the mixed variety (32%) with vagal being the least common (10%). There is not a great deal of difference in episode severity between vagal, adrenergic and mixed LAF. Digestive problems are common affecting from 56% of afibbers with the vagal variety to 32% among permanent afibbers. A daily aspirin is the most popular stroke prevention measure taken by paroxysmal afibbers while warfarin is the choice among permanent afibbers. Over 50% of adrenergic afibbers and 40% of mixed do not take anti-coagulation medication on a regular basis.

Although the overall difference in episode severity between the various forms of LAF would appear to be small it is clear that choice of preventive drug (antiarrhythmic) can have a profound effect on episode severity.

Triggers

The most important trigger of an atrial fibrillation episode was found, as in the 2001 survey, to be emotional or work-related stress. Forty-six percent of the 133 respondents who listed their triggers had stress on their list. It was by far the most important trigger for adrenergic afibbers (94%) and mixed afibbers (56%), but of less importance for vagal afibbers (29%). Overall, the following triggers were most important.

Triggers for Paroxysmal Afib Episodes				
Trigger	Vagal, %	Adrenergic, %	Mixed, %	All Types, %
Stress and anxiety	29	94	56	46
Alcohol consumption	33	19	36	32
Digestive problems/overeating	28	6	33	27
Exercise	17	44	36	26
Specific foods ad additives*	25	38	20	25
Caffeine	22	31	20	23
Resting/sleeping	33	0	7	20
Cold and cold drinks	7	6	11	8
Other causes**	22	25	33	26
*cheese, spicy foods, rice, chocolate, sugar, wheat, MSG ** overwork, inflammation, viral infection, dehydration, medications, hypoglycemia, bending over, sleeping on left side, air travel, migraine, sex				

Please note that the percentages do not add up to 100% as most respondents listed more than one trigger.

It is clear that adrenergic and mixed afibbers in particular could benefit substantially from getting their stress level under control and going easy on the exercise. Vagal afibbers, on the other hand, could probably avoid a fair number of episodes by taking it a bit easier, getting adequate sleep, cutting back on alcohol, and avoiding overeating.

Interventions

Radiofrequency ablation
Eight vagal afibbers have undergone radiofrequency ablation. Three of the procedures were successful with the patients completely eliminating their atrial fibrillation and no longer requiring antiarrhythmics to prevent further episodes. The successful procedures were done by Dr. Robert Bock at the Presbyterian Hospital (?), at the Good Samaritan Hospital in San Jose (Dr. Coggins), and at the Cleveland Clinic (Dr. Natale); this last procedure had to be repeated.

Three vagal afibbers underwent ablation for atrial flutter; they also had atrial fibrillation so an attempt was made to eliminate the fibrillation foci at the same time. The flutter ablations were successful in all cases. One of the fibrillation ablations, done at the Virginia Mason Hospital in Seattle (Dr. Chris Fellow), was successful but the patient is still taking beta-blockers to prevent further afib episodes. The remaining two afib ablations were not successful and the patients are still taking antiarrhythmics to prevent episodes. These last two procedures were done at the Seton Medical Center in Austin and the Ottawa Heart Institute in Canada.

Two of the procedures involving vagal afibbers were done within the last six months. One, done at Johns Hopkins (Dr. Calkins), appears to have been at least partly successful although the patient is still on Tambocor. The other has, so far, not been successful and the patient is still on antiarrhythmics.

No adrenergic afibbers reported ablation therapy. It is not clear whether this is because they did not attempt it or because the electrophysiologist could not find an active area to ablate.

Five afibbers with the mixed variety of LAF underwent ablation. Two of these operations were clearly not successful; one was performed at Saint Joseph's Hospital in Tampa, and one at St. Thomas Hospital in London, England. It is too early to tell whether the remaining three were successful, but a least one, done at the Cleveland Clinic (Dr. Natale) appears to have been.

Two permanent afibbers had ablation therapy. One operation, done at the Duke Medical Center (Dr. Marcus Wharton), was successful. The other was done very recently and it is not clear whether it was successful or not.
In conclusion, four of the 15 ablation procedures reported were completely successful and the patients are off all antiarrhythmics. One procedure was successful, but the patient is still on beta- blockers. Four operations were clearly not successful, and six were done so recently that it is difficult to say whether they were successful. It is not clear whether the lack of success with ablation for atrial fibrillation was due to poor procedure or because there was nothing to ablate (no focal points).

Maze procedure

Two afibbers with mixed LAF had undergone maze surgery. Both operations were completely successful and the patients are no longer taking antiarrhythmics. The procedures were performed at the Cleveland Clinic (Dr. Patrick McCarthy) and at St. Joseph's Hospital (Dr. Enrique Cuenza Lopez).

Amalgam replacement

The question as to whether afibbers without amalgam dental fillings have fewer or less severe episodes then do those with amalgam fillings is not clear. One major reason for this is the difficulty in sorting out the individual effects of age, drug use, and other preventive treatments with that of having amalgam fillings. Nevertheless, there does not appear to be any significant amalgam-related difference in number and severity of episodes as far as adrenergic and mixed afibbers are concerned. There is, however, an indication that vagal afibbers with amalgam fillings have more episodes (median of 4 versus 2 per 6 months) and spend more time in fibrillation per month (median of 5 hours versus 1.7 hours for those without amalgams). This possible effect needs to be confirmed in a detailed correlation analysis.

A total of 10 people (6 vagal, 3 mixed, 1 adrenergic) with paroxysmal LAF have had their amalgam fillings replaced. Five of them underwent proper detoxification while four did not. The detoxification status of the remaining person is unknown. Detoxification did not seem to affect the number of episodes, but did affect their duration. The average time spent in fibrillation for the detox group was 3 hours per month versus 21 hours for those who had not detoxified. Considerable caution is needed though in interpreting these numbers since the sample size is very small.

Subjectively, some people felt that amalgam removal had been highly beneficial whilst others had observed no benefits. Here are their comments:

- "I have had no afib episodes since removal of my amalgam fillings and gold alloy bridges in December 2000. I would absolutely recommend this procedure to other afibbers provided it is carried out by an outstanding holistic dentist and is followed up by complete detoxification. Watch out for residual amalgam under old bridges and crowns." – *vagal afibber*
- "I have had no episodes since June 2001 when I had all my amalgam (silver) fillings replaced. I am still undergoing detoxification, but hope to stop this once my mercury levels are back to normal. I feel the replacement has been beneficial." – *vagal afibber*
- "I had all my amalgam fillings replaced in 1992, but did not undergo detoxification. I still have dissimilar metals in my mouth. I have had no episodes in the past 6 months, but do not believe that this is due to the replacement. Nevertheless, I would, for other reasons, recommend replacement." – *vagal afibber*
- "I had all my amalgam fillings replaced in 1995 and followed up with chelation therapy. I did not find the amalgam replacement beneficial." – *mixed afibber*

- "I had all my amalgam fillings replaced in 1997 and am now doing detoxification. I feel this was beneficial and would recommend the procedure to other afibbers." – *mixed afibber*
- "I had all my amalgam fillings replaced in 2000 followed by detoxification. I have not noticed much difference in the number and severity of episodes." – *mixed afibber*
- "I had all my amalgam fillings replaced in the latter part of 2001. I did not follow up with detoxification and am not sure the replacement has made any difference." – *vagal afibber*
- "I had my fillings replaced in September 2000. No detoxification though. The frequency of episodes did not decrease, but the duration did. I think the procedure was beneficial and would recommend it to other afibbers." – *vagal afibber*
- "I had my fillings replaced in November 2001. I am not sure yet whether it has decreased my episode severity. So I cannot yet recommend the procedure for atrial fibrillation relief, but I am sure my general all round health will be improved." – *vagal afibber*
- "I had all my fillings replaced in July 1999 and followed up with partial detoxification – not long enough though to bring my mercury levels to normal. I don't think the removal helped a lot." – *adrenergic afibber*

So, a fairly mixed bag of results. Amalgam replacement and detoxification would likely have overall health benefits including a reduction in the risk of developing neurodegenerative diseases such as Alzheimer's and Parkinson's. However, it is not clear that it should be the first measure taken against lone atrial fibrillation unless you have proven toxic levels of mercury in your body and/or are especially sensitive to mercury. In any case, amalgam replacement should always be performed under strictly controlled conditions and followed up by thorough detoxification.

Anti-inflammation protocol
Four people had tried the anti-inflammatory protocol (The AFIB Report, September 2001 www.afibbers.org/S/afib9.htm). Here are their comments:

- "When I started the anti-inflammation protocol both my allergies and my adrenergic afib disappeared and I was able to work out again. But it seems like when you think it's gone it comes back. Now I have vagal instead; it comes on right after a meal. I do believe the protocol helped though." – *vagal/mixed afibber*
- "It certainly helped for the first couple of months and according to my C-reactive protein test I no longer have an inflammation. It did not completely eliminate my afib episodes." – *adrenergic afibber*
- "I started the anti-inflammation protocol in September 2001. I has definitely helped and I would recommend it to other afibbers." – *mixed afibber*
- "I started the protocol in December 2001 using just the Moducare. I have not had an episode since so I think it would be worth a try." – *vagal afibber*

I would conclude that the anti-inflammation protocol is worth a try if a C-reactive protein (CRP) test shows a higher than normal value indicating the presence of inflammation.

Antiarrhythmic drugs

I have taken a two-pronged approach in evaluating the effectiveness of antiarrhythmics and beta and calcium channel blockers. First, I have compared the overall episode frequency and duration in afibbers taking these drugs with the frequency and duration among afibbers not taking drugs. This comparison is further stratified by type of afib (vagal, adrenergic, and mixed) and by major subgroup of drugs.

Second, I have compiled and evaluated 211 responses regarding the effectiveness of individual drugs by the 115 respondents who had tried them. Most afibbers have tried several drugs thus there are many more individual responses than there are actual respondents.

I believe this subjective evaluation of drug effectiveness is extremely revealing and worthwhile. The individual afibber is, by far, the best judge of what works and what doesn't. If a drug reduces the frequency or duration of episodes without significant side effects then the afibber will declare it a success and be keen to continue on it. If, on the other hand, the drug does not produce noticeable benefits or has horrendous side effects then the afibber trying it will get off it and declare it a failure.

Before we get into the actual evaluation it may be worthwhile to just briefly recap the properties and mode of action of the drugs evaluated.

How antiarrhythmics work

The very first thing to realize is that no drug has ever been developed specifically for the treatment of LAF. All antiarrhythmics currently available were expressly developed for the treatment of arrhythmias associated with cardiovascular disease and heart attacks. The second thing to bear in mind is that ALL arrhythmias connected with heart disease are adrenergic in nature. As a consequence there is very little research on the use of antiarrhythmics in the management of vagally mediated LAF.

Antiarrhythmic drugs are divided into 4 classes depending on their mode of action. To understand how they work let us take a brief look at the modus operandi of an individual heart muscle cell (myocyte). The membranes of myocytes act as small pumps that pump sodium, potassium and, to a lesser extent, calcium and magnesium ions in and out of the cells. When the cell is at rest the concentration of potassium is high inside the cell and the concentration of sodium is high outside the cell. At certain times the ion channels which allow entry of sodium into the cell open and sodium ions rush into the cell causing it to generate an electric charge (depolarization) and contract. The contractions proceed from cell to cell making the whole muscle fiber contract and ultimately making the whole atria contract.

Potassium leaks out of the cell during the depolarization period, but as soon as the depolarization is over it begins to flow back into the cell during what is called the rest or refractory period. Atrial fibrillation is characterized by a total lack of refractory periods. Calcium and magnesium ions follow the sodium and potassium ions respectively, but at a slower rate. Thus sodium and calcium are "excitatory" ions while potassium and magnesium can be viewed as "calming" ions. This underscores the importance of having adequate intracellular levels of both potassium and magnesium and also explains why a magnesium infusion often halts AF. It is likely that a potassium infusion would have a similar effect, but it would be far too dangerous because of the much faster action of potassium ions.

The rate of the fibrillating heart can be slowed by partially blocking the ion channels that allow the influx of sodium or calcium or the outflow of potassium. Antiarrhythmic drugs owe their effectiveness to their capability to block ion channels. Class I drugs such as quinidine, disopyramide, flecainide and propafenone primarily block the sodium channels, but also have some potassium blocking effect. Class III drugs such as sotalol, amiodarone and dofetilide primarily block the potassium channels and class IV drugs such as verapamil and diltiazem block the inward movement of calcium. Class II drugs, the so-called beta-blockers, have no direct effect on the heart cells, but slow the heart rate by blunting the stimulatory effects of norepinephrine on the sympathetic nervous system.

Beta-blockers such as atenolol and propranolol, and antiarrhythmics like flecainide, propafenone, sotalol, amiodarone, verapamil, and diltiazem are the drugs most often prescribed for LAF. Digoxin (Lanoxin) used to be widely used, but has now been totally discredited. Several clinical trials have shown that it can lengthen attacks and even cause the LAF to become permanent. Verapamil and diltiazem are useful in lowering the heart rate during an attack, but do not prevent attacks or speed up the conversion to sinus rhythm. Flecainide is useful in converting afib to sinus rhythm and somewhat useful in preventing attacks. It can, however, have some rather nasty side effects in patients with compromised heart function. It, like other antiarrhythmic drugs, can also be pro-arrhythmic.

It is easy to see why drugs like flecainide can have serious side effects. Their action is not limited to the atria. They also slow down the action of the ventricles – sometimes with disastrous results. Propafenone is somewhat similar to flecainide; however, it also has slight beta-blocking properties making it a poor choice for afibbers with vagal LAF. Sotalol is not effective in converting to normal sinus rhythm, but supposedly has some preventive action. It also has beta-blocking properties. Amiodarone is used in patients with serious ventricular arrhythmias and is generally not recommended for LAF due to its potentially serious adverse effects.

Antiarrhythmic use vs. episode frequency and duration
A total of 179 respondents submitted data concerning drug use and episode severity. Of the 148 paroxysmal afibbers 77 had the vagal variety, 20 the

adrenergic, and the remaining 51 the mixed form of LAF. Thirty-one were in permanent afib; these respondents are omitted from the following evaluation as drugs would clearly not affect the frequency and duration of episodes although they may affect heart rate and general feeling of well-being.

Eighty-seven (59%) of aroxysmal afibbers were currently using a pharmaceutical drug to ward off or shorten episodes while 61 (41%) were not taking any such drugs. The average number of episodes over a six-month period was 11 for drug takers and 8 for non-drug takers; this difference was not statistically significant.

The average duration of an episode was 9 hours for both drug takers and non-drug takers and there was no significant difference in the total time spent in fibrillation over the six-month survey period (79 hours versus 75 hours).

There were no differences between drug takers and non-drug takers as far as average age, gender distribution or total years of LAF. The finding that, overall, afibbers who take antiarrhythmics are no better off than afibbers who do not is indeed surprising; however, it should be kept firmly in mind that none of the drugs prescribed for LAF have been specifically developed to deal with this condition and, as a matter of fact, some of them are not even approved for the treatment of paroxysmal atrial fibrillation as such. So essentially whenever a LAF patient is prescribed an antiarrhythmic it is a trial and error procedure – there is no guarantee of success. This is compounded by the fact that many afibbers are clearly receiving the wrong drugs for their particular condition. This is particularly pronounced among vagal afibbers.

Drugs in vagal LAF
Forty-eight of the 77 vagal afibbers (62%) were taking antiarrhythmics or other drugs to prevent or ameliorate episodes. The average number of episodes over a six-month period was 12 for drug takers and 10 for non-drug takers. The average duration of an episode for drug takers was 9 hours as compared to 11 hours for those not on drugs. None of these differences were statistically significant.

A closer look at the collected data shows that the seeming overall lack of effect of drugs is actually caused by the fact that some drug takers are on drugs that are clearly contraindicated for their condition while others are on drugs that are beneficial. There is ample evidence that vagal afibbers should not take digoxin (Lanoxin), beta-blockers or antiarrhythmics with beta-blocking properties as these drugs are known to markedly worsen their condition. Yet, of the 48 vagal afibbers on drugs 24 (50%) were on beta-blockers or drugs with beta-blocking properties. These people had an average of 9 episodes lasting 12 hours over the six-month survey period. In comparison, vagal afibbers on the drugs best suited for them flecainide (Tambocor) or disopyramide (Norpace, Rythmodan) had 17 episodes lasting an average of only 4 hours over the survey period. Vagal afibbers on contraindicated drugs spent an average of 106 hours in afib over the period as compared to 41 hours for those on flecainide or disopyramide and 116 hours for those taking no drugs at all. The number of afibbers having no episodes at all was 7 (41%) in the flecainide/disopyramide group, 3 (12%) in the beta-blocking group, 1 (17%) in the group on a variety of other drugs, and 7 (24%) in the group taking no drugs.

The conclusion from this data is that vagal afibbers who cannot tolerate flecainide or disopyramide are better off taking no drugs at all.

Drugs in adrenergic LAF
Eleven of the 20 adrenergic afibbers, for which complete data is available, took drugs while 9 (45%) did not. Afibbers on drugs had an average of 2 episodes over the six months while those not on drugs had 6. The duration of episodes was 13 and 17 hours respectively. Although these differences were not statistically significant due to the small sample size, there is a trend for some drugs to be beneficial for adrenergic afibbers. The most successful would appear to be metoprolol (Lopressor, Toprol).

Drugs in mixed LAF
Twenty-eight (55%) of the 51 mixed afibbers took drugs while the remaining 23 (45%) did not. Those on drugs had an average of 15 episodes lasting 9 hours during the six months as compared to 7 episodes lasting 5 hours for the non-drug group. Overall, the drug group spent an average 107 hours in afib over the period compared to 29 hours for the non-drug group. This difference is statistically significant (p=0.04) and indicates that mixed afibbers may be better off not taking any drugs. This finding is perhaps not too surprising as most of the drug group were taking drugs (beta-blocking), which would aggravate the vagal component of their condition.

Drugs in permanent LAF
Eleven (35%) of permanent afibbers took no drugs while the remaining 20 were on a variety of beta- blockers and other drugs. Most popular were amiodarone (5 respondents), diltiazem (5 respondents), verapamil (3 respondents), sotalol (2 respondents), and flecainide (2 respondents). It is not immediately clear why some permanent afibbers are on antiarrhythmics (amiodarone, sotalol, flecainide) as there is no evidence that this will help them convert to sinus rhythm unless they are being prepared for cardioversion – none of these respondents were. It would make more sense just to take diltiazem or verapamil to keep the heart rate under control and avoid potentially dangerous drugs like amiodarone and flecainide.

In conclusion, the data collected in the survey does not support the assumption that treatment with antiarrhythmics is generally beneficial to people with lone atrial fibrillation. There are clearly cases where afibbers have been helped by these drugs, e.g. flecainide or disopyramide for vagal afibbers, but in general terms they do not seem to be helpful and, in many cases, are clearly detrimental. It would appear to be up to each individual, in cooperation with his or her physician, to find the right drug or to forego antiarrhythmics altogether. Remember that LAF is not life- threatening, but antiarrhythmics can be. The best and safest approach for many afibbers may well be to just take verapamil or diltiazem during an episode to keep the heart rate under control.

Subjective Evaluation of Drug Performance

A total of 115 respondents reported on the various drugs they had tried and provided their judgment as to which ones were beneficial and what side effects were observed. The results are as follows:

Atenolol (Tenormin)
A total of 22 afibbers (7 vagal, 7 adrenergic, 7 mixed and 1 permanent) had tried atenolol. None of the vagal afibbers had found it beneficial when taken continuously, but one respondent had found if useful to take periodically when under stress. Only 2 out of 7 adrenergic afibbers had found it useful with one entering a "maybe". Again, only 2 of the mixed afibbers had found it useful while the remaining 5 had not. One permanent afibber thought that it may be beneficial. Thirteen of the atenolol users (59%) reported one or more side effects with fatigue being reported by 7 respondents, slow heart rate and low blood pressure by 4, and dizziness by 3. The most common dosage was 25 mg once a day with a range of 12.5 to 100 mg/day. Overall benefit rate with daily use of atenolol was 0% for vagal and 29% each for adrenergic and mixed afibbers.

Metoprolol (Toprol, Lopressor)
A total of 21 afibbers (11 vagal, 5 adrenergic and 5 mixed) had tried metoprolol. None of the vagal afibbers had found it beneficial. Two of the adrenergic afibbers had found it beneficial, 2 had not, and 1 had entered a "maybe". Four mixed afibbers had found metoprolol useful while 1 had not. Fifteen (71%) of users reported side effects with fatigue being reported by 7 respondents and slow heart rate and low blood pressure reported by 4. The most common dosages were 25 or 50 mg once or twice a day, but 2 respondents took 200 mg/day. Overall benefit rate with daily use of metoprolol was 0% for vagal, 40% for adrenergic, and 80% for mixed afibbers.

Other beta-blockers (bisoprolol, propranolol)
Four afibbers (3 vagal and 1 adrenergic) had tried bisoprolol or propranolol. None had found these beta-blockers beneficial, but one vagal afibber had entered a "maybe". Two of the respondents reported fatigue as a side effect. Overall benefit rate with daily use of bisoprolol or propranolol was 0% for both vagal and adrenergic afibbers. Please note that this conclusion is based on data from only 3 afibbers.

Amiodarone (Cordarone, Pacerone)
Seventeen afibbers (8 vagal, 1 adrenergic, 4 mixed and 4 permanent) had tried amiodarone. Four vagal afibbers had found it beneficial while 4 had not. One adrenergic had found it beneficial, but none of the 4 mixed afibbers had done so. Two (50%) of the permanent afibbers had found amiodarone to be of no benefit while 1 had found it beneficial and one was not sure. Ten users (59%) reported side effects with thyrotoxicosis being experienced by 5 users. The most common dosage was 200 mg once a day. Overall benefit rate with daily use of amiodarone was 50% for vagal, 100% for adrenergic, 0% for mixed, and 25% for permanent afibbers.

Disopyramide (Norpace, Rythmodan)
Eight afibbers (5 vagal and 3 mixed) had tried disopyramide. Four (80%) of vagal and 2 (67%) of mixed afibbers had found the drug beneficial. The most common side effects were urinary problems and dry mouth, which was experienced by 38% of all afibbers taking disopyramide. Overall benefit rate with daily use was 80% for vagal and 67% for mixed afibbers.

Flecainide (Tambocor)
Twenty-six (19 vagal, 1 adrenergic and 6 mixed) had tried flecainide. Twelve (63%) of vagal afibbers had found it beneficial while 6 (32%) had not. The lone adrenergic respondent had not found it beneficial, but 4 out of 6 (67%) of mixed afibbers had. Twelve (46%) of all users reported side effects with fatigue being the most common. The most common dosage was 100 mg twice a day ranging from 50 mg to 300 mg/day. Overall benefit rate was 63% for vagal, 0% for adrenergic, and 67% for mixed afibbers.

Propafenone (Rythmol)
Nineteen (8 vagal, 2 adrenergic, 7 mixed and 2 permanent) afibbers had tried propafenone. Three (38%) of vagal afibbers, one (50%) of adrenergic, and 2 (29%) of mixed had found it beneficial. The 2 permanent ones were not sure about the benefits. Nine (47%) of all users reported side effects with fatigue being the most common. The most common dosage was 150 or 225 mg 3 times a day ranging from 100 mg to 300 mg 3 times a day. Overall benefit rate was 38% for vagal, 50% for adrenergic, and 29% for mixed afibbers.

Sotalol (Betapace, Sotacor)
Thirty-eight (22 vagal, 3 adrenergic, 11 mixed and 2 permanent) afibbers had tried sotalol. Not one (0%) had found it beneficial although one vagal afibber thought it might have reduced severity, but not frequency of episodes. Twenty-nine (76%) of all users reported side effects with 11 actually reporting heart palpitations or fibrillation as the main side effect. Another 7 reported increased fatigue. The most common dosage was 80 mg twice a day. With a success rate of 0% and side effects occurring in 76% of patients sotalol is easily classified as the most useless drug for lone afib. Unfortunately, it is the most frequently prescribed one.

Digoxin (Lanoxin)
Twenty-two (12 vagal, 1 adrenergic and 9 mixed) afibbers had tried digoxin. Only 1 mixed afibber had found it useful in keeping heart rate under control. The remaining 21 (95%) had found no benefits from taking the drug. Seventeen (77%) of all users reported side effects with the most common being palpitations and atrial fibrillation (32%) and fatigue (23%). The most common dosage was 0.25 mg daily. With only one respondent out of 22 finding some benefit from digoxin and 77% experiencing serious side effects digoxin clearly ranks right alongside sotalol as the most useless drug for LAF.

Diltiazem (Cardizem, Tiazac)
Eleven (5 vagal, 1 adrenergic, 2 mixed and 3 permanent) afibbers reported that they had tried diltiazem. None of the paroxysmal afibbers had found it useful in

preventing episodes. The 3 permanent afibbers were not sure if it had been beneficial. Five users (45%) reported unspecified side effects. The most common dosage was 240 mg once a day. While it is not surprising that diltiazem was not found to prevent episodes it is somewhat surprising that nobody found it beneficial in other ways (keeping heart rate down).

Verapamil (Veramil)
Twelve (6 vagal, 1 adrenergic, 3 mixed and 1 permanent) afibbers had tried verapamil. Only 1 vagal, 1 mixed and 1 permanent afibber had found it beneficial in reducing symptoms (not frequency) of episodes. Eight (67%) users reported side effects with fatigue being the most common. Most common dosage was 240 mg once a day, but dosages of 80 mg 4 times a day and 120 mg once a day were also reported.

Drug combinations
Five afibbers had tried a combination of flecainide and a beta-blocker or calcium channel blocker. One mixed afibber had found this combination beneficial [using 100 mg/day flecainide and 10 mg/day propranolol (Inderal)] and one vagal afibber had found a combination of 200 mg/day of flecainide and 10 mg/day of nadolol to be of benefit. The remaining 3 had found no benefit of the combinations although one mixed afibber on 50 mg flecainide and 50 mg atenolol twice daily thought it might be somewhat beneficial. Side effects were few.

Three afibbers had tried a combination of propafenone and beta-blockers. One adrenergic afibber had found a combination of 150 mg propafenone and 50 mg metoprolol twice a day to be beneficial. The other 2 found no benefits.

One mixed afibber had found a combination of 25 mg metoprolol and .125 mg digoxin daily to be of benefit.

Drugs for conversion only
One vagal afibber has found that taking 225 mg of propafenone at the beginning of an episode helps speed up conversion – usually converts within a few hours. One mixed afibber has found that taking flecainide at the onset of an episode speeds up conversion. Both of these findings are in accordance with the results of clinical trials aimed at testing the efficacy of flecainide and propafenone for conversion.

Conclusion
It is clear that the most effective drugs for vagal afib are flecainide and disopyramide. Although not terribly effective the best drugs for adrenergic afibbers would appear to be metoprolol and propafenone either singly or in combination. Mixed afibbers may do well on metoprolol with flecainide and disopyramide either singly or in combination with metoprolol also showing some effectiveness. No drug except perhaps verapamil was deemed to be of benefit for permanent afibbers. Sotalol and digoxin are not effective and have serious side effects. Amiodarone has been beneficial to some afibbers, but its

potential for serious long-term adverse effects rules it out as a viable drug for a non-life-threatening condition such as LAF.

Although the above conclusions are based on subjective evaluations by 115 afibbers they are in remarkably good agreement with clinical experience and with the conclusions reached by relating actual episode severity to drug use. I believe these conclusions can be used as guidelines if you want to try a drug to reduce the number or duration of LAF episodes. Bear in mind though that both flecainide and disopyramide are very powerful and should only be used by afibbers with structurally sound hearts; they also tend to lose their effectiveness over time.

Finally, do keep in mind that 40% of all afibbers participating in our survey use no drugs to prevent episodes and, on aggregate, have no more episodes than do afibbers on drugs. Whether or not drugs help is clearly a highly individual matter and much experimentation will likely be required to find the optimum one for you – if indeed there is one.

Supplements
Sixty-two per cent of 153 respondents took one or more supplements. There was not a great deal of difference in the preponderance of supplement use between vagal (62%), adrenergic (71%), mixed (59%), and permanent (71%) afibbers. As was the case for pharmaceutical drugs there was no statistically significant overall difference in episode severity (hours spent in afib) between those who took supplements and those who did not.

There was, however, a statistically significant trend for vagal afibbers who took supplements to have significantly shorter episodes (p=0.04). This effect was independent of age. There was also a trend for people who took multivitamins to have longer lasting episodes; however, this trend could be confounded by the fact that afibbers who took multivitamins were less likely to take magnesium as well. Respondents who took large amounts of calcium tended to have more severe episodes; however, these people also tended to be older thus possibly confounding this finding.

Sixty-four respondents with paroxysmal afib gave an opinion as to whether they had, subjectively, found supplementation to be beneficial – 44% said "Yes", 19% "No", and 37% were not sure. Somewhat surprisingly, there was a statistically significant correlation between how respondents felt about the benefits of supplementation and how severe their afib was. Afibbers who felt that supplements were beneficial spent an average of 50 hours in afib during the six-month survey period. This was almost 4 times less than the 194 hours spent in afib by those who did not believe supplementation was beneficial. Respondents who were not sure whether supplements had helped spent an intermediate 76 hours in afib. These differences were statistically significant (p=0.02). Afibbers who had experienced afib for a long time were more likely to say that supplements were beneficial (p=0.005) and older afibbers were less likely to take multivitamins (p=0.04). Fifty-three per cent of permanent afibbers found supplements beneficial even though they did not affect their afib.

53

The finding that there is a statistically significant correlation between how afibbers feel about supplementation and their episode severity may indicate that most afibbers are very observant as to what works and what doesn't work. On the other hand, the finding could also be interpreted to mean that afibbers who believe something works will actually make it work – in other words, a very strong placebo effect. A fascinating subject for a future clinical trial!

Sixty-four per cent of adrenergic afibbers felt that supplements were helpful as compared to 42% of vagal, 36% of mixed, and 53% of permanent afibbers.

The following supplements were used by more than 10% of respondents who reported use of supplements:

Supplement	Used By	Daily Dose (Average)	Dose (Range)
Magnesium	72%	520 mg	100-1600 mg
Multivitamin	51%	-	-
Vitamin E	41%	500 IU	160-1450 IU
Vitamin C	35%	1000 mg	250-3000 mg
Coenzyme Q10	35%	100 mg	30-320 mg
Fish oil	35%	2 grams	-
Calcium	25%	500 mg	80-2000 mg
L-carnitine	17%	750 mg	25-1500 mg
B-complex	16%	50 mg	25-100 mg
Hawthorn	16%	700 mg	10-1500 mg
Selenium	12%	150 mcg	25-200 mcg

The following supplements were used by less than 10% of respondents:

Supplement	Used By	Supplement	Used By
Alpha-lipoic acid	9%	Ginkgo biloba	5%
Flaxseed	8%	Niacin	5%
Digestive enzymes	8%	Potassium	5%
Vitamin D	8%	Beta-carotene	4%
Garlic	7%	Cod liver oil	4%
Taurine	7%	Zinc	4%
Vitamin B12	7%	Ginseng	1%
Folic acid	5%	-	-

Adrenergic and mixed afibbers who took multivitamins tended to have longer lasting episodes ($p=0.02$) independent of age. There was a highly significant trend for vagal afibbers who took calcium to have longer episodes ($p=0.002$); this effect increased with larger dosages ($p=0.001$).

There were trends (statistically non-significant) for vitamin E to decrease episode frequency and severity ($p=0.08$) and for high calcium intakes to be detrimental ($p=0.08$); this was especially true for vagal afibbers. Mixed afibbers tended to have shorter episodes and spent less time in afib if they supplemented with magnesium ($p=0.06$).

Afibbers who believed that supplements were helpful were more likely to take vitamin C, B-complex, and magnesium and less likely to take calcium than were those who did not believe supplements to be helpful. These differences, however, were not statistically significant.

Permanent afibbers were less likely to take multivitamins and magnesium, but generally took higher dosages of vitamin C and calcium than did paroxysmal afibbers. These differences again were not statistically significant.

Conclusion
Vagal afibbers who took supplements had significantly shorter episodes than did vagal afibbers who did not and this effect was independent of age and years of afib. No overall benefits of supplementation were observed for adrenergic and mixed afibbers. The effect of supplementation on episode severity could not, for obvious reasons, be determined for permanent afibbers. There was a significant trend for all types of afibbers, most pronounced for adrenergic, who felt that they benefited from supplementation to actually do so. Adrenergic and mixed afibbers who took multivitamins tended to have longer lasting episodes. Vagal afibbers who supplemented with calcium had longer episodes while mixed afibbers tended to have shorter episodes if they took magnesium.

In contemplating these findings it should be kept in mind that some sample groups were small and that the possibility of confounding by other variables is likely. I hope to eventually be able to put all the questionnaire data through a more powerful statistics program that will sort this out. Nevertheless, I believe it is safe to conclude that this survey does not support the idea that there is any one supplement that will "magically" reduce episode severity for all afibbers. This does not mean that supplementing is not beneficial. Many respondents commented that their overall health and well-being had improved since they began supplementing even though their afib burden had not changed.

Relaxation/breathing therapies
Thirty out of 124 paroxysmal afibbers (24%) had tried one or more relaxation, breathing or meditation techniques. There was no statistically significant indication that using these therapies reduced afib frequency or duration. Nevertheless, 80% of the users reported that they had found at least one therapy to be beneficial. In contrast to the supplement study results there was no indication that believing a technique to be beneficial actually translated into less severe afib. Six out of 15 adrenergic afibbers (40%) had tried one or more techniques and 80% had found them beneficial. Sixteen of 67 vagal afibbers (24%) had done likewise and 80% reported beneficial results. Eight out of 42 mixed afibbers (19%) had tried various techniques and 75% had found them beneficial. The most commonly used therapies were:

Therapy	Used By	Success, %
Deep breathing	15%	78
Meditation	9%	64
Yoga	7%	56
Acupuncture	6%	43
Relaxation	5%	83

One respondent had found walking to be beneficial, one had found prayer to be effective, and one reported benefits from using the Heart Lock-In technique developed by the Heart Math Institute. Two respondents had tried hypnosis but did not find it useful. Three had tried biofeedback with two observing some benefit and one reporting no benefit.

Closer scrutiny of the collected data revealed some intriguing correlations. Although these were statistically significant they should, because of the very small sample sizes, be taken with a very large grain of salt.

- Older men were more likely to believe meditation to be beneficial (p=0.04)
- Older men and women were more likely to believe yoga to be beneficial (p=0.05)
- People who had experienced afib for many years were less likely to find relaxation therapies beneficial (p=0.004), but more likely to find meditation beneficial (p=0.04).

Conclusion

Although many respondents had found one or more relaxation/breathing therapies to be beneficial there was no statistically significant correlation between the use of these techniques and reduced episode frequency or duration. In other words, the survey did not uncover a universal therapy that would benefit everyone. This does not mean that some individual afibbers may not find real benefit from using one of these therapies. It just means that the therapy may not be beneficial for everyone. As we all know, one size definitely does not fit all when it comes to dealing with lone atrial fibrillation.

Follow-up on Ablation Procedures

In the May 2002 issue of *The AFIB Report* we reported on the results of 15 ablation procedures. Four had been completely successful, 4 were clearly not successful, and 6 were done so recently (November 2001 – January 2002) that it was too early to tell whether they had been successful or not. One of the respondents was still on beta-blockers after the operation.

We have now followed up on the recently performed procedures and can report that we have heard from 4 of the afibbers who underwent ablation therapy late last year or early this year. Three of the procedures were completely successful and one was not. This brings the final score to:

- Vagal – 4 successful; 3 not
- Adrenergic – No procedures done
- Mixed – 2 successful; 3 not
- Permanent – 1 successful; 1 not

The successful procedures were done at the Cleveland Clinic (3), Presbyterian Hospital (1), Duke Medical Center (1), and Virginia Mason in Seattle (1).

Hunting for Clues

By Hans R. Larsen [2002]

The May 2002 survey yielded 105 responses of which 36 were from afibbers who had not previously participated in a survey. This brings our total database to 236 respondents with lone atrial fibrillation.

The majority (42%) of these 236 respondents have the vagal variety of LAF, 30% the mixed form, and 11% the adrenergic. The remaining 17% have permanent LAF. The average (mean) age of respondents with paroxysmal LAF is 53 years (54 years for adrenergic, 56 for mixed and 51 for vagal) with a range from 19 years to 81 years. The average age of permanent afibbers is 57 years with a range of 34 to 82 years. The average age at diagnosis for paroxysmal (intermittent) afibbers is 46 years (48 years for adrenergic, 49 for mixed and 45 for vagal) with a range of 14 to 80 years. The average age at diagnosis for permanent afibbers is 48 years with a range of 8 to 72 years. Fifty per cent of respondents were between the ages of 40 and 55 years when first diagnosed and only 7% were 65 years or older. This finding clearly refutes the generally held belief that lone atrial fibrillation is an "old age" disease.

Afib burden
Adrenergic afibbers had an average (median) of 4 episodes (0-68) lasting an average (median) of 12 hours (0-72) resulting in an average (median) 24 hours being spent in afib during the 6-month survey period [afib burden]. Corresponding numbers for mixed afibbers were 5 episodes of 3 hours duration for a total afib burden of 22 hours. Vagal afibbers, on average, had the most episodes (6) lasting the longest (6 hours) resulting in an average 48 hours being spent in afib over the period. This observation can, in part, be explained by the fact that many vagal afibbers are on the wrong drugs (beta-blockers and antiarrhythmics with beta-blocking properties) for their condition.

There was a clear association between time spent in fibrillation and both the number of episodes and the average duration of each episode (p=0.0001). This association was particularly strong for vagal afibbers with the correlation between episode duration and afib burden being the most pronounced (r=0.7026 p=0.0001).

Afib burden increased significantly with age from an average (mean) of 26 hours per 6 months at age 30 years to 80 hours at age 60 years. This age effect was particularly strong for vagal afibbers who spent an average 109 hours in afib at age 60 years.

Afib burden also increased with the number of years since diagnosis. A recently diagnosed afibber had an average afib burden of 53 hours while someone diagnosed 10 years ago spent an average of 81 hours in afib over a 6-month period.

There was a trend for afibbers who reported bowel problems to have fewer episodes and mixed afibbers with bowel problems also spent less time in fibrillation. This finding could, however, be confounded by the fact that women, who do spend less time in fibrillation, also are more likely to have bowel problems.

Gender
The majority (81%) of respondents are male. Whether this actually reflects the distribution of LAF in the general population or is an indication of the relative use of the Internet among men and women is not clear. Only 11% of female respondents had the vagal variety while 30% had the mixed type. Adrenergic and permanent each had a 20% female component. The median age at diagnosis was 52 years (range of 22 to 70) for women and 47 years for men. This difference is statistically significant.

Women, particularly with the mixed variety, tended to have significantly shorter episodes than did men and spent less time in fibrillation. Women were more likely to have a bowel disorder and were less likely to have engaged in prolonged strenuous physical activity than were men. Women were also more likely to be suffering from an autoimmune disorder.

Possible Causal Associations [Questionnaire Responses]

Have you ever been told that you have an enlarged left atrium?
Twenty-four or 23% of respondents had been told that they had an enlarged left atrium. This diagnosis was most common among adrenergic afibbers (46%) and permanent afibbers (33%) and less common among mixed (14%) and vagal (17%) afibbers. The size range for an enlarged atrium was 42 to 50 mm. An enlarged left atrium was associated with advanced age and the use of vitamin E and beta-carotene. However, the use of vitamin E is also strongly associated with advanced age so this no doubt confounds this finding. The finding regarding beta-carotene is puzzling but fairly robust (r=0.37 p=0.0001). An enlarged atrium was not associated with increased episode severity and physical activity did not correlate with an enlarged atrium.

Were you a smoker when you experienced your first episode?
Only 13 or 13% of respondents answered yes to this question (20% among vagal afibbers, 8% among adrenergic, 7% among mixed, and 6% among permanent). Smokers were more likely to have had a dysfunctional childhood (p=0.01). Smoking at the time of the first episode was not associated with an increased episode severity.

Are you now a smoker?
Only 5 or 5% of respondents answered yes to this question (4% among vagal afibbers, 8% among adrenergic, 7% among mixed, and 0% among permanent). Almost 80% of vagal afibbers had thus given up smoking after experiencing their first episode. With only 5 smokers in a population of 103 respondents it

is not possible to draw statistically valid conclusions regarding possible associations. However, there was a trend for current smokers to be younger, to have been on Valium, and to have been brought up in a dysfunctional home. Considering that about 30% of the male American adult population are smokers the proportion of smokers among afibbers (5%) is clearly exceptionally low. Is this part of the generally healthy lifestyle of afibbers or could smoking actually be protective?

Smoking is primarily a nicotine delivery system. Nicotine is known to increase circulating levels of cortisol, DHEA, norepinephrine (noradrenaline) and epinephrine (adrenaline) [1-3]. While this would be bad news for adrenergic afibbers and possibly for mixed afibbers it could be helpful for vagal afibbers. Norepinephrine and epinephrine increase sympathetic nervous activity. Vagal afibbers have an excess of parasympathetic activity so increasing the sympathetic activity (through smoking) would tend to balance their autonomic nervous system and may help prevent vagally-mediated afib episodes.

A nicotine patch, chewing nicotine gum or, for fast action, using a nicotine nasal spray are all efficient ways of delivering nicotine to the circulation [4]. It is conceivable that a vagal afibber could cut down on the number of episodes or avoid them altogether by using a slow, continuous delivery system such as a 2 mg nicotine patch or nicotine gum. Using a nasal spray after dinner might prevent post-prandial episodes. I want to emphasize that this is all pure speculation on my part. I have no scientific evidence to support it. However, if I had the vagal kind of LAF (I am adrenergic) I would definitely give it a try. Although not without long-term side effects, the nicotine approach would probably still be safer than amiodarone and some of the other antiarrhythmics and, if it works, could pave the way for the development of a novel class of drugs to treat vagal LAF.

Have you ever been diagnosed with a bowel disorder?
Twenty-five or 25% of respondents answered yes to this question (32% among vagal, 25% among mixed, 17% among adrenergic, and 11% among permanent). Women were more likely to have bowel problems and there was also a significant association between taking beta-carotene and having bowel problems. Afibbers with a bowel disorder were also significantly more likely to have an autoimmune disorder and a dysfunctional childhood. Sixteen (67%) of the 24 respondents who specified their disease had irritable bowel syndrome (IBS), seven (29%) had diverticulitis, and one (4%) had Crohn's disease. IBS was particularly common among vagal afibbers. Seventeen respondents specified how long they had had the disorder; 13 years was the average with a range from 1 to 40 years.

The estimated prevalence of IBS in the general population is 15 to 20%. The confirmed incidence among our 102 respondents is 16%; thus it would appear that the IBS incidence among afibbers is not abnormally high. The confirmed incidence of diverticulitis is 7%, which again is not out of line with the prevalence in the general population. So overall our survey data does not support the contention that bowel disorders are more common among afibbers than in the general population.

Do you suffer from acid reflux or have you ever been diagnosed with GERD (gastroesophageal reflux disease)?

Thirty-eight or 37% of respondents answered yes to this question (40% among vagal, 38% among mixed, 33% among adrenergic, and 28% among permanent). Respondents who had answered yes were also more likely to report a correlation between an afib episode and a flare-up of GERD as well as an association between diet and episode severity. Eighteen (51%) of the 35 respondents who specified their disease had GERD, 29% reported acid reflux, 11% a hernia, and the remaining 9% described their condition as heartburn. Thirty respondents specified how long they had had the disorder; 11 years was the average with a range from 1 to 30 years. Heartburn and acid reflux are common symptoms of GERD so it is reasonable to conclude that 34 of the 104 respondents could be classified as having GERD. This gives an incidence of 33%. GERD, heartburn and acid reflux are not steady conditions, which makes it difficult to estimate the prevalence in the general population. The overall prevalence may be around 7 to 10%, but up to 50% of Americans report at least one episode of heartburn per month [5]. In retrospect it is clear that the questionnaire should have been more specific in regards to frequency of symptoms. Nevertheless, GERD could be an important afib factor.

Do you suffer from acid reflux or have you ever been diagnosed with GERD (gastroesophageal reflux disease)? [Follow-up]

I covered the responses to this question in the above paragraph. However, it became clear that it was not possible to draw a conclusion as to whether or not afibbers were more likely to have GERD than was the "normal" population because I had not asked about the frequency of GERD episodes. I have now received the responses to my supplementary questionnaire and can report that 10% of respondents have daily episodes, 14% have weekly, and 10% have monthly episodes for a total of 34%. This compares to the following values reported in the literature: Daily episodes= 11%, weekly (one or more per week, but not daily) =12%, and monthly episodes =15% for a total of 38% [5]. Thus it would not appear that afibbers are significantly different from the rest of the population when it comes to the incidence of GERD. I found no correlation between H. *pylori* eradication and GERD incidence or between childhood antibiotics exposure and GERD.

Have you noticed any correlation between episodes and a flare-up of GERD or a bowel disorder?

Twenty-six (41%) of the 63 respondents reporting either GERD (including heartburn and reflux) or a bowel disorder had noticed a correlation between a flare-up of their condition and worsening LAF symptoms. By far the most common correlation was between GERD and the initiation of an episode or a worsening of chronic symptoms. Eighteen of the 26 respondents (69%) reported this correlation while 3 respondents (12%) felt there was a connection with an IBS flare-up. Adding this evidence to the finding that some afibbers with GERD or reflux symptoms have found relief by taking the prescription medicine

Nexium would indicate that GERD could be an important trigger for LAF and its elimination could materially improve the condition in some afibbers.

Have you ever taken tranquillizers (valium, ativan, xanax, etc.) for an extended period of time?
Eleven or 11% of respondents answered yes to this question (25% among adrenergic, 17% among mixed, 11% among permanent, and 2% among vagal). It is interesting to note the difference in tranquillizer use between adrenergic and vagal afibbers. It is likely that tranquillizers would tend to benefit adrenergic afibbers more because of their greater level of sympathetic nervous activity and accompanying anxiety. Considering that more than 60 million prescriptions are written every year for minor tranquillizers in the United States alone a use rate of 11% is probably normal and does not support the idea that past tranquillizer use could be an important cause of LAF. Respondents who had used tranquillizers were more likely to be current smokers, to have a high CRP level, and to have had a dysfunctional childhood (r=0.38 p=0.0001).

Do you feel more upbeat on a sunny day (high barometric pressure) than on a rainy day (low barometric pressure)?
One respondent answered yes with the comment "Doesn't everyone?" Well as a matter of fact not all afibbers feel more upbeat on a sunny day (high barometric pressure). Fifty-five (62%) of the 89 respondents who answered this question did answer yes (91% among adrenergic, 70% among mixed, 59% among permanent, and 50% among vagal). However, a sizeable proportion (38%) did not feel more upbeat on a sunny day (50% among vagal, 41% among permanent, 30% among mixed, 9% among adrenergic). Research has shown that cortisol levels are lower at high barometric pressures and that lower levels are associated with a lessening of depression [6, 7]. So conceivably a person with elevated cortisol levels might feel better on a sunny day. A person who already has an excessively low level may feel worse because low cortisol levels diminish the ability to handle stress. At this point all this is pure speculation though. Obviously more research is required on a potential cortisol/LAF connection. There was tendency for women to be more likely to feel upbeat on a sunny day.

Have you had your tonsils removed?
Sixty or 58% of respondents had had their tonsils removed (72% among permanent, 62% among mixed, 53% among vagal, and 42% among adrenergic). Tonsils are an integral part of the immune system and serve an important function in fighting infections. During this process they can become inflamed and sometimes infected. When this happens they are often surgically removed [tonsillectomy]. The annual rate of tonsillectomy [pediatric and adolescent] in Canada in 1996 was 38 per 10,000 population or 0.38% [8]. Most tonsils are removed before the age of 15 years so applying the 0.38% annual removal rate over 15 years would give a total "lifetime" removal rate of about 6%. This estimated rate is clearly significantly lower than that experienced among our survey participants. If it is correct and comparable then having a tonsillectomy could be an important cause of the development of LAF.

If this is indeed so, then taking steps to make up for the loss of ones tonsils may be beneficial.

There was a significant correlation between present age (and age at diagnosis) and the likelihood of having had a tonsillectomy. Older people were more likely to have had one than were younger people indicating that the practice is becoming less prevalent.

Do you consider yourself sedentary, somewhat active or highly active and in strong physical shape?

Forty (38%) of the 105 respondents considered themselves to be highly active and in strong physical shape (50% among adrenergic, 43% among vagal, 39% among permanent, and 24% among mixed). Fifty-six (53%) considered themselves somewhat active (62% among mixed, 50% among vagal, 50% among adrenergic, and 50% among permanent). Only 9 or 9% described themselves as being sedentary, again confirming that afibbers tend to lead a healthy lifestyle. Men tended to be more physically active than women. Afibbers who were highly active were also more likely to have engaged in strenuous physical activity in the past. Highly active afibbers were less likely to have an autoimmune disease.

Do you or did you in the past engage in strenuous physical activity for extended periods (longer than 40 minutes at a time)?

Research has shown that regularly engaging in vigorous exercise for 40 minutes or more will raise cortisol levels. Eighty-three (79%) of the respondents answered yes to this question (92% among adrenergic, 87 among vagal, 69% among mixed, and 67% among permanent) again proving that afibbers are highly active people. The level of strenuous activity did decline with age and was higher among men than among women.

Do you regularly supplement with vitamin E (alpha-tocopherol)?

Ninety-two (43%) of the 212 respondents who answered this question answered yes (62% among permanent, 54% among adrenergic, 47% among mixed, and 31% among vagal). The use of vitamin E increased sharply with age ($r=0.44$ $p=0.0001$) and people taking beta-carotene were also more likely to take vitamin E. There was no indication that vitamin E supplementation was either beneficial or detrimental. However, as vitamin E supplementation is very strongly associated with age a more sophisticated statistical analysis is required in order to say for certain. Vitamin E has been found beneficial in the prevention of many conditions so supplementation is a good idea especially if using a mixed tocopherol preparation rich in gamma-tocopherol. The most common daily dosage of vitamin E was 400 IU ranging from 200 to 1600 IU/day and some respondents had been supplementing for 30 years or more.

Do you regularly supplement with beta-carotene?

Forty (20%) of the 204 respondents answering this question took beta-carotene (29% among permanent, 24% among adrenergic, 19% among vagal, and 13% among mixed). Most got the beta-carotene from a multivitamin so the most common dosage was 15,000 IU/day ranging from 7500 to 30,000 IU/day.

Some users had supplemented for as long as 30 years. People who supplemented with beta-carotene (multivitamin?) were more likely to have a bowel disorder. There was no indication that beta- carotene supplementation was either beneficial or detrimental in regard to episode severity.

Has anyone else in your close family (parents, grandparents, and siblings) been diagnosed with arrhythmias?
Forty-three or 43% of respondents had a close relative with cardiac arrhythmia (54% among mixed, 44% among permanent, 40% among vagal, and 25% among adrenergic). The most common "carriers" were the mother who accounted for 13 of the relatives (30%), siblings who accounted for 11 (26%), the father who accounted for 10 (23%), and grandparents who accounted for 3 (7%). Permanent afibbers reported the mother to be the "carrier" in 71% of cases. For adrenergic afibbers the mother was implicated in 50% of cases. The father was the predominant "carrier" among mixed afibbers (27%) and mothers, fathers and siblings shared the "honours" among vagal afibbers at 28% each.

The estimated overall prevalence of all cardiac arrhythmias in the United States is about 1% with atrial fibrillation accounting for about half of this [9, 10]. Cardiac arrhythmias are generally more common among older people. With only 1% of the general population having arrhythmia is it odd that 43% of the survey respondents had a close relative with arrhythmia? This question can really only be answered definitely by comparing the rate of arrhythmia among close relatives of a group of lone afibbers with the rate in a group of age- and sex-matched controls. Too major a project for my limited resources.

Nevertheless, it is possible to get some idea about the likelihood of a genetic connection. Although we afibbers tend to be an odd bunch, it is probably safe to assume that we each had two biological parents?! This means that there could have been from 10 to 23 cardiac arrhythmia cases among the 202 parents included in the survey or a rate between 5 and 11% - in other words, considerably higher than the 1% that would have been expected. This finding does not prove that LAF can be inherited, but it certainly supports the possibility.

The possibility of a genetic connection is supported by work done by Dr. Ramon Brugada and his colleagues at Baylor College of Medicine and University of Barcelona [11]. These researchers located three families in Spain in which 21 of 49 family members had lone atrial fibrillation. They mapped their genes and concluded that in these families a mutation in a specific chromosome region (10q22-q24) was the cause of their atrial fibrillation. Dr. Maurits Allessie, MD of the University of Maastricht in the Netherlands makes several very interesting observations concerning these findings [12]:

- If, as in the three Spanish families, lone atrial fibrillation in the general population is also caused by a genetic mutation, then Brugada's findings are of paramount importance.
- The possibility that small molecular defects in DNA can cause changes in the electrophysiological properties of the atria that, in turn, create a

substrate for chronic atrial fibrillation is not unlikely. NOTE: The term chronic used in this statement does not mean permanent as opposed to paroxysmal, but rather that LAF is a long-term rather than an acute condition.

- The genes that encode adrenergic receptors are located at the observed mutation site on chromosome 10q. This means that the basis for familial atrial fibrillation could lie in abnormal atrial triggering mechanisms.

Dr. Allessie concludes, "The anatomical and electrophysiological features of the atria are such that there is only a narrow margin of safety between normal sinus rhythm and chronic atrial fibrillation." Our survey findings of a possible genetic connection and the fascinating discoveries of Dr. Brugada and colleagues together with Dr. Allessie's profound observations certainly provide much food for thought and will hopefully be followed up by additional research.

Have you ever been diagnosed as having a high CRP (C-reactive protein) level and if so, what was the level?

Only 5 (7%) of the 75 respondents who answered this question had been diagnosed with a high CRP value. The values considered high were 0.6, 1.0, 2.2, and 4.0 mg/L. The 5 respondents were more likely to have taken Valium and to have had a dysfunctional childhood, but these observations must, due to the small sample size, be taken with a very large grain of salt. It is also not clear whether the respondents who answered "No" to this question did so because they had never had their CRP level tested or because their level was low. So from this data it is not possible to deduce whether high CRP levels are associated with atrial fibrillation

.

What is your basal body temperature?

Twenty-two respondents answered this question. Nine (41%) had a normal value (97.6 - 98.2 degrees F or 36.4 - 36.8 degrees C), 10 (45%) had a low value and the remaining 3 had a high value. Of the 10 with low values 4 had actually been diagnosed with hypothyroidism; their basal temperatures were 96.5, 97.0, 97.1 and 97.3 degrees F respectively. The 6 undiagnosed respondents with low values had values of 96.4, 96.8, 97.0, 97.1, 97.2 and 97.3. This may indicate that the 6 respondents with low values also have hypothyroidism.

The 3 respondents with high values had basal temperatures of 98.6, 98.8 and 100.0 degrees F. This may indicate an overactive thyroid gland (hyperthyroidism). Hyperthyroidism is a recognized trigger of atrial fibrillation and it is possible, but to my knowledge yet unproven, that hypothyroidism could also be a trigger.

Four of the respondents had no data for episode severity so was left out of the following analysis. The remaining 18 respondents consisted of 2 adrenergic, 8 mixed, 6 vagal and 2 permanent afibbers. The 16 paroxysmal afibbers were separated into 3 groups – those with low basal temperatures, those with normal and those with high. There was a clear difference between the 3 groups in the number of episodes over the 6-month study period. The normal group had an average of 4 episodes lasting 7 hours and spent 29 hours in fibrillation. The low temperature group had an average of 8 episodes lasting 7 hours and spent 53 hours in afib. The high temperature group had an average of 9 episodes lasting 22 hours and spent 249 hours in fibrillation. The 2 permanent afibbers both had abnormally low basal temperatures.

This analysis implies that both low (hypothyroidism) and high (hyperthyroidism) basal temperatures worsen the severity of LAF. Unfortunately, the analysis was only based on 18 data points so it must be viewed with considerable caution. Nevertheless, the result is intriguing and certainly worthy of further investigation.

Have you noticed any correlation between your diet and the severity of your episodes?
Forty-eight (47%) of the 102 respondents had noticed a correlation (52% among vagal, 48% among mixed, 41% among permanent and 33% among adrenergic). The most common factors that seemed to initiate or prolong an episode were:

- A large meal [reported by 44%]
- High glycemic index food [reported by 10%]
- Eating as such [reported by 10%]
- Alcohol [reported by 8%]
- MSG [reported by 8%]
- Starchy meal [reported by 5%]
- Salmon [reported by 5%]

Gluten, salt and a fatty meal were each mentioned by one respondent. There was no indication that afibbers who had noticed a correlation between their diet and afib had more or fewer episodes or shorter or longer ones than fibbers who had not noticed a correlation. Afibbers who had noticed a dietary correlation were also more likely to have been diagnosed with a bowel disorder or GERD.

Do you have rheumatoid arthritis, fibromyalgia, chronic fatigue or thyroid problems?
Sixteen (15%) of 105 respondents (21% among mixed, 17% among adrenergic, 13% among vagal and 11% among permanent) reported that they had one of the above disorders. Six had thyroid problems (4 specified hypothyroidism), 4 fibromyalgia, 3 osteoporosis, and 1 each had arthritis or chronic fatigue. Osteoporosis, depression, and irritable bowel syndrome have all been linked to elevated cortisol levels while low levels have been linked to rheumatoid arthritis, fibromyalgia and permanent fatigue syndrome [13-20]. It is thus possible that these disorders could affect LAF severity through the cortisol connection, but there was no statistically significant indication that afibbers with these disorders have more or less episodes than those without. There is also no indication that any of the above disorders, with the exception of thyroid problems, could be an important underlying cause of LAF.

Were you brought up in a dysfunctional home (alcoholism, frequent parental fights, etc.) or were you physically or sexually abused as a child?
At least 2 studies have found that adverse conditions that produced frequent elevated cortisol levels in childhood may contribute to low levels in adulthood and that these low levels may make the adult hypersensitive to stress and thus a good candidate for LAF [21, 22].

Twenty-six (25%) of 104 respondents (28% among mixed, 28% among vagal, 25% among adrenergic and 12% among permanent) reported that they had been brought up in a dysfunctional home. Is this high when compared with the general population? I have been unable to find out, but my guess would be that it probably is not. There was no indication that being raised in a dysfunctional home affected LAF severity, however, it did affect other parameters. Afibbers brought up in a dysfunctional home were more likely to be women. They were also more likely to smoke, have a bowel disorder, have been on Valium, and have a high CRP level. Quite a legacy!

Conclusions

This completes the evaluation of the results of our third LAF survey. It has certainly turned up some interesting clues, but most of them will need to be verified by larger studies with matched, afib-free controls. Our 3rd LAF survey confirmed the main findings of the previous two surveys.

- The vagal variety of LAF is the most common followed by mixed, adrenergic and permanent.
- Vagal afibbers tend to develop LAF at a slightly younger age.
- Fifty per cent of lone afibbers have their first episode between the ages of 40 and 55 years. Only 7% are diagnosed at age 65 or older.
- Women tend to be diagnosed with LAF at a later age than men and tend to have less severe episodes.
- Afib burden tends to increase with age and number of years since diagnosis.
- About a quarter of the respondents have an enlarged atrium (42-50 mm), but this was not associated with increased episode severity.
- Bowel disorders and GERD (gastroesophageal reflux disease) are common among afibbers. Flare-ups of GERD could be an important trigger of LAF.
- The prevalence of previous tonsil removal was considerably higher among the survey respondents than would have been expected. It is thus possible that tonsillectomy could predispose to the later development of LAF; this, however, needs to be confirmed in a much larger study comparing age and sex-matched afibbers with afib-free controls.
- Over 90% of respondents considered themselves highly or somewhat physically active.
- Cardiac arrhythmias were more common among close relatives of afibbers than would be expected. However, a much larger study

involving afib-free controls is needed to confirm or disprove a possible genetic connection.

- There is some indication that hypothyroidism (low basal temperature) could be an afib trigger just as hyperthyroidism is. Again, this needs to be confirmed in a larger survey.
- Almost half of all respondents had noticed an association between their diet and LAF episodes. A large meal was the most common trigger.
- About a quarter of all respondents had a dysfunctional childhood. This did not significantly affect episode severity, but did have an impact on several other parameters.

REFERENCES

1. Pomerleau, O.F. Nicotine and the central nervous system: biobehavioral effects of cigarette smoking. American Journal of Medicine, Vol. 93 (1A), July 15, 1992, pp. 2S-7S
2. Baron, J.A., et al. The effect of cigarette smoking on adrenal cortical hormones. J Pharmacol Exp Ther, Vol. 272, January 1995, pp. 151-55
3. Gilbert, D.G., et al. Effects of nicotine and caffeine, separately and in combination, on EEG topography, mood, heart rate, cortisol, and vigilance. Psychophysiology, Vol. 37, No. 5, September 2000, pp. 583-95
4. Benowitz, N.L., et al. Cardiovascular effects of nasal and transdermal nicotine and cigarette smoking. Hypertension, Vol. 39, June 2002, pp. 1107-12
5. Bloom, Bernard S. and Glise, Hans. What do we know about gastroesophageal reflux disease? American Journal of Gastroenterology, Vol. 96 (suppl), August 2001, pp. S1-S5
6. Khraisha, S. Comparative study of serum insulin, glucose, growth hormone and cortisol of students at 794.7 mm Hg (Dead Sea level) and 697.5 mm Hg (Amman) barometric pressures. Aviat Space Environ Med, Vol. 61, February 1990, pp. 145-47
7. Young, A.H., et al. Elevation of the cortisol-dehydroepiandrosterone ratio in drug-free depressed patients. American Journal of Psychiatry, Vol. 159, July 2002, pp. 1237-39
8. Van Den Akker E.H., et al. Large international differences in (adeno) tonsillectomy rates. Clin Otolaryngol Allied Sci, Vol. 29, April 2004, pp. 161-4
9. Kottkamp, Hans, et al. Atrial fibrillation: epidemiology, etiology, and symptoms, Chapter 9. From Atrial Flutter and Fibrillation, edited by N. Saoudi, et al. Armonk, NY, Futura Publishing Company, 1998, pp. 135-51
10. Hall, Burr W., et al. Hospitalizations for arrhythmias in the United States, 1985 through 1999: Importance of atrial fibrillation. American College of Cardiologists, Georgia World Congress, March 2002 (abstract)

11. Brugada, Ramon, et al. Identification of a genetic locus for familial atrial fibrillation. New England Journal of Medicine, Vol. 336, March 27, 1997, pp. 905-11

12. Allessie, Maurits A. Is atrial fibrillation sometimes a genetic disease? New England Journal of Medicine, Vol. 336, March 27, 1997, pp. 950-52

13. Klinkenberg-Knol, Elizabeth and Castell, Donald O. Clinical spectrum and diagnosis of gastroesophageal reflux disease, Chapter 19. In The Esophagus, edited by D.O. Castell and J.E. Richter. Philadelphia, PA, Lippincott Williams & Wilkins, 1999

14. Heitkemper, M., et al. Increased urine catecholamines and cortisol in women with irritable bowel syndrome. American Journal of Gastroenterology, Vol. 91, May 1996, pp. 906-13

15. Patacchioli, F.R., et al. Actual stress, psychopathology and salivary cortisol levels in the irritable bowel syndrome (IBS). Journal of Endocrinology Investigations, Vol. 24, March 2001, pp. 173-77

16. Putignano, P., et al. Salivary cortisol measurement in normal-weight, obese and anorexic women: comparison with plasma cortisol. European Journal of Endocrinology, Vol. 145, No. 2, August 2001, pp. 165-71

17. Stein, Jay H., Editor-in-Chief. Internal Medicine, 3rd edition, 1990, Little, Brown and Company, Boston, MA, p. 2194

18. Parker, A.J., et al. The neuroendocrinology of permanent fatigue syndrome and fibromyalgia. Psychol Medicine, Vol. 31, No. 8, November 2001, pp. 1331-45

19. Catley, D., et al. A naturalistic evaluation of cortisol secretion in persons with fibromyalgia and rheumatoid arthritis. Arthritis Care and Research, Vol. 13, No. 1, February 2000, pp. 51-61

20. Chrousos, George P. Stress, permanent inflammation, and emotional and physical well-being: concurrent effects and permanent sequelae. Journal of Allergy and Clinical Immunology, Vol. 106, November 2000, pp. S275-91

21. Small, Meredith F. Trouble in paradise. New Scientist, December 16, 2000, pp. 34-38

22. Gunnar, M.R. and Vazquez, D.M. Low cortisol and a flattening of expected daytime rhythm: potential indices of risk in human development. Developmental Psychopathology, Vol. 3, No. 3, summer 2001, pp. 515-38

2003 Ablation/Maze Surveys

By Hans R. Larsen [2003]

The **January 2003** survey attracted 42 responses from afibbers who had undergone focal point ablation, pulmonary vein isolation, or a combination of both. The overall success rate was 46%, but varied widely depending on the type of procedure and the type of afib (adrenergic, mixed, vagal or permanent).

Demographics

The majority (48%) of respondents had the mixed variety of LAF prior to their ablation. 38% had vagal LAF, 2% had adrenergic, and the remaining 12% had permanent LAF. These percentages are somewhat different from the percentages among our full database of 236 afibbers. Here 30% have the mixed form, 42% the vagal, 11% the adrenergic, and 17% the permanent form of LAF. The most striking difference is the low percentage of adrenergic afibbers who reported having an ablation. Is this coincidence, or is there some underlying reason why adrenergic afibbers are not considered good candidates for ablation?

The average age of the respondents was 55 years (52 for adrenergic and mixed, 54 for vagal, and 55 for permanent). The average age at diagnosis was 46 years (47 for adrenergic, 43 for mixed, 47 for vagal, and 53 for permanent). Thus the average number of years that the respondents had experienced LAF was 9 years with paroxysmal afibbers averaging 8 years and permanent afibbers averaging 11 years. These numbers are not significantly different from the averages obtained by considering all the entries in our main database, so there is no reason to believe that the respondents to the ablation survey were either younger or older than the general population of afibbers.

76% of respondents were male (71% adrenergic or mixed, 69% vagal, and 80% permanent). This again, is not significantly different from the gender distribution within our entire database.

Effectiveness by Procedure

Focal point ablation

Focal point ablation is the original method for ablating the inside of the atrium so as to isolate or destroy the areas of heart tissue producing the ectopic beats that initiate an afib episode. The procedure begins with an electrophysiology study (EPS), a test designed to map the electrical activity of the heart during fibrillation. Small tubes (catheters) are inserted into the veins in the groin, arms or neck, or under the collarbone, and then directed into the heart. Once the measuring electrodes are in place fibrillation is induced (if not already present), and the electrophysiologist is then able to pinpoint the areas where the rogue (ectopic) beats originate. These areas are often found at the junction between the left atrium and the pulmonary veins. The study is performed under mild sedation, but can still be somewhat uncomfortable and can last from 1 to 3 hours. At the end the electrophysiologist may report nothing to ablate if they have not located any foci of rogue cells, or they may go directly to the next step and ablate the active area(s).

Radiofrequency (RF) ablation utilizes radio frequency energy to heat the tip of a special catheter inserted through one of the tubes used in the EPS. The cardiologist or electrophysiologist places the catheter next to the area initiating the fibrillation and then "zaps" this area. This produces a scar, which destroys the offending area or prevents impulses originating in it from going anywhere.

The ablation procedure is generally fairly painless and lasts 4 hours or less. Nineteen afibbers reported that they had undergone focal point ablation. The average age of this group was 52 years (range of 36-70) with age at diagnosis being 42 years (range of 23-55). The average number of months since the ablation was 25 with a range of 5 to 67 months. There were 10 mixed, 5 vagal, and 4 permanent afibbers in the group. Most of the 19 respondents had had only one ablation, but one had undergone 3 and three had undergone 2 focal point ablations.

The **success** of the ablation procedure can be expressed in three ways:

- A subjective impression by the afibber;
- Complete absence of afib episodes with or without medication;
- Complete absence of afib episodes without medication.

Procedures	#	Subjective Evaluation	No Episodes*	No Episodes**
All procedures	19	21%	24%	16%
Paroxysmal	15	23%	20%	13%
Recent only	11	27%	36%	27%

Medication includes antiarrhytmics, beta-blockers, and warfarin
* With or without medication ** Without medication

The results may be somewhat biased by the fact that the series included 4 ablations done on permanent afibbers. However, considering only procedures done on paroxysmal afibbers did not improve the success rate.

The possibility that procedures done 3 or 4 years ago might have brought down the average was also considered. Taking just the 11 procedures done within the last 2 years the success rate did indeed improve, but was still not exactly spectacular.

So, the conclusion from this survey of 19 afibbers who have undergone focal point ablation is that the success rate is poor – only about 25%.

The successful procedures were done by Dr. Andrea Natale at the Cleveland Clinic, Dr. Chun Hwang at the Utah Valley Regional Medical Center, Dr. Robert

Bock at the Presbyterian Hospital, and Dr. Ron Berger at the Johns Hopkins University Electrophysiology Service.

Stenosis (narrowing of the opening of the pulmonary veins) is usually not a problem with focal point ablation. Only one of the 19 afibbers was checked for stenosis and did not have any signs of it. 68% of the group remained on antiarrhythmics or beta-blockers after the procedure and 32% continued on warfarin. Those of the respondents whose ablations were unsuccessful did not see an improvement in their frequency or duration of episodes.

Pulmonary vein isolation

This procedure involves the creation of a ring of scar tissue in the left superior, left inferior and right superior pulmonary veins. Electrophysiological studies have shown that these 3 veins are the most likely sources of the ectopic beats that generate AF. By isolating them from the left atrium via the scar tissue AF is prevented. Some cardiologists now also isolate the right inferior vein. Pulmonary vein isolation is much less effective for permanent AF indicating that most of the offending foci are located in the atrium rather than in the pulmonary veins [1]. Of particular interest to afibbers contemplating ablation is the fact the researchers have found no correlation between left atrial size and the success of the procedure [1].

Stenosis can be a problem with the pulmonary vein isolation procedure. Research is ongoing in an effort to solve this problem by using ultrasound or laser technology rather than the standard radiofrequency electrode. Cryosurgery is also being considered.

Seventeen afibbers reported that they had undergone pulmonary vein isolation. The average age of this group was 55 years (range of 37-71) with age at diagnosis being 49 years (range of 36-67). The average number of months since the ablation was 10 with a range of 2 to 33 months. This is a significant difference from the focal point ablation group and reflects the fact that pulmonary vein isolation is a more recent procedure. There was 1 adrenergic, 6 mixed, 9 vagal, and 1 permanent afibber in the group. Most of the 17 respondents had undergone only one ablation, but 4 had undergone the procedure twice. The **success** rates were as follows:

Procedures	Subjective Evaluation	No Episodes*	No Episodes**
17 procedures	71%	59%	47%

Medication includes antiarrhytmics, beta-blockers, and warfarin
* With or without medication ** Without medication

It is clear that the pulmonary vein isolation procedure is more successful than the focal point ablation. However, part of this improved success rate would appear to be connected with the continued use of drugs after the ablation.

Six of the completely successful procedures were performed by Dr. Andrea Natale at the Cleveland Clinic (100% success rate). Other successful procedures were done by Dr. Steve Furniss at the Freeman Road Hospital in Newcastle-upon-Tyne in the UK and Dr. P. Chang-Sing at the Santa Rosa Memorial Hospital in California. The remainder of the successful procedures involved continued drug use.

47% of the pulmonary vein isolation group remained on antiarrhythmics or beta-blockers after the procedure and 44% continued on warfarin.

Respondents whose ablations were unsuccessful did not see an improvement in their frequency or duration of episodes.

Fifteen of the 17 respondents had gone longer than 3 months since their ablation and therefore should have been checked for pulmonary vein **stenosis** via a special CT scan. Only 6 or 43% of them had actually been checked and 50% of those checked showed signs of stenosis.

Severe stenosis, i.e. greater than 70% narrowing of a pulmonary vein, is treated much the same way as blocked arteries. The vein is expanded with a balloon catheter and a large coated stent is inserted to keep the vein from closing up again (restenosis). It is likely that the development of stenosis depends on many factors, especially the skill of the surgeon performing the procedure. However, I don't believe that the possibility of stenosis should be taken lightly. Here is what one afibber had to say about his experience after undergoing an ablation:

"I had an upper body CT scan in which a radioactive dye is used to check the condition of the pulmonary veins. I was shocked and very disturbed to learn that two of the four pulmonary veins had severe stenosis as a result of the procedure. The right superior pulmonary vein has three branches, one far larger than the other two. That branch was completely closed and the doctor thought it was unlikely that it could be reopened by balloon angioplasty or a stent. The left inferior vein is 80% closed and likely to close further. One of the other two is somewhat narrowed and the last was not affected by the procedure. If all four veins close, you die! If three close you are in real trouble. So far I am not experiencing notable symptoms, but, at best, I can look forward to one or more stents, a lifetime of continued Coumadin use with a stroke risk at least as high as from AF and, of course, a lot of worry.

Would I do the procedure over if I know this would be the outcome? No, even though I have been very pleased with the relief from AF symptoms for almost six months. The risks are not worth it. Perhaps in a year or so, the problem of PV stenosis will be better understood and the ablation techniques will avoid this complication. I was told before the procedure that the chance of stenosis was less than 5%, but I think that is a great exaggeration. There is also an issue of the long-term consequences of the scarring in the areas where the ablations are done, especially when they are done up in the veins. At the very least, prospective candidates for the procedure should investigate not only the probability of complications like PV stenosis, but the seriousness of those consequences and the available therapies for dealing with them."

Focal point and pulmonary vein ablation
This procedure combines pulmonary vein isolation with the ablation of focal points in the left atrium.

Five afibbers had undergone the procedure. The average age of this group was 52 years (range of 47-54) with age at diagnosis being 42 years (range of 39-45). The average number of months since the ablation was 15 with a range of 5 to 24. There were 3 mixed and 2 vagal afibbers in the group. Three had had only one ablation, but one had undergone the procedure twice, and one 3 times.

Procedure	#	Subjective Evaluation	No Episodes*	No Episodes**
Combined	5	60%	60%	20%

Medication includes antiarrhytmics, beta-blockers, and warfarin
*With or without medication ** Without medication

The low success rate in the "no episodes without medications" is due to the fact that 2 of the successful afibbers were kept on warfarin even though they had no episodes.

The successful procedures were done in Bordeaux by Dr. Haissaguerre, by Dr. Dwayne Coggins at Good Samaritan Hospital, and by Dr. Paul Friedman at the Mayo Clinic.

Only 2 out of 5 (40%) had been checked for stenosis and both were found to have some degree of it.

Effectiveness by Afib Type

Twenty **mixed** afibbers had undergone ablation therapy with 53% having had focal point ablation, 32% pulmonary vein isolation, and 16% the combined procedure. One respondent did not know which procedure they had undergone.

Sixteen **vagal** afibbers had undergone ablation with 31% having had focal point ablation, 56% pulmonary vein isolation, and 13% the combined procedure.

Five **permanent** afibbers had undergone ablation with 80% having had focal point ablation and 20% having had pulmonary vein ablation. Only one procedure out of the five (a focal point ablation) was successful. This result, although based on a very small sample, confirms the belief that ablation is less successful with permanent afibbers than with paroxysmal ones.

The single **adrenergic** afibber who had undergone ablation had had the pulmonary vein isolation procedure. The procedure, done 5 months ago, was completely successful with the person having had no episodes and being off all medications.

Subjective success rates were as follows:

Procedure	Mixed	Vagal	Adrenergic	Permanent
Focal point ablation	40%	20%	-	20%
Pulmonary vein isolation	67%	80%	100%	0%
Combined procedure	33%	100%	-	-

Pulmonary vein ablation by itself is clearly the procedure most likely to be judged successful by paroxysmal afibbers while ablation involving permanent afibbers is still a challenge.

New Developments in Ablation Therapy

Dr. Andrea Natale and colleagues at the Cleveland Clinic recently released a comprehensive report describing their experience with pulmonary vein ablation in 211 atrial fibrillation [AF] patients. Most of the patients (54%) had paroxysmal AF, 16% had persistent AF, and the remaining 30% had permanent AF. Seventy-six per cent of the patients had **lone** atrial fibrillation. [2]

The Cleveland researchers evaluated two different ablation procedures and three different ablation catheters. The patients were first put into atrial fibrillation through the use of an isoproterenol infusion – assuming, of course, that they were not already fibrillating when they entered the operating room. The area around the pulmonary veins was then mapped using the circular mapping technique in order to locate the focal points from which the PACs and fibrillation originated.

The patients had originally been divided into two groups. Group 1 (21 patients) was scheduled to undergo distal isolation, that is, creation of scar tissue more than 5 mm into the pulmonary vein. The remaining 190 patients were scheduled for ostial ablation, that is, ablation right at the openings in the atrium where the pulmonary veins terminate. All ablations in group 1 were done with a quadripolar 4 mm tip. The ablations in the second group were done using 3 different tips – the quadripolar 4 mm (47 patients), an 8 mm tip (21 patients), and a cooled tip catheter (122 patients).

The researchers found the distal procedure to be relatively ineffective. Only six (29%) of the patients in group 1 experienced complete relief from PACs and AF. The patients in the second group had their pulmonary veins completely isolated at the ostium regardless of the mapping information. The success rate was 79% for the conventional 4 mm tip, 85% for the cooled tip, and 100% for the 8 mm tip. The time on the operating table was 3 hours with the 8 mm tip, 4.6 hours with the cooled tip, and 5.5 hours with the 4 mm tip, again showing the superiority of the 8 mm tip.

The researchers confirmed that an enlarged left atrium does not affect the success rate and that the ostial isolation procedure is highly effective even for permanent afibbers (success rate at 7.5 months of follow-up – 89%).

The rate of severe stenosis was 14% in group 1, but only 1% in the second group. Other researchers have reported stenosis rates of from 3 to 42%. Only 8 out of the 211 patients had significant complications from the procedures [2].

It is clear that ablation technology is improving at a rapid pace and that Dr. Natale and his group are now pretty close to achieving a 95-100% success rate using the 8 mm tip catheter and ostial ablation. However, the fact that this group has achieved this kind of success does not mean that every other cardiologist or electrophysiologist will achieve the same favourable outcome. New technology takes time to become standard practice, so unless you have a surgeon with a top notch track record such as Dr. Natale perform your ablation you may be better off waiting a bit longer so as to give the new technology a better chance to become more widely accepted.

September 2003 Survey

The September 2003 ablation survey attracted 59 responses from afibbers who had undergone focal point ablation, pulmonary vein ablation, or a combination of both. The overall success rate was 54%, but varied considerably depending on the type of procedure, the skills of the EP performing the procedure, and the year in which the procedure was done.

Demographics

The majority of the 59 respondents (83%) had the paroxysmal form of LAF, 10% had the permanent form, and the remaining 7% (all vagal) had persistent afib prior to their ablation. Among the paroxysmal afibbers 3 (6%) were adrenergic, 28 (57%) were mixed, and 18 (37%) were vagal. These percentages are somewhat different from the overall make-up of our current database of 341 afibbers (14% adrenergic, 37% mixed, and 49% vagal). This may reflect the fact that mixed LAF generally responds poorly to pharmacological treatment.

The average age of the respondents was 54 years with a range of 33 to 76 years. The average age at diagnosis was 46 years with a range of 23 to 75 years. Thus the average number of years that LAF had been present was 8 years with a range of 1 to 30 years. These numbers are not significantly different from the averages obtained by considering all the entries in our main database, so there is no reason to believe that the respondents to the ablation survey were either younger or older than the general population of afibbers.

Twenty-seven per cent of respondents were female, again not significantly different from the proportion in our total database.

Demographics * mean			
#	SUCCESSFUL GROUP	UNSUCCESSFUL GROUP	TOTAL RESPONDENTS
Total in group	32	27	59
Paroxysmal	28	21	49
Persistent	2	2	4
Permanent	2	4	6
Adrenergic	1	2	3
Mixed	13	15	28
Vagal	16	6	22
Average age*	54	54	54
Age at diagnosis*	47	46	46
Years of afib*	7	9	8
Females	26%	28%	27%

Success Rates by Afib Type		
AFIB TYPE	SUCCESS RATE	# IN SAMPLE
Overall	54%	59
Paroxysmal	57%	49
Persistent	50%	4
Permanent	33%	6
Adrenergic	33%	3
Mixed	46%	28
Vagal	73%	22

The observed differences in success rates were not statistically different although the difference between mixed and vagal afibbers approached significance (p=0.06). However, evidence in the literature suggests that ablation in permanent afibbers is usually less successful than ablation in paroxysmal afibbers.

Procedures

The most common procedure was pulmonary vein ablation (PVA) performed on 37 afibbers (63%) followed by focal point ablation on 16 (27%), and a combination of both performed on the remaining 6 (10%). The overall success rate for the PVA procedure was 62%, for the focal point ablation 25%, and for the combined procedure 83%. It should be pointed out that the success rate was dependent on how recently the procedure had been performed. For the 38 procedures performed in 2002 or 2003 the overall success rate was 66% and the success rate for PVA, focal point and combined was 68%, 40%, and 100% (only 2 procedures) respectively. The overall success rate of 66% and the 68% success rate for PVA procedures performed during 2002-2003 found in our survey is well within the range reported in the literature of 47% to 80% [3]. These success rates include 20-40% of patients still taking antiarrhythmic drugs and 10-30% requiring a second procedure [3]. In our survey 10 out of 59 respondents (17%) had undergone more than one ablation procedure. The repeat procedure rate was particularly high (25%) in the unsuccessful group. One afibber in the successful group later developed left atrial flutter.

There was a highly significant correlation between success rate and the year in which the procedure was performed (r=0.43, p=0.0008) with success steadily improving since 1999 to the present. This improvement is no doubt due to a combination of improved technology and equipment and greater EP skills.

Eighteen or 75% of 24 respondents who knew their ablation site had undergone PV ablation in the area of the atrium adjoining the pulmonary veins (ostial ablation) while the remaining 6 (25%) had their ablation inside the veins. The success rates for the ostial ablation were 67% as compared to 33% for the vein ablation.

Sixteen ablated afibbers submitted information regarding the catheter size used in their procedure. An 8 mm catheter was used in 8 cases, a 4 mm in 7 cases, and a 5 mm in 1 case. The success rate with the 8 mm catheter was 75%. (NOTE: All but one of these procedures were performed at the Cleveland Clinic). The success rate with the 4 mm catheter was 57%, but neither rate should be considered definitive due to the small sample size (8 and 7 respondents respectively).

Procedure Details and Success Rates				
DETAILS	TOTAL #	SUCCESSFUL GROUP #	UNSUCCESSFUL GROUP #	SUCCESS RATE %
Total ablations	59	32	27	54%
Pulmonary vein (PVA)	37	23	14	62%
Focal point	16	4	12	25%
Combined ablations	6	5	1	83%
PVA in ostial area	18	12	6	67%
PVA in veins	6	2	4	33%
PVA (site unknown)	13	9	4	69%
8 mm catheter used	8	6	2	75%
4 mm catheter used	7	4	3	57%
On afib drugs	46%	12%	85%	
On warfarin	38%	23%	56%	
All ablations 2002-03	38	25	13	66%
PVAs 2002-03	31	21	10	68%
Multiple ablations	10	3	7	

Recovery time, drug use, and stenosis

Even successful ablations were not always instantly successful. The average time span from ablation to full return to continuous sinus rhythm was about 7 weeks with a range of 1 day to 3 months. Afibbers who had been successfully ablated were significantly less likely to be on antiarrhythmics or blockers than were non-successful ones (12% versus 85%) and their use of antiarrhythmics was often short-term - just post ablation. The majority (56%) of afibbers in the unsuccessful group were on warfarin (Coumadin) as compared to 23% in the successful group. Most of the warfarin users in the successful group had undergone their ablation very recently so the warfarin use is likely to be a temporary measure only.

Only 3 of the 8 afibbers (38%) who had an ablation inside the pulmonary veins had been checked for stenosis and none was found. Thirty-eight per cent of those undergoing ostial ablation had also been checked for stenosis and none had shown any sign of it. While stenosis should not be a factor in ostial ablation it could be in vein ablation. Of the 22 afibbers who did not specify the area ablated 9 or 41% had been checked for stenosis and 3 (33%) had shown signs of it.

Supplementation, diet and ablation outcome

It is conceivable that supplementation, especially with vitamin C and vitamin E could affect the healing process of the ablation scars and thus alter the outcome of an ablation. Fifty-one per cent of respondents supplemented with vitamin C (average daily intake of 1425 mg) and 53% with vitamin E (average daily intake of 475 IU) in the time period before and after the ablation.

Most (74%) of the 38 respondents who specified their diet consumed a standard American diet, while 14% ate a vegetarian or partly vegetarian diet.

Supplementation and Diet			
DETAILS	SUCCESSFUL GROUP	UNSUCCESSFUL GROUP	TOTAL RESPONDENTS
Vitamin E	65%	35%	53%
Mean daily dosage, IU	435	600	475
Vitamin C	62%	35%	51%
Mean daily dosage, mg	1585	970	1425
Multivitamin	65%	35%	53%
Standard American diet	76%	71%	74%
Vegetarian diet	16%	12%	14%
Other diet	8%	17%	12%

There was a trend for afibbers who supplemented with vitamins C and E in the weeks preceding and the weeks following their ablation to be more likely to be in the successful group (based on a total sample of 26). Although the trend was not statistically significant (p=0.1) there is certainly no indication that taking vitamins C and E or a multivitamin affects the ablation outcome in a negative way. There was no indication that diet affected the outcome.

Blood pressure changes after ablation

Atrial fibrillation episodes release copious amounts of atrial natriuretic peptide (ANP) as a result of the rapid movement of the walls of the atria. ANP is a powerful diuretic and helps lower blood pressure by suppressing the release of aldosterone. It is conceivable that eliminating the periodic release of ANP through a successful ablation could affect blood pressure. Three afibbers reported a slightly lower pressure after the ablation while 2 reported a slight increase. However, 88% reported no change. Average blood pressure for afibbers in the successful group was 116/73 as compared to 117/72 for those in the unsuccessful group.

Sequel to unsuccessful ablation

A question uppermost in the minds of afibbers considering an ablation is, "Will I be worse off if the ablation fails?" Fifteen afibbers who had undergone an unsuccessful ablation reported on their episode severity after the ablation. Twelve (80%) felt that their episode severity was the same or less than before the procedure, two felt the situation had gotten worse, and one felt it had gotten much worse. The median number of episodes for 24 non-successes was 24 over a 6-month period and the median duration of these episodes was 8 hours. The number of episodes reported is substantially higher than that observed in the general afib population (median of 6 over a 6-month period), but may not represent a worsening for the specific afibbers who underwent an unsuccessful ablation. It should also be kept in mind that a group of "heavy hitter" paroxysmal afibbers experienced a median of 84 episodes over a 6-month period. Thus it is not clear whether one is better or worse off after an unsuccessful ablation, but the majority of afibbers actually experiencing a failed ablation did not feel they were worse off.

Rhythm Parameters			
DETAILS	SUCCESSFUL GROUP	UNSUCCESSFUL GROUP	TOTAL RESPONDENTS
# of respondents	15	6	21
# of adrenergic	0	2	2
# of mixed	8	3	11
# of vagal	7	1	8
# of permanent	0	0	0
Ectopic beats noticed	71%	100%	75%
Ectopic beats a nuisance	20%	-	20%
PACs predominant*	89%	50%	82%
PVCs predominant*	11%	50%	18%
Atrial runs*	75%	100%	80%
Periods of bradycardia*	57%	-	57%

*on Holter monitor recording

The response rate regarding rhythm parameters was too low to draw meaningful conclusions. There was some indication that respondents who underwent both successful and unsuccessful ablations continued to experience ectopic beats after the procedure, but few considered them a major nuisance. PACs (prior to ablation) were predominant in the successful group and atrial runs (during Holter monitoring) were common in both groups.

Perhaps the most interesting observation was that an increase in pulse rate following the ablation was quite common. Ten out of 19 respondents reported an increase in rate, eight reported no change, and one reported a decrease. The average (mean) increase was 12 bpm with a range of 7 to 29 bpm. Three respondents reported that their pulse rate reverted to normal after about a year, but another 4 had experienced no reversal after a year or longer. The remaining 3 were too close time-wise to their ablation to conclude whether their pulse rate would return to normal. I have been unable to find any studies that have investigated the possible long-term consequences of an increased heart rate subsequent to ablation therapy.

Successful ablations

The 32 successful ablations were performed by 20 different electrophysiologists (EPs) at 15 different institutions.

Electrophysiologist	Institution/Location	# of Procedures	Type of Procedure
Dr. Andrea Natale	Cleveland Clinic	9	PVA
Dr. Walid Saliba	Cleveland Clinic	2	PVA & Combined
Dr. Robert Schweikert	Cleveland Clinic	1	PVA
Dr. Chun Hwang	Utah Valley	2	Focal
Dr. Pierre Jais	Bordeaux, France	2	PVA
Dr. M. Haissaguerre	Bordeaux, France	1	Combined
Dr. Ron Berger	Johns Hopkins	1	Focal
Dr. Hugh Calkins	Johns Hopkins	1	PVA
Dr. Robert Bock	Charlotte, NC	1	PVA
Dr. Larry Chinitz	NYU Medical Center	1	PVA
Dr. Bhandan	Good Samaritan	1	PVA
Dr. Dwain Coggins	Good Samaritan	1	PVA
Dr. Paul Friedman	Mayo Clinic	1	Combined
Dr. K. Nademanee	Pacific Rim	1	Combined
Dr. Marcus Wharton	U of SC	1	PVA
Dr. David Wilber	Loyola University	1	PVA
Dr. Charlie Young	Kaiser, Stanford	1	PVA
Dr. Richard Leather	Victoria, Canada	1	PVA
Dr. Steve Furniss	Newcastle, UK	1	PVA
Dr. Ian Melton	New Zealand	1	PVA

Conclusions

- Mixed afibbers have the highest overall number of ectopic beats on an average day while vagal afibbers have the lowest.
- PACs are 3 times more prevalent than PVCs on Holter monitor recordings of lone afibbers.
- Runs of ectopic beats are more common than single beats.
- Most afibbers (53%) have not observed any change in ectopic beat frequency prior to an episode, but 42% have noted an increase.
- A change in position is associated with an increase in ectopic beats among 25% of all afibbers. Time of day and exposure to stress also influence ectopic beat frequency.
- There is a strong association between the frequency of PACs on an average day and the number of episodes over a 6-month period.
- A total of 37 out of 161 respondents (23%) have atrial flutter. Thirty-five per cent have undergone an ablation for the flutter with an average success rate of 62%. Afibbers with atrial flutter are more likely to experience hypoglycemia (idiopathic postprandial syndrome).

- Fifty-nine respondents have undergone radiofrequency ablation with an overall success rate of 54% (66% if performed in 2002 or 2003). Pulmonary vein ablation is the most common procedure with a success rate of 68% if performed within the last couple of years (2002 and 2003).
- The average time from ablation to the achievement of continuous sinus rhythm is 7 weeks ranging from 1 day to 3 months.
- Supplementation with multivitamins or vitamins C and E prior to and after the ablation procedure did not affect the outcome in a negative way, but could perhaps be beneficial.
- No changes in blood pressure were observed as a result of the ablation.
- Most afibbers (80%) who had a failed ablation did not feel that their episode severity had worsened after the procedure. However, afibbers experiencing a failed ablation did have substantially more episodes than the general population of afibbers.
- Most (75%) of ablated afibbers continued to experience ectopic beats after the procedure irrespective of whether it had been successful or not.
- A significant increase in heart rate (mean 12 bpm) was quite common (experienced by 53% of all ablated afibbers) after the ablation. In some cases the pulse rate returned to normal within a year, in other cases it remained elevated.
- The 32 successful ablations were performed by 20 different electrophysiologists at 15 different institutions.

Maze surgery, ICD implantation, AV node ablation

Only two afibbers, both vagal, had undergone the maze procedure and in both cases the procedure was a success. One adrenergic and one vagal afibber had had an ICD (implantable cardioverter defibrillator) installed and both were successful in eliminating episodes. None of the respondents had undergone AV node ablation and subsequent implantation of a pacemaker.

REFERENCES

1. Oral, Hakan, et al. Pulmonary vein isolation for paroxysmal and persistent atrial fibrillation. Circulation, Vol. 105, March 5, 2002, pp. 1077-81
2. Marrouche, Nassir F., et al. Circular mapping and ablation of the pulmonary vein for treatment of atrial fibrillation. Journal of the American College of Cardiology, Vol. 40, No. 3, August 7, 2002, pp. 464-74
3. Ellenbogen, KA and Wood, MA. Ablation of atrial fibrillation: Awaiting the new paradigm. Journal of the American College of Cardiology, Vol. 42, July 16, 2003, pp. 198-200

2003 General Survey

By Hans R. Larsen [2003]

Statistics

The **September 2003 General Survey** yielded 166 responses. Combining these responses with those from previous surveys results in a total database of 352 afibbers. Thus it is possible to establish the values of common variables such as present age, age at diagnosis, gender, number of episodes in the last 6 months, etc. with a fair degree of reliability as the means and distribution of these variables are based on a sample size of around 350.

Answers to questions such as "Have you been diagnosed with diabetes", which was only asked in this survey and in our very first survey can be answered with a somewhat lesser degree of reliability due to the smaller sample size. The reliability is further reduced when it comes to evaluating the prevalence of diabetes in a subgroup of afibbers (adrenergic, mixed, vagal or permanent). Thus in order to arrive at meaningful conclusions it is essential to use the proper statistical techniques to evaluate the survey responses.

The evaluation of the survey results involves three different approaches:

1. Conclusions drawn from a simple study of averages (means and medians) and range of the variables.
2. Conclusions drawn by comparing the prevalence of a particular condition among afibbers to that found in the general population.
3. Conclusions drawn from performing an analysis of the correlation between 2 sets of variables.

All statistical tests are carried out using the GraphPad Instat program (GraphPad Software Inc., San Diego, USA).

Averages and ranges
An example of this type of study would be the evaluation of episode duration. A close look at the results for mixed afibbers shows that the average (mean) duration of episodes is 4.7 hours (median 2.5 hours) for women and 11.6 hours (median 6 hours) for men. Also, that the range of episode duration is 0-48 hours for men and 0-21 hours for women. A comparison of the means for men and women shows that the difference in episode duration is statistically significant with a probability (p) value of 0.03. This means that there is less than a 3 in a hundred (3%) chance that the finding that the means are different is due to chance. In this study differences between means will be considered significant if the value of the two-tailed t-test (p) is 0.05 or less.

The comparison of afib burden between different groups of afibbers poses a particular problem.

The number and duration of afib episodes and the total time spent in fibrillation over a 3 or 6 month period [afib burden] is our "gold standard" measure of the severity of paroxysmal LAF. It is an essential component in evaluating the effectiveness of drugs, supplements and other interventions. It is, unfortunately, difficult to calculate a meaningful average of these values for a group of afibbers. The problem is that most respondents have fairly low values, but a small minority has greatly elevated values, which essentially makes a normal average (mean) quite meaningless in describing the overall severity for a particular group. For example, the calculated average time spent in afib per month for paroxysmal afibbers is 15 hours despite the fact the 81% of them spend less than 15 hours in afib. The average is skewed because a small group spends between 50 and 120 hours in fibrillation per month. I have, therefore, decided to use **median** rather than **mean** (average) values in describing group averages related to episode severity. The **median** is the value in the middle, i.e. the value above which half of all individual values can be found and below which the remaining 50% can be found. Using the median eliminates the bias introduced by a small group of "heavy hitters".

Prevalence of conditions

Several questions in this survey relate to the prevalence of conditions such as diabetes, hypertension, congestive heart failure, etc. The percentage of mixed afibbers diagnosed with diabetes is 1.8% (sample size N=57). The prevalence in the general population (aged 30 to 64 years) is between 3 and 9%. Thus the prevalence of diabetes among mixed afibbers is well below that found in the general population.

Correlation analysis

The discovery of correlations between variables is perhaps the most exciting part of the survey data evaluation. Two measures are used in determining whether one set of variables is correlated with another, the correlation coefficient and the probability of significance.

The correlation coefficient (calculated by the GraphPad program) is expressed as a number between minus one and plus one. A minus one indicates a perfect negative correlation, while a plus one indicates a perfect positive correlation. A correlation of zero means there is no relationship between the two variables. When there is a negative correlation between two variables, as the value of one variable increases, the value of the other variable decreases, and vice versa. In other words, for a negative correlation, the variables work opposite each other. When there is a positive correlation between two variables, as the value of one variable increases, the value of the other variable increases. The variables move together.

In the case of mixed afibbers the correlation coefficient between the average duration of episodes experienced over a 6-month period and the number of years since diagnosis is 0.3677 (sample size N=77). The **probability of** this correlation being due to chance (**p**) is 0.001; in other words, there is only a one in a thousand chance that the observed correlation is due to chance. We would say that the correlation between years of AF and episode duration is moderate.

83

In other words, the longer you have experienced afib the longer the episodes tend to last.

Generally, a correlation coefficient greater than 0.7 indicates a strong correlation, a value between 0.4 and 0.7 a moderate degree of correlation, and a value between 0.2 and 0.4 a weak one. However, a correlation coefficient of say 0.3500 for a large sample of 50 or more is considered a stronger indicator of correlation than is the same correlation coefficient if observed for a sample of only 15 participants. For the purpose of this survey, no correlation will be considered statistically significant unless p is equal to or less than 0.05.

The correlation coefficient also provides a measure of the percentage of variation of a dependent variable that is due to variation in its associated independent variable. The coefficient of determination (r-squared) is the square of the correlation coefficient. Taking the correlation between years of afib and duration of episodes as an example, the correlation coefficient "r" is 0.3677. The coefficient of determination (r-squared) is thus 0.135 meaning that 13.5% of the variation in episode duration can be explained by the variation in number of years of AF. This finding, of course, is both good news and bad news. The good news is that the number of years of AF is only a minor element in determining the duration of episodes and the bad news is that we still need to discover what lies behind the remaining 86.5% of variation in episode duration.

The presence of a few "heavy hitters" poses a problem when it comes to evaluating possible correlations between episode frequency and duration and other variables. In order to ensure valid correlations the analysis is performed on two sets of data. One containing all data and one with the "heavy hitters" omitted. "Heavy hitters" are defined as follows:

- Episode frequencies greater than the mean plus two standard deviations (of the complete data set).
- Episode durations greater than one week (168 hours)
- Total time spent in afib greater than the mean plus two standard deviations (of the complete data set).

Thus correlations involving episode severity is performed on both the complete data set and the data set with "heavy hitters" omitted. All other correlation analyses are performed on the full data set only.

Correlation is determined by using the Pearson or Spearman correlation coefficients or the Chi Square test as appropriate.

Finally, it should always be kept in mind that a high correlation coefficient is not enough to establish cause and effect. It also has to be scientifically plausible that an association exists. For example, a strong correlation between regular aspirin usage and nighttime leg cramps must have a plausible scientific explanation before it can be considered valid.

Demographics

A total of 341 afibbers (40 adrenergic, 108 mixed, 146 vagal, and 47 permanent) have now answered questions regarding their present age, their age at diagnosis, and their gender. A total of 9 afibbers with underlying heart disease also participated in the survey. Their responses, however, will be treated separately. The **present average age of respondents** was as follows:

Adrenergic	55.0 (mean)	53 (median)	range: 25-83 years
Mixed	54.5 (mean)	56 (median)	range: 31-73 years
Vagal	53.0 (mean)	54 (median)	range: 19-74 years
Permanent	57.7 (mean)	57 (median)	range: 34-82 years
Total paroxysmal	53.8 (mean)	54 (median)	range: 19-83 years
All participants	54.3 (mean)	55 (median)	range: 19-83 years

The difference in present age between the paroxysmal group and the permanent group was statistically significant as was the difference in age between vagal and permanent afibbers. The **average age at diagnosis** was as follows:

Adrenergic	49.6 (mean)	48 (median)	range: 22-80 years
Mixed	46.3 (mean)	48 (median)	range: 17-71 years
Vagal	46.6 (mean)	48 (median)	range: 14-73 years
Permanent	48.1 (mean)	48 (median)	range: 8-75 years
Total paroxysmal	46.9 (mean)	48 (median)	range: 14-80 years
All participants	47.0 (mean)	48 (median)	range: 8-80 years

There were no statistically significant differences in age at diagnosis. The finding that the average age at diagnosis among 341 lone afibbers is 47 years (median 48 years) should hopefully put a serious dent in the myth that lone atrial fibrillation is an "old age" disease. It clearly is not – quite the contrary, it tends to strike men and women at their most productive age. As a matter of fact, well over 50% of all afibbers were between the ages of 40 and 55 years when first diagnosed and over 16% were at or below the age of 35 when first diagnosed. Only 6.5% were 65 years of age or older when first diagnosed.

Years of afib
The average number of years that the survey respondents had experienced LAF episodes was as follows:

Adrenergic	5.4 (mean)	3 (median)	range: 1-15 years
Mixed	8.2 (mean)	7 (median)	range: 1-39 years
Vagal	6.5 (mean)	4 (median)	range: 1-40 years
Permanent	9.0 (mean)	5 (median)	range: 1-65 years
Total paroxysmal	7.0 (mean)	5 (median)	range: 1-40 years
All participants	7.3 (mean)	5 (median)	range: 1-65 years

Although the years of afib and the present age of respondents are not really that indicative of anything other than as a measure of how long the afibber had suffered with afib before finding *www.afibbers.org* and participating in the survey, it is interesting to note that it is indeed possible to live with LAF for a very long time – up to 40 years for paroxysmal afibbers and 65 years for permanent. As a matter of fact, 25% of paroxysmal afibbers had lived with afib for 10 years or more. I am not sure whether this is good news or bad. Living with this condition for 65 years sure seems like a very, very long time indeed! But, unless we come up with a solution that is exactly what some of us may just have to do.

Number of episodes during first year

This question was answered by 141 afibbers (15 adrenergic, 51 mixed, 67 vagal and 8 permanent).

Adrenergic	4.7 (mean)	3.0 (median)	range: 1-18
Mixed	15.5 (mean)	3.0 (median)	range: 1-225
Vagal	15.3 (mean)	4.0 (median)	range: 1-365
Permanent	13.0 (mean)	7.5 (median)	range: 1-52
Total paroxysmal	14.2 (mean)	3.0 (median)	range: 1-365
All participants	14.1 (mean)	3.0 (median)	range: 1-365

Clearly there is a vast variation in the number of episodes during the first year of afib. However, 50% of all afibbers experienced 3 or fewer episodes during the first year while 68% had 6 or fewer. There was no statistically significant difference between the numbers of first-year episodes for the various types of afib.

There was, however, a very significant correlation between the number of episodes experienced during the first year and the use of pharmaceutical drugs during the first year. Sixty-seven respondents (49%) had not taken any drugs (antiarrhythmics or beta-blockers) while the remaining 71 respondents (51%) had taken drugs. The non-drug takers experienced an average (mean) number of episodes of 4.7 during the year (median=2) while drug takers experienced an average (mean) number of episodes of 13.9 (median=6). This difference was highly significant ($p<0.0001$). The detrimental effects of drugs applied to all types of paroxysmal afib. There were too few responses from permanent fibbers to draw valid conclusions.

Adrenergic	27% no drugs	mean 1.8 episodes (median 2)	range: 1-3
Adrenergic	73% drugs	mean 5.7 episodes (median 4)	range: 1-18
Mixed	63% no drugs	mean 4.6 episodes (median 2)	range: 1-50
Mixed	37% drugs	mean 18 episodes (median 8)	range: 1-72
Vagal	44% no drugs	mean 5.5 episodes (median 2)	range: 1-57
Vagal	56% drugs	mean 13.5 episodes (median 5)	range: 1-52

All observed differences in episode frequency between drug and non-drug users were statistically highly significant.

It is clear that taking antiarrhythmics or beta-blockers during the first year of afib is detrimental. This could well be because the first choice in drugs is often digoxin or sotalol or a beta-blocker. All are directly detrimental to vagal afibbers and of dubious, if any, value for mixed and adrenergic afibbers. So based on this statistically highly significant finding the conclusion is to stay away from antiarrhythmics and beta-blockers for at least the first year of your afib career unless your heart rate goes so high during an episode that you need to slow it down by taking a calcium channel blocker or a beta-blocker during the actual episode only.

Conversion to permanent afib

Only 15 permanent afibbers provided a complete or partial answer to this question. The majority (73%) had developed permanent afib from the paroxysmal form while the remaining 27% (4 respondents) had been diagnosed with permanent afib when the condition was first discovered. Only 7 of the 11 respondents who had progressed to permanent were aware of what kind of paroxysmal afib they had. The majority (57%) believed they had progressed from mixed while the remaining 43% (3 respondents) believed they had progressed from vagal. The small sample size clearly makes any conclusions on this aspect very tenuous to say the least. However, it does appear that vagal afibbers can indeed become permanent. It took an average 3 years (range 1-8 years) for the condition to turn permanent, but again these numbers are based on a very small sample size (11 respondents) so should be taken with a large grain of salt.

Gender differences

The majority (80.4%) of all afibbers were male. There was a statistically non-significant trend for female afibbers to be diagnosed somewhat later than males.

Adrenergic	17.5% female	median age at diagnosis	M=49	F=47
Mixed	27.8% female	median age at diagnosis	M=46	F=53
Vagal	14.4% female	median age at diagnosis	M=46	F=54
Permanent	19.1% female	median age at diagnosis	M=47	F=60
All afibbers	19.6% female	median age at diagnosis	M=47	F=53

Only the 8-year difference in median age at diagnosis between male and female vagal afibbers was statistically significant ($p < 0.02$). Is it possible that the delay in females developing vagal afib could be due to a protective effect of estrogen? Tantalizing possibility, but as far as I know, pure speculation on my part.

Number of episodes during first year [revisited]

I earlier concluded that afibbers who took preventive drugs (antiarrhythmics or beta-blockers) during their first year of afib had significantly more episodes (median=6) than did those who did not take drugs (median=2). From this response I further concluded that taking these drugs during the first year is detrimental. I surmised that this could well be because the first choice in drugs is often digoxin, sotalol or beta-blockers. All are directly detrimental to vagal afibbers and of dubious value to mixed and adrenergic afibbers.

Several afibbers pointed out that the data could also be interpreted to mean that afibbers with frequent episodes are more likely to be prescribed drugs. Of course, this is correct. In order to attempt to settle the question of the effect of drugs during the first year I sent another questionnaire to the 72 afibbers who had indicated that they had taken drugs during their first year of afib. The questions were:

1. Did you start therapy with antiarrhythmics, beta-blockers or digoxin immediately after your first or second episode or did you only begin therapy after it became clear that you had an abnormally high frequency of episodes?
2. Which drug(s) did you take during your first year?

Thirty-seven (51%) of the 72 original respondents answered the second questionnaire. There was no statistically significant difference between the numbers of episodes experienced in the two groups within the first year. Thus the responses from the second group can be considered representative of the whole group.

An evaluation of the results of the second questionnaire produced the following results:

- 87% of all respondents were prescribed drugs after their first or second episode; in other words, they were not prescribed drugs because it had been established that they had frequent episodes.
- 81% were prescribed either digoxin, beta-blockers or sotalol after their first or second episode.
- 75% of vagal afibbers took digoxin, beta-blockers or sotalol after their first or second episode. These drugs are clearly contraindicated for vagal afibbers. The average (mean) number of episodes for this group was 12.0 (median=6.5).
- 49% of all afibbers took beta-blockers either alone or in combination with digoxin during their first year. The average (mean) number of episodes for this group was 16.6 (median=12).
- 38% of all afibbers took digoxin either alone or in combination with beta-blockers. The average (mean) number of episodes for this group during the first year was 20.0 (median=8).
- 19% of all afibbers took sotalol. The average (mean) number of episodes for this group during the first year was 12.7 (median=8).
- Only four out of 37 (11%) of survey respondents had taken antiarrhythmics as their sole medication during their first year. The average (mean) number of episodes for this small group was 2.0 (median = 2). Although the small data set precludes any firm conclusions it would appear that properly prescribed antiarrhythmics (flecainide, disopyramide, propafenone and amiodarone) on their own

may be beneficial, neutral or at least not detrimental during the first year.

Considering that the average (mean) number of episodes for those not taking any drugs during their first year was 4.7 (median=2) it is probably fair to say that digoxin, beta-blockers, and sotalol during the first year are generally not helpful and may indeed be detrimental. It is, of course, impossible to say if the people who took drugs during their first year would have been better off if they had not done so. However, the evidence from the survey certainly indicates that they might have been.

In conclusion, I believe it would be prudent to follow the advice given in the 2001 Guidelines for the Management of Patients with Atrial Fibrillation [1]:

"Prophylactic drug treatment is seldom indicated in case of a first-detected episode of AF and can also be avoided in patients with infrequent and well-tolerated paroxysmal AF".

In other words, do not begin drug treatment until it is clear that your episodes are frequent or intolerable. It is also prudent to postpone drug treatment until you are reasonably sure which type of AF you have (adrenergic, mixed or vagal). Digoxin should be avoided by all afibbers and beta-blockers and sotalol should be avoided by vagal afibbers. Properly prescribed antiarrhythmics, on their own, may be helpful in dealing with frequent or intolerable episodes during the first year.

Afib Severity

The severity of paroxysmal (intermittent) LAF is measured by four parameters – episode frequency over a 3 or 6-month period, average duration of episodes, total time spent in fibrillation over a 3 or 6-month period [afib burden], and intensity of episodes (extent of discomfort). A total of 255 paroxysmal afibbers (33 adrenergic, 94 mixed and 128 vagal) supplied data regarding episode frequency and duration and 148 supplied information about intensity.

A preliminary review of the data revealed that the sample population was far from homogenous. It was clear that there was a distinct group of "heavy hitters" who had far more frequent or far longer lasting episodes than did the majority of afibbers. The presence of this group led to a significant skewing of results and could result in erroneous conclusions being drawn regarding correlations with other variables. The "heavy hitter" group consisted of 25 afibbers (1 adrenergic, 14 mixed and 10 vagal) or 10% of the total sample. The members of this group fulfilled one or more of the following criteria:

- Number of episodes greater than total group mean plus two standard deviations;
- Average episode duration longer than 168 hours (1 week);

- Total time spent in fibrillation longer than total group mean plus two standard deviations.

The mean values for episode frequency, episode duration, and time spent in fibrillation differed significantly between the "heavy hitter" group and the group containing the remaining 230 afibbers (main group). The following statistical analyses were carried out on both of these groups individually as well as on the total group of 255 paroxysmal afibbers.

Episode frequency
The median number of episodes experienced by the main group over a 6-month period was 5. Further analysis produced the following results:

Afib Type	Respondents #	Mean	Median	Range
Whole Group	255	17	**6.0**	0-180
Adrenergic	33	9	4.0	0-68
Mixed	94	22	9.0	0-176
Vagal	128	16	5.0	0-180
Males	206	17	6.0	0-180
Females	49	18	8.0	0-180
Main Group	230	10	**5.0**	0-70
Adrenergic	32	7	4.0	0-68
Mixed	80	12	6.0	0-70
Vagal	118	10	4.0	0-70
Males	187	11	5.0	0-70
Females	43	8	5.5	0-25
Heavy Hitters	25	81	**84.0**	6-180

Episode frequency was significantly different between adrenergic and mixed afibbers in the whole group, but not between adrenergic and vagal or between mixed and vagal. The difference between adrenergic and mixed was no longer statistically significant when considering only the main group (omitting the "heavy hitters").

In conclusion then, for the main group the median number of episodes over a 6-month period is 5 with a mean of 10 and a range of 0-70. There is no statistically significant difference in the frequency of episodes between adrenergic, mixed and vagal afibbers when ignoring the heavy hitters. No statistically significant difference was found in episode frequency between men and women neither in the whole group nor in the main group considered by itself.

Correlations

- 55% of respondents were taking one or more drugs in an attempt to manage their afib while 45% were not taking any preventive drugs. There was no difference in episode frequency between the two groups. The effectiveness of drugs will be covered in considerably more detail later in this survey

- Somewhat surprisingly, no correlation was observed between frequency of episodes and age or number of years since first diagnosed. However, when only drug-free afibbers were considered there was a moderate positive correlation between age and increased frequency of episodes. No correlation was observed with number of years since diagnosis.
- Afibbers whose episodes occurred at regular intervals tended to have more episodes than those whose episodes occurred irregularly (median of 16 episodes versus 6 episodes per 6 months).
- There was a modest negative correlation for mixed afibbers only between the frequency of episodes and a high heart rate during an episode. This can either mean that mixed afibbers with less frequent episodes tend to have higher heart rates during their episodes or that those with a high heart rate during their episodes tend to have fewer episodes.
- There was a moderate to strong positive correlation for vagal afibbers only to have a higher episode frequency with a high intake of elemental magnesium. This is certainly an unexpected finding and clearly needs to be investigated further.

Episode duration

The median duration of episodes experienced by both the main group and the whole group was 6 hours as compared to 12 hours for the "Heavy Hitters".

Afib Type	Respondents #	Mean (hrs)	Median (hrs)	Range (hrs)
Whole Group	255	14	**6**	0-168
Adrenergic	33	16	8	0-72
Mixed	94	15	6	0-168
Vagal	128	12	6	0-168
Males	206	15	6	0-168
Females	49	7	4	0-48
Main Group	230	11	**6**	0-84
Adrenergic	32	15	8	0-72
Mixed	80	10	5	0-48
Vagal	118	10	6	0-84
Males	187	12	6	0-84
Females	43	6	4	0-48
Heavy Hitters	25	40	**12**	0-168

The difference in episode duration between adrenergic, mixed and vagal was not significant in the whole group or in the main group. The difference in episode duration between male and female afibbers was, however, highly significant with men tending to have longer episodes than did women.

Correlations

- There was no significant difference in the whole group in episode duration between afibbers taking preventive drugs and drug-free afibbers. The effectiveness of drugs will be covered in considerably more detail in a future issue.

- There was a modest, but statistically highly significant correlation between exposure to pesticides and solvents and duration of episodes with afibbers who had been exposed having longer episodes. This correlation was most apparent in the main group where afibbers with no solvent exposure had a median episode duration of 6 hours as compared to 15 hours for exposed afibbers. This finding raises the intriguing possibility that afibbers with long lasting episodes may benefit from a detoxification program.
- Adrenergic afibbers who were able to terminate their episodes with rest tended to have significantly shorter episodes.
- There was a modest positive correlation for vagal afibbers between the amount of elemental calcium absorbed and duration of episodes. This confirms earlier findings indicating that supplementation with large amounts of calcium may be detrimental for vagal afibbers.

Time spent in atrial fibrillation [Afib burden]
The median time spent in atrial fibrillation for the main group was 30 hours over a 6-month period [afib burden]. Further analysis produced the following results:

Afib Type	Respondents #	Mean (hrs)	Median (hrs)	Range (hrs)
Whole Group	255	261	**45**	0-3960
Adrenergic	33	201	24	0-3300
Mixed	94	400	45	0-3960
Vagal	128	175	47	0-1920
Males	206	270	48	0-3960
Females	49	222	24	0-3888
Main Group	230	123	**30**	0-1428
Adrenergic	32	105	24	0-1224
Mixed	80	139	29	0-1200
Vagal	118	119	36	0-1428
Males	187	139	36	0-1428
Females	43	57	22	0-399
Heavy Hitters	25	1526	**1144**	10-3960

The differences in time spent in fibrillation between adrenergic, mixed and vagal were not statistically significant in the whole group or in the main group. The difference observed between male and female afibbers was barely significant in the main group, but not significant in the whole group.

Correlations

- There was no significant difference in the whole group in time spent in fibrillation between afibbers taking preventive drugs and drug-free afibbers. The effectiveness of drugs will be covered in considerably more detail in a future issue.

- Not surprisingly, there was a strong, extremely significant correlation within all groups between episode frequency and time spent in fibrillation and between episode duration and time spent in fibrillation.
- There was a strong, positive significant correlation between time spent in afib and previous exposure to solvents or pesticides in both the main and whole groups.
- Afibbers whose episodes occurred at regular intervals tended to spend considerably longer in afib than did those whose episodes occurred at irregular intervals (150 hours versus 48 hours over a 6-month period).

Intensity of episodes

Episode intensity was judged subjectively by 148 respondents (18 adrenergic, 52 mixed and 78 vagal). Intensity was rated on a scale from 1 to 5 where 1 is barely noticeable while 5 is akin to World War III erupting in the chest area. The average (median) intensity for the whole group was 2.5. Specific values were as follows:

Afib Type	Respondents #	Mean	Median	Range
Whole Group	148	2.6	2.5	1-5
Adrenergic	18	2.0	2.0	1-4
Mixed	52	2.7	3.0	1-4.5
Vagal	78	2.7	2.75	1-5

Adrenergic afibbers judged their episodes to be significantly less intense than did mixed and vagal afibbers. There was no significant difference between mixed and vagal afibbers as far as intensity is concerned.

Sixty-seven (47%) of 143 respondents felt their episodes had decreased in intensity over time, 55 (38%) reported no change, and 21 (15%) felt they had increased in intensity over time. So the good news is that episode intensity is likely to decrease over time or at least remain constant. Adrenergic afibbers showed the largest decrease in intensity.

Correlations

- There was a highly significant negative correlation between intensity of episodes and present age confirming the earlier observation that intensity lessens with age. This effect is independent of how many years afib has been present indicating that aging, as such, is what tends to lessen episode severity.
- There was a modest, but highly significant positive correlation between intensity and maximum heart rate during an episode, indicating that a rapid heartbeat contributes significantly to the feeling of discomfort during an episode.
- Surprisingly, no correlation was observed between reported intensity and the use of a calcium channel or beta-blocker during the episode.

Initiation of episodes

A distinct difference was observed between the timing of the onset of an episode and type of LAF. Adrenergic afibbers had most of their episodes begin during the day, mixed had mostly an evening onset, and episodes for vagal afibbers began most often during the night. This is perhaps not surprising as adrenergic (sympathetic) tone is higher during the day while vagal (parasympathetic) tone predominates during rest and sleep.

Episode Onset						
AFIB TYPE	RESPONDENTS	AM	PM	EVENING	NIGHT	ANYTIME
Adrenergic	17	29%	29%	6%	6%	30%
Mixed	59	12%	19%	29%	14%	26%
Vagal	74	7%	5%	22%	61%	5%
All	150	11%	13%	23%	36%	17%

LAF episodes among adrenergic afibbers were all initiated by events that tend to increase adrenergic tone such as exercise or emotional or work-related stress. Vagal episodes were initiated by events that increase vagal tone such as rest, sleep, digestion or winding down after exercise. Mixed episodes were initiated by either an increase in adrenergic or vagal tone with no special preference for either one.

About 26% of all vagal afibbers noted that they were more likely to have an episode during the evening or night if they had experienced a stressful day. Prof. Coumel has described this phenomenon as "vagal rebound" and suggests that it may be possible to avoid it by taking a small amount of beta-blocker (atenolol) first thing in the morning if a stressful day or event is anticipated.

Almost two thirds (64%) of all paroxysmal afibbers reported frequent urination at the onset of an episode. This phenomenon was most pronounced among vagal afibbers where 72% experienced it versus 50% in the adrenergic group and 59% in the mixed group. The frequent urination is caused by the release of the diuretic hormone atrial natriuretic peptide (ANP) in the walls of the atria during chaotic beating.

Termination of episodes

Fifty-three per cent of all afibbers had observed that light exercise partway through an episode helped terminate it while 34% felt that resting helped speed conversion to normal sinus rhythm. Vagal afibbers were more likely to find exercise beneficial while adrenergic ones found rest to be more effective. Adrenergic afibbers who had found rest beneficial in terminating episodes actually did have significantly shorter episodes. Afibbers who were able to terminate their episodes with rest tended to be older than those who had found no benefit from rest.

Earlier Termination With			
AFIB TYPE	EXERCISE	REST	NEITHER
Adrenergic	31%	53%	16%
Mixed	39%	47%	14%
Vagal	67%	21%	12%
All	53%	34%	13%

Twenty per cent of all respondents felt that they had more than normal difficulty in sleeping during the nights following an episode. This problem was most pronounced among mixed (22%) and vagal afibbers (20%), but not of major concern among adrenergic afibbers (6%).

Repeated sneezing after the termination of an episode was reported by 5% of paroxysmal afibbers with 11% of adrenergic, 7% of vagal afibbers and none in the mixed group reporting this problem. Sneezing could be an indication of heightened vagal tone.

Pattern of episodes

About one third (35% adrenergic, 33% mixed, 34% vagal) of 142 respondents reported a distinct pattern to their episodes. The average (mean) number of days between episodes was 13 (median: 10, range: 1-42 days). There was no correlation between living a routine life and having episodes at regular rather than random intervals. However, afibbers with a regular pattern to their episodes tended to have more frequent and longer lasting episodes than did afibbers with no pattern. Could it be that afibbers with a regular pattern tend to be exposed continually to an environmental, dietary, or emotional irritant?

There was also a strong negative correlation (not too surprisingly) between the number of days between episodes and the frequency of episodes; i.e. afibbers with a short interval between episodes tended to have more frequent episodes over a 6-month period. There was, however, no correlation between the duration of episodes and the interval between episodes neither for all paroxysmal afibbers nor for drug-free paroxysmal afibbers.

Heart rate during episodes

Heart Rate During Episodes				
AFIB TYPE	MAXIMUM	RANGE	MINIMUM	RANGE
Adrenergic	148	85-230	81	45-140
Mixed	143	70-200	75	40-139
Vagal	133	55-280	76	35-140
Paroxysmal	139	55-280	76	35-140
Permanent	136	100-178	68	50-90

The average maximum heart rate during an episode was 139 bpm (range 55-280) for all paroxysmal afibbers (132 respondents). The minimum was 76 bpm (range 35-140) for 86 respondents.

The average maximum heart rate did not differ between afibbers continuously on antiarrhythmics or beta-blockers and those not on drugs nor was there any statistically significant effect in maximum heart rate between those taking beta-blockers or calcium channel blockers on demand and those that did not. This latter finding is counter-intuitive and needs further investigation.

There was no statistically significant difference in maximum episode heart rate between men and women; however, there was a slight, statistically significant trend for the maximum heart rate to decrease with age. No correlation was observed between maximum heart rate and length of time since first diagnosis of afib; nor was there any correlation between resting heart rate and maximum heart rate during an episode.

Main symptoms during episodes

The most common symptom experienced in an afib episode was palpitations. Other symptoms were breathlessness, fatigue, and dizziness. Some afibbers felt more than one of these symptoms.

Main Episode Symptoms				
AFIB TYPE	PALPITATIONS	BREATHLESSNESS	FATIGUE	OTHER
Adrenergic	78%	6%	-	16%
Mixed	79%	2%	12%	7%
Vagal	71%	9%	11%	9%
All paroxysmal	74%	6%	10%	10%

Cardiovascular health

Blood pressure and pulse rate

The average resting pulse rate for all paroxysmal afibbers was 60 bpm (170 respondents) and the average resting blood pressure readings were 124/76 mm Hg (153 respondents).

Pulse Rate and Blood Pressure (all respondents)						
	MEAN		MEAN		MEAN	
AFIB TYPE	PULSE RATE	RANGE	SYSTOLIC BP	RANGE	DIASTOLIC BP	RANGE
Adrenergic	63	48-80	122	98-153	73	60-87
Mixed	61	43-88	122	95-140	77	60-100
Vagal	60	40-80	126	90-180	76	60-105
Paroxysmal	60	40-88	124	90-180	76	60-105
Permanent	n/a	n/a	124	104-150	77	70-90

Beta-blockers, calcium channel blockers and some antiarrhythmics may influence pulse rate and blood pressure. A table showing pulse rate and blood pressure for afibbers not on any drugs is presented below (83 respondents for pulse rate, 72 for blood pressure).

Mean Pulse Rate and Blood Pressure (non-drug afibbers)						
AFIB TYPE	PULSE RATE	RANGE	SYSTOLIC BP	RANGE	DIASTOLIC BP	RANGE
Adrenergic	63	48-80	125	100-153	75	60-90
Mixed	59	43-83	122	95-140	75	60-90
Vagal	60	40-80	126	90-180	77	60-105
Paroxysmal	60	43-80	125	90-180	76	60-105
Permanent	n/a	n/a	118	104-130	72	70-86

There were no significant differences between pulse rates or blood pressure of adrenergic, mixed, and vagal afibbers, nor was there any significant differences in these parameters between afibbers taking drugs and those not. However, there was a statistically significant correlation between resting pulse rate and gender with women tending to have higher pulse rates than men. There was also a highly significant inverse correlation (not too surprisingly) between resting pulse rate and level of physical activity with highly active afibbers having lower resting pulse rate than sedentary ones. There was no correlation between resting pulse rate and frequency or duration of episodes.

Systolic blood pressure correlated moderately with the presence of diagnosed hypertension (this correlation is no doubt weakened by the use of antihypertensive drugs) and also with the perceived exposure to emotional or work-related stress. Afibbers who felt stressed had higher systolic blood pressures than those who did not feel stressed.

Diastolic blood pressure correlated weakly with the presence of diagnosed hypertension (this correlation is no doubt weakened by the use of antihypertensive drugs) and also with the perceived exposure to emotional or work-related stress with stressed afibbers having higher diastolic pressures.

Hypertension

Thirty-one paroxysmal afibbers had been diagnosed with hypertension and 3 additional respondents qualified as hypertensive because of a systolic pressure over 140 mm Hg or a diastolic pressure above 90 mm Hg. Thus a total of 20% of all paroxysmal afibbers (171 respondents) had excessively high blood pressure (hypertension).

Prevalence of Hypertension		
AFIB TYPE	NUMBER	PER CENT
Adrenergic	5/24	21%
Mixed	10/59	17%
Vagal	19/88	22%
Paroxysmal	34/171	20%
Permanent	6/21	29%

The prevalence of hypertension was significantly higher among permanent than among paroxysmal afibbers (29% versus 20%). The prevalence of hypertension in the general population varies with age, sex and race. Overall estimates are as follows [2]:

Prevalence of Hypertension, %			
AGE	WHITES	BLACKS	ALL RACES
45-54	39%	62%	41%
55-64	51%	71%	53%
65-74	63%	76%	64%

Considering that the average age of all paroxysmal afibbers is 54 years a prevalence of 20% is clearly well below the norm. This is probably a result of the generally high health level and fitness of afibbers. A more speculative reason could perhaps be that the diuretic action of the periodic release of atrial natriuretic peptide (ANP) during afib episodes prevents hypertension from taking hold.

Sixty-five per cent of paroxysmal afibbers used drugs to control their hypertension (60% among adrenergic, 60% among mixed, and 68% among vagal). The most popular drugs were atenolol (Tenormin), diltiazem (Cardizem), quinapril (Accupril), followed by metoprolol (Toprol XL), hydrochlorothiazide, and amlodipine (Norvasc).

There was a strong correlation between age and the presence of hypertension with hypertensive afibbers tending to be significantly older.

Congestive heart failure
Congestive heart failure (CHF) is a serious condition in which the heart is weakened to the point that it can no longer pump sufficient blood to meet the body's requirements for oxygen and nutrients. CHF is a major health problem in the United States and Western Europe where about 10 million people are now affected. CHF is a highly lethal condition with one 1 of 5 patients dying within the first year after diagnosis. The prevalence of CHF increases with age and is about 2% among people aged 40-59 years, over 5% among those aged 60-69, and over 10% in people aged 70 years or older. The prevalence among blacks is at least 25% greater than among whites. The incidence of CHF is twice as high in hypertensives as in people with normal blood pressure and having had a heart attack increases risk by a factor of five. Type 2 diabetes is associated with a two-fold increase in the risk of CHF [3].

Our survey of 66 lone afibbers showed that not a single one had been diagnosed with CHF and only one (a 12-year veteran of permanent afib) had been diagnosed with a left ventricular ejection fraction below 0.35. An LVEF below 0.35 is considered a precursor to CHF. Thus it would seem that lone afibbers are at a particular low risk of developing CHF. This is perhaps not too surprising in view of the fact that lone afibbers are generally healthy and fit and have a low incidence of hypertension and diabetes.

Stroke
Stroke (cerebral infarction, cerebrovascular event) is the third leading cause of death in the United States. It strikes about half a million Americans and kills upwards of 150,000 every year. A stroke involves a sudden interruption of blood flow to the brain. This interruption can be caused by a blood clot (thrombus) or a segment of arterial plaque that lodges in a small artery in the brain (ischemic stroke) or by the rupture of an artery wall (hemorrhagic stroke). An ischemic stroke is sometimes referred to as a "heart attack of the brain". The interrupted blood flow results in brain cells being starved of oxygen; if the interruption last more than 4 or 5 minutes the cells will die and irreversible damage will occur. If the cells that die are the ones that control your speech or your left arm then these functions will become impaired. If enough cells die (massive stroke) then so will you.

The risk of a stroke increases with age; it is estimated that 5% of the population over 65 years of age will suffer a stroke. A prior stroke, heart disease, diabetes, hypertension, atrial fibrillation, high homocysteine levels, and a bacterial infection of the lining of the heart cavity (endocarditis) are significant risk factors. Major surgery accounts for a large number of ischemic strokes. It is estimated that as many as 25,000 people suffer a stroke every year as a sequel to coronary bypass surgery [4-8].

Atrial fibrillation is a risk factor for ischemic stroke because of the inefficient pumping action of the atria during fibrillation. The fibrillating atrium basically sits and quivers like a bowl of jelly. This can cause blood to stagnate and if the fibrillation goes on long enough to coagulate and form blood clots (thrombi). If one of these blood clots finds its way to a small artery in the brain a stroke may result. The danger of this happening is actually highest when the fibrillation ceases. The increased pumping action, once the atria gets back to normal, flushes out the heart chamber and with it any newly formed blood clots. This is why anticoagulation with warfarin (Coumadin) and/or heparin is essential prior to cardioversion and for about 3 weeks after.

Lone atrial fibrillation, by definition, means that there are no underlying heart problems present. So unless you have hypertension, diabetes, are over 75 years of age or have suffered a previous stroke or TIA you are at no greater risk for stroke than is the general population [9]. Medical experts are pretty unanimous on this point. Dr. Rodney Falk, MD of Boston University, a world-renowned expert on atrial fibrillation, says that the stroke risk in patients with lone atrial fibrillation is minimal [8]. Professor Michael D. Ezekowitz, MD of the Veterans Administration says, "patients with lone atrial fibrillation are not at higher risk for thromboembolism than the general population and can be managed without anticoagulation or anti-platelet therapy" [10]. Dr. Stephen L. Kopecky of the Mayo Clinic did the first study regarding stroke risk in patients with lone atrial fibrillation. He found that lone afibbers under the age of 60 years had an exceptionally low stroke risk (0.55%) and that this risk varied little whether the fibrillation was paroxysmal or permanent [11].

More recently Canadian researchers evaluated the stroke risk among 2500 atrial fibrillation (non-valvular AF) patients who were treated with a daily aspirin. Twenty-four per cent of the group was considered at low risk for stroke because of the absence of hypertension (systolic blood pressure below 140 mm Hg), no history of stroke or TIA, no symptomatic coronary artery disease, and no diabetes. In this low-risk group the incidence of stroke was 1.0 per 100 person years as compared to 1.2 per 100 person years in an age- and sex-matched group of people with no atrial fibrillation. Low risk patients who were randomized to oral anticoagulation (warfarin) experienced 1.5 strokes per 100 person years. Strokes included both ischemic and hemorrhagic. The researchers conclude, "Irrespective of age, patients with AF and none of the above four clinical features and who take aspirin have stroke rates comparable to those of age-matched community cohorts and would not benefit substantially from anticoagulation."[12]

Our survey included 159 lone afibbers. Not one had suffered a stroke of any kind. Interpretation of this finding must, of course, be approached with extreme caution. Clearly afibbers having suffered a fatal or severely disabling stroke would be unlikely to have participated in the survey. However, there is no reason why afibbers who have suffered a mild stroke or a transient ischemic attack (TIA) should not have participated. A TIA involves a temporary blockage of blood flow to the brain. Effects are usually reversible within 24 hours. A TIA is followed by a stroke in about 1 out of 3 cases [13].

A total of 5 TIAs (3 among permanent afibbers) were reported in the survey. These were in a sample covering 1145 person years of exposure (years of afib). So the incidence is 0.4 per 100 person years. Is this normal or abnormal?

Dr. Jerome FX Naradzay of the Samaritan Medical Center estimates a TIA incidence rate of 0.4 to 0.8 cases per 100 person years in the general population aged 50-59 years and a recent study carried out at the Ottawa Heart Institute found a combined stroke rate of 1.0 per 100 person years in afibbers treated with aspirin [12,14].

So overall the TIA rate found in our survey would appear to be fairly normal except in the case of permanent afibbers where the rate was 2.6 per 100 person years. The sample was, however, quite small (15 people) so the results must be taken with a grain of salt. The ages of the 3 permanent afibbers who had suffered a TIA were 59, 63 and 65 years respectively. One was on aspirin or warfarin at the time of the TIA while one was not on stroke prevention medicine. The medication status of the third one is unknown.

Electrolyte levels
Electrolyte levels, that is, the intracellular levels of potassium (K), sodium (Na), magnesium (Mg), and calcium, are important for proper functioning of the heart. Low levels of potassium and magnesium, in particular, may predispose to ectopic beats and afib.

Thirty-seven out of 159 respondents had had their intracellular electrolyte levels checked and 23 (62%) had abnormal levels. Low magnesium levels were found in 6, low potassium in 4, high calcium in 3, and one each of low and high phosphorous levels.

Conclusion
Lone afibbers would appear to have excellent cardiovascular health with normal resting pulse rate, normal blood pressure, and a low incidence of hypertension. There were no cases of congestive heart failure in our survey group (166 afibbers) even though a prevalence of 2-5% would have been expected. No strokes were reported by 159 afibbers (this observation must be viewed with caution as afibbers who have suffered a stroke may be less likely to participate in the survey). There were 5 reported cases of transient ischemic attack (TIA) in the group (3 among permanent afibbers). This is probably in the normal range except among the small sample of permanent afibbers (15 respondents) where the incidence was 2.6 per 100 person years. A majority

(62%) of afibbers who had been tested for intracellular electrolyte levels had abnormal levels, most often, low magnesium, low potassium or high calcium. It is not known how this finding compares to what would be expected in the general population.

Our finding that lone afibbers have excellent cardiovascular health supports those made in 1998 by researchers at the University of Helsinki [15]. Their study concluded that men who engaged in long-term vigorous exercise (as many afibbers do) have a 5 times greater risk of developing LAF, but a 3 times lower risk of developing coronary heart disease and 5 times lower overall premature mortality than less active men.

General Health

Diabetes/Hypoglycemia
The overall prevalence of diabetes among 202 afibbers surveyed was slightly less than 1%. This is clearly substantially lower than the overall prevalence of type 2 diabetes in the United States, which is now estimated at 6% (approaching 8% in New York City) [16]. The prevalence of glucose intolerance or insulin resistance among 159 afibbers was 4.4%, again substantially lower than the 6% estimated for the US population as a whole [16]. The prevalence of hypoglycemia or idiopathic postprandial syndrome among 184 afibbers was 26%, which is probably somewhat higher than that found in the general population.

Diabetes and Hypoglycemia			
AFIB TYPE	DIABETES	GLUCOSE INTOLERANCE	HYPOGLYCEMIA
Adrenergic	0/24 (0%)	0/18 (0%)	10/24 (41.7%)
Mixed	1/59 (1.7%)	1/52 (1.9%)	14/57 (24.6%)
Vagal	0/96 (0%)	2/75 (2.7%)	20/83 (24.1%)
Paroxysmal	1/179 (0.6%)	3/145 (2.0%)	44/164 (26.8%)
Permanent	1/23 (4.3%)	1/14 (7.1%)	3/20 (15.0%)
TOTAL	2/202 (1.0%)	7/159 (4.4%)	47/184 (25.5%)

The low prevalence of diabetes among afibbers is a welcome surprise. I don't know whether having afib in itself or a genetic abnormality underlying afib prevents the development of diabetes, but this is clearly an area where more in-depth research may prove fruitful. Afibbers though, in an attempt to avoid frequent episodes, tend to take many of the measures that have been proven effective in the prevention of diabetes and glucose intolerance. Among these are:
- Regular exercise
- Healthy diet
- Decreased fat intake (total and saturated)
- Avoidance of trans-fatty acids
- Increased fiber intake
- Maintenance of ideal weight
- Vitamin and mineral supplementation (particularly vitamin E)

The prevalence of hypoglycemia (idiopathic postprandial syndrome) among afibbers is probably somewhat high at 26% although I have not been able to find any official prevalence figures. The prevalence among adrenergic afibbers (42%) is almost certainly abnormally high. Postprandial hypoglycemia involves epinephrine (adrenaline) release (adrenergic stimulation) which is known to cause palpitations and full-blown AF.

It is also possible that a glutamate/MSG sensitivity could explain the absence of diabetes and the prevalence of hypoglycemia as glutamate stimulates insulin release. The high prevalence of hypoglycemia and low prevalence of diabetes could, of course, both point to an oversensitive insulin response. This can be attenuated by emphasizing foods with a low glycemic load and by ensuring that each meal and snack contains some protein.

There was a slight, but statistically highly significant association between having hypoglycemia and having been diagnosed with atrial flutter. There was also a moderate, but statistically significant correlation between having hypoglycemia and having a high maximum heart rate during an episode.

Leg cramps
Leg cramps during the night or after exercise is a fairly common complaint among afibbers. A survey of 166 afibbers showed that 35 (21%) experienced leg cramps mostly (9%) occurring at night.

Leg Cramps				
AFIB TYPE	AT NIGHT	AFTER EXERCISE	OTHER	TOTAL
Adrenergic	3/19 (15.8%)	0/19 (0%)	1/19 (5.3%)	4/19 (21.1%)
Mixed	6/53 (11.3%)	4/53 (7.5%)	4/53 (7.5%)	14/53 (26.4%)
Vagal	5/79 (6.3%)	4/79 (5.1%)	4/79 (5.1%)	13/79 (16.5%)
Paroxysmal	14/151 (9.3%)	8/151 (5.3%)	9/151 (5.9%)	31/151 (20.5%)
Permanent	1/15 (6.7%)	2/15 (13.3%)	1/15 (6.7%)	4/15 (26.7%)
TOTAL	15/166 (9.0%)	10/166 (6.0%)	10/166 (6.0%)	35/166 (21.1%)

Leg cramps sometimes involve a magnesium deficiency, but the survey did not find any correlation between magnesium intake from supplements and the presence of leg cramps. Leg cramps, particularly at night, are quite common among elderly people. A British study involving 365 people aged 65 years or older found that 50% of them experienced leg cramps regularly. The researchers point out that the risk of leg cramps increases with the presence of arthritis and peripheral vascular disease [17].

Premenstrual syndrome (PMS)
Only 30 respondents answered the question about experiencing PMS (2 adrenergic, 13 mixed, 12 vagal and 3 permanent). Five of the 30 (17%) reported suffering from PMS (1 adrenergic, 3 mixed, 1 vagal). The number of data points was too small to draw any conclusions regarding possible correlations with other variables.

Asthma

The current prevalence of asthma among adults in the United States is 7.2% [18]. We found a prevalence of 8.0% among 162 respondents in the 5th LAF survey. Thus there is no indication that asthma rates among afibbers are significantly different from that in the general population and no reason to suspect a connection between asthma and AF.

Asthma		
AFIB TYPE	NUMBER	PER CENT
Adrenergic	3/19	15.8
Mixed	5/52	9.6
Vagal	5/76	6.6
Paroxysmal	13/147	8.8
Permanent	0/15	0
TOTAL	13/162	8.0

The difference in prevalence among adrenergic and vagal afibbers is not statistically significant.

Common cold/Runny nose

The average number of colds experienced by 165 respondents was 1.2/year. The National Institutes of Health estimates the average incidence of colds among adults in the United States to be 3/year [19]. Thus there is no reason to suspect that afibbers have a weakened immune system, perhaps rather the opposite.

AFIB TYPE	# COLDS/YEAR	RUNNY NOSE WITHOUT COLD
Adrenergic	0.9	5/19 (26.3%)
Mixed	1.3	23/53 (43.4%)
Vagal	1.2	28/75 (37.3%)
Paroxysmal	1.2	56/147 (38.0%)
Permanent	0.9	8/15 (53.3%)
TOTAL	1.2	64/162 (40.0%)

There was a moderate, but extremely statistically significant inverse correlation between present age of respondents and the number of colds per year with older people tending to have fewer colds. There was no correlation between the number of colds and episode frequency or duration.

A total of 40% of 162 respondents answered "yes" to the question "Do you often suffer from a runny nose without having a cold?" I have not been able to find an official estimate of the prevalence of runny noses in the general population, but 40% does seem rather high. A non-cold related runny nose could be a sign of an allergy, excessive vagal domination or a glutamate/MSG sensitivity. Adrenergic afibbers had a slightly lower prevalence than did mixed, vagal and permanent afibbers, but these differences were not statistically significant. There was no correlation between a tendency to runny nose and self-reported MSG sensitivity or between a tendency to runny nose and episode frequency or duration. It is possible that the high prevalence of runny noses among afibbers is an important clue, but clearly more research would be required to ascertain this.

Environmental Factors

Solvent and pesticide exposure
A total of 33 afibbers (20%) reported exposure to volatile industrial solvents, pesticides, crop-dusting chemicals or Agent Orange prior to their LAF diagnosis. There was a very significant correlation between prior solvent/pesticide exposure and duration of afib episodes among paroxysmal afibbers. Those who had been exposed to solvents/pesticides had significantly longer episodes (23 hours versus 9 hours mean; 15 hours versus 6 hours median).

Solvent and Pesticide Exposure		
AFIB TYPE	# EXPOSED	% EXPOSED
Adrenergic	4/18	22
Mixed	7/52	14
Vagal	19/78	24
Paroxysmal	30/148	20
Permanent	3/14	21
TOTAL	33/162	20

There was no correlation between present age and solvent exposure or between gender and incidence of solvent exposure. There was, however, a significant association between solvent exposure and self-reported MSG sensitivity with afibbers exposed to solvents being more likely to report MSG sensitivity. There was a slight, but statistically not quite significant (P=0.07) trend for solvent-exposed afibbers to have hypoglycemia. Solvent-exposed afibbers were more likely to take magnesium supplements, perhaps reflecting the more serious nature of their LAF (longer episode duration).

Sensitivity to gasoline smell
Only 5 out of 140 respondents (3 mixed, 2 vagal) reported that exposure to the smell of gasoline (petrol) was likely to precipitate an episode. Four of these 5 had prior exposure to solvents or pesticides and 3 had MSG sensitivity as well. There were not enough data points to establish the statistical significance of this or other possible correlations.

Dietary Factors

Sensitivity to MSG
Twenty-one of 120 respondents (17.5%) reported that exposure to MSG (monosodium glutamate) was likely to trigger an episode.

MSG Sensitivity		
AFIB TYPE	# SENSITIVE	% SENSITIVE
Adrenergic	2/15	13.3
Mixed	5/53	9.4
Vagal	14/52	26.9
Paroxysmal	21/120	17.5

The fact that only 17.5% of respondents reported that MSG exposure would set off an afib episode does not mean that only 17.5% are actually sensitive to MSG or glutamate exposure. It could well be that many more have a "subclinical" sensitivity that requires an accumulation of MSG exposure rather than just a single exposure to initiate an episode. Afibbers with acute MSG sensitivity were significantly more likely to have been exposed to solvents and pesticides prior to their diagnosis of LAF. Perhaps prior solvent/pesticide exposure sensitizes one to later MSG exposure. There was a trend (P=0.06) for afibbers taking bulk-forming laxatives (psyllium, Metamucil) to be more likely to report MSG sensitivity.

Regular use of bulk-forming laxatives

Bulk-forming laxatives, such as psyllium and Metamucil, were used regularly by 22 out of 163 respondents (13.5%). The difference in usage between adrenergic, mixed and vagal afibbers is not statistically significant.

Use of Laxatives		
AFIB TYPE	NUMBER	PER CENT
Adrenergic	1/19	5.3
Mixed	13/52	25.0
Vagal	6/77	7.8
Paroxysmal	20/148	13.5
Permanent	2/15	13.3
TOTAL	22/163	13.5

There was no correlation between the use of bulk-forming laxatives and episode frequency or duration; however, there was a trend for laxative users to be sensitive to MSG.

Consumption of licorice

Only 3 out of 164 respondents (1.8%) reported regular consumption of licorice or licorice root. Thus there is no reason to suspect a connection between licorice consumption and LAF. Licorice contains a component, glycyrrhizic acid, which is known to inhibit 11-beta-hydroxysteroid dehydrogenase type 2, the enzyme responsible for the conversion of cortisol to its inactive form (cortisone).

Daily water consumption

The average daily drinking water consumption among 160 respondents was about five 8-oz glasses.

Average Daily Water Consumption		
AFIB TYPE	# OF 8-OZ GLASSES	RESPONDENTS
Adrenergic	3.6	19
Mixed	4.8	51
Vagal	4.7	76
Paroxysmal	4.7	146
Permanent	5.4	14
TOTAL	4.8	160

There was no correlation between episode frequency and duration and daily water consumption. There was a statistically significant slight trend for heavy water drinkers to have vagally induced episodes. There was a moderate statistically significant association between a high daily water intake and a high intake of calcium from supplements. There was also a slight trend for heavy water drinkers to report frequent emotional or work-related stress or, equally plausible, for emotionally stressed afibbers to drink more water.

Lifestyle Factors

Sleep pattern
There were no significant differences in the average sleep pattern of adrenergic, mixed, vagal and permanent afibbers. Most (77%) slept in a completely dark room (important for proper melatonin synthesis), went to bed around 11 pm, and got a little more than 7 hours of sleep every night.

Sleep Pattern				
AFIB TYPE	RESPONDENTS	DARK ROOM YES	BEDTIME (PM)	HRS. SLEEP
Adrenergic	18	67%	11:00	7.7
Mixed	52	75%	11:00	7.2
Vagal	78	82%	11:00	7.0
Paroxysmal	148	78%	11:00	7.2
Permanent	15	67%	10.45	7.5
TOTAL	163	77%	11:00	7.2

There were no associations between episode frequency or duration and bedtime, hours of sleep or sleeping in a dark room. However, there was a slight to moderate statistically highly significant association between hours of sleep and leading a routine life with afibbers leading a routine life tending to sleep longer. Those who slept longer were also more likely to be able to terminate their episodes with rest.

Level of physical activity
The majority of 201 respondents (62%) considered themselves somewhat physically active, 28% considered themselves very physically active, and only 10% considered themselves to be sedentary.

Physical Activity Level				
AFIB TYPE	RESPONDENTS	SEDENTARY	SOMEWHAT ACTIVE	VERY ACTIVE
Adrenergic	29	3%	66%	31%
Mixed	59	15%	53%	32%
Vagal	92	9%	65%	26%
Paroxysmal	180	10%	61%	29%
Permanent	21	10%	67%	23%
TOTAL	201	10%	62%	28%

There was no association between physical activity level and episode frequency, duration or intensity. There was an extremely significant correlation between gender and physical activity level with women tending to be less physically active than men. There was also a significant correlation between the regular use of beta- blockers and physical activity with afibbers on beta-blockers tending to be less physically active. Not surprisingly, there was an extremely significant correlation between physical activity level and resting heart rate with more physically active afibbers having significantly lower resting heart rates.

Stress level

The majority (58%) of 165 respondents reported frequent exposure to emotional or work-related stress again underscoring the major role played by psychological stress in the etiology of afib.

Stress Level		
AFIB TYPE	# RESPONDENTS	FREQUENTLY EXPOSED TO STRESS
Adrenergic	19	63%
Mixed	53	57%
Vagal	78	60%
Paroxysmal	150	59%
Permanent	15	47%
TOTAL	165	58%

It is tempting to speculate that permanent afibbers are less stressed then paroxysmal afibbers because they are not always anxiously awaiting the next episode; however, the observed difference in perceived stress exposure is not significantly different.

There was no correlation between episode frequency and level of stress exposure; however, there was a statistically significant trend for stressed afibbers to have longer lasting and more intensely felt episodes. There was also a significant inverse correlation between leading a routine life and feeling stressed. Afibbers who lead a routine life were less likely to report emotional or work-related stress.

There was a highly significant correlation between stress level and systolic blood pressure. Afibbers who reported frequent exposure to stress had an average systolic blood pressure of 125 mm Hg while unstressed afibbers averaged 120 mm Hg. There was also a significant trend for stressed afibbers to drink more water during the day.

Conclusions

- Afibbers have a very low prevalence of diabetes and perhaps a higher than normal prevalence of hypoglycemia (idiopathic postprandial syndrome). It is possible that afibbers have a heightened insulin response perhaps stimulated by glutamate or high glycemic index foods.
- Afibbers are no more likely to have asthma than is the general population and tend to have significantly fewer colds than observed in the general population.
- Experiencing a runny nose without having a cold was quite common among afibbers and could indicate the presence of an allergy, excessive vagal domination or a glutamate/MSG sensitivity.
- Twenty per cent of all afibbers (out of 162) reported exposure to solvents, pesticides, crop-dusting chemicals or Agent Orange prior to their diagnosis of LAF. These afibbers had significantly longer episodes and were more likely to report a sensitivity to MSG.
- There were no significant differences in sleep patterns between adrenergic, mixed, vagal, and permanent afibbers and no indication that sleep pattern (bedtime, hours of sleep, sleeping in a dark room) had any association with episode frequency and duration. However, afibbers with longer hours of sleep were more likely to lead a routine life and to be more likely to be able to terminate their episodes with rest.
- Most afibbers considered themselves physically active or very physically active. There was no correlation between physical activity level and episode frequency, duration or intensity. Women and afibbers on beta- blockers tended to be less physically active and not surprisingly, there was an extremely significant correlation between physical activity level and resting heart rate with more physically active afibbers having significantly lower resting heart rates.
- Emotional or work-related stress was regularly experienced by 58% of all afibbers underscoring the major role played by psychological stress in the etiology of afib. There was no correlation between episode frequency and stress level, but stressed afibbers did tend to have longer lasting and more intensely felt episodes. Stressed afibbers were also less likely to lead a routine life and tended to have significantly higher systolic blood pressure than did non-stressed afibbers.

Use of Pharmaceutical Drugs

Fifty-five per cent of 326 afibbers surveyed used pharmaceutical drugs in the management of their condition. Twenty-six per cent used antiarrhythmics on a continuous basis to prevent afib episodes (rhythm control) while 19 per cent used beta or calcium channel blockers on a continuous basis to control their heart rate. Eleven per cent used both antiarrhythmics and blockers.

AFIB TYPE	#	NO DRUGS	DRUGS	ANTI-ARRHYTHMICS	BLOCKERS	COMBO
Adrenergic	38	39%	61%	21%	34%	8%
Mixed	97	46%	54%	24%	16%	14%
Vagal	145	48%	52%	32%	11%	10%
Paroxysmal	280	46%	54%	28%	16%	11%
Permanent	46	37%	63%	14%	35%	14%
TOTAL	326	45%	55%	26%	19%	11%
Men	260	47%	53%	25%	17%	11%
Women	66	36%	64%	25%	23%	17%

Use of Pharmaceutical Drugs

Women were slightly more likely to be using pharmaceutical drugs than were men, however, the difference in usage was not statistically significant. There was no statistical difference in age between users and non-users of drugs. Adrenergic afibbers were significantly more likely to be using beta or calcium channel blockers than were vagal afibbers. Other differences in observed drug use among the various afib types were not statistically significant.

The most widely used antiarrhythmic drug was flecainide while atenolol was the most used beta-blocker and diltiazem was the most used calcium channel blocker.

DRUG NAME	TRADE NAME	COMMON DOSE mg/day	RANGE mg/day
Flecainide	Tambocor	200	50-300
Atenolol	Tenormin	37	6-100
Diltiazem	Cardizem	180	120-480
Sotalol	Betapace	160	80-480
Amiodarone	Cordarone	200	150-600
Disopyramide	Norpace	300	150-600
Propafenone	Rythmol	450	300-675
Metoprolol	Toprol	50	25-100
Metoprolol XL	Toprol XL	25	12-200
Verapamil	Veralan	240	180-360
Digoxin	Lanoxin	-	-
Dofetilide	Tikosyn	-	-
Propranolol	Inderal	-	-
Procainamide	Procan	-	-
Other	-	-	-

Pharmaceutical Drugs Used

Number of Respondents Using Indicated Drugs						
DRUG NAME	ADREN	MIXED	VAGAL	PAROX	PERM	TOTAL
Flecainide	1	13	24	38	1	39 (19%)
Atenolol	5	9	10	24	3	27 (13%)
Diltiazem	2	5	6	13	6	19 (9%)
Sotalol	2	6	7	15	3	18 (9%)
Amiodarone	4	1	7	12	5	17 (8%)
Disopyramide	1	5	11	17	0	17 (8%)
Propafenone	2	4	6	12	2	14 (7%)
Metoprolol	4	2	5	11	1	12 (6%)
Metoprolol XL	3	5	2	10	1	11 (5%)
Verapamil	0	4	4	8	2	10 (5%)
Digoxin	1	4	1	6	2	8 (4%)
Dofetilide	0	3	2	5	1	6 (3%)
Propranolol	0	2	1	3	0	3 (1%)
Procainamide	1	0	1	2	0	2 (1%)
Other	0	2	1	3	1	4 (2%)
TOTAL	26	65	88	179	28	207 (100%)

The most notable finding from this tabulation is that 36% of the drugs used to treat vagal afibbers were beta-blockers (20%) or drugs with beta-blocking properties (16%). These drugs are not recommended for vagally mediated afib. These findings support those of our first drug survey in which 50% of all vagal afibbers had been prescribed drugs contraindicated for their condition. About half of the vagal afibbers who were on beta-blocking drugs also took an antiarrhythmic, which may have ameliorated somewhat the negative effects of the beta- blocking drug. Nevertheless, it is possible that a sizeable proportion of vagal afibbers could significantly improve their situation by optimizing their drug regimen.

It is encouraging that the current use of digoxin, a drug contraindicated for all afibbers, is only 4% - a level well below that observed in our first drug survey. Nevertheless, 30% of 180 respondents reported that they had been taking digoxin for an extended period (3 months or longer) at some point during their afib "career".

It is puzzling that 28% of permanent afibbers were taking an antiarrhythmic drug, as there is no indication that this would be helpful except in preparation for electrical cardioversion.

There was a slight [not statistically significant] trend for afibbers with a regular pattern to their episodes to be less likely to use drugs.

Efficacy by afib type
The average [median] number of afib episodes during a 6-month period among 223 paroxysmal afibbers was 5 for non-drug users and 4 for drug users. This difference was not statistically significant. The average [median] duration of episodes among 223 paroxysmal afibbers was 6 hours for non-drug users and 6 hours for drug users.

AFIB TYPE	#	Frequency NO DRUGS	Frequency DRUGS	Duration NO DRUGS	Duration DRUGS
Adrenergic	30	4	3	3 hrs	12 hrs
Mixed	74	5	9	4 hrs	7 hrs
Vagal	119	6	4	7 hrs	5 hrs
Paroxysmal	223	5	4	6 hrs	6 hrs

The average median time [hours] spent in afib over a 6-month period [afib burden] among 223 paroxysmal afibbers was 30 hours for non-drug users and 37 hours for drug users. This difference was not statistically significant.

Drug Efficacy by Afib Type – Afib Burden [6 months]			
AFIB TYPE	#	Afib Burden NO DRUGS	Afib Burden DRUGS
Adrenergic	30	15 hrs	24 hrs
Mixed	74	22 hrs	69 hrs
Vagal	119	45 hrs	30 hrs
Paroxysmal	223	30 hrs	37 hrs

Frequency: Median number of episodes over a 6-month period
Duration: Median duration of episodes in hours over a 6-month period

There were no statistically significant differences in episode frequency or duration or in total time spent in afib over a 6-month period among non-drug users and drug users when viewed by afib category (adrenergic, mixed, vagal). There was a slight, statistically non-significant trend ($p=0.06$) for non-drug treated adrenergic afibbers to spend less time in afib than did non-drug treated vagal afibbers.

Efficacy by drug type
Drug therapy aimed at preventing or shortening afib episodes was generally found not to be effective. Disopyramide (Norpace) showed a trend towards fewer episodes, but this trend was not quite statistically significant ($p=0.08$). Sotalol (Betapace), on the other hand, confirmed its reputation as possibly the worst drug for afibbers. All differences observed between individual drugs and no drugs were not statistically significant.

Efficacy by Drug Type			
DRUG	# OF USERS	EPISODES(1)	DURATION(2) Hrs	AFIB BURDEN (3)
No drug	96	5	6	30
Flecainide	22	5	4	29
Disopyramide	12	2	4	15
Atenolol	12	4	11	39
Sotalol	10	19	12	48
Metoprolol*	9	3	4	10
Propafenone	7	2	6	12
Amiodarone	7	8	15	100
Diltiazem	5	4	4	22
Verapamil	5	9	10	90
Combination	28	4	8	24

*including Toprol XL
(1) median number of episodes over a 6-month period
(2) median duration of episodes in hours over a 6-month period
(3) total time [hrs] spent in afib over a 6-month period

The use of beta or calcium channel blockers on their own on a continuous basis did not shorten episode duration, did not decrease intensity of episodes nor did it, somewhat surprisingly, reduce the maximum reported heart rate during an episode.

There was no indication that amiodarone, as prescribed among these survey respondents, was effective in preventing or shortening episodes.

Drugs in vagal Afib

The problem of finding the appropriate drug for an individual afibber is particularly difficult in the case of vagally-mediated afibbers where beta-blocking drugs should be avoided. An evaluation of drugs used in the treatment of vagal afibbers shows this.

Flecainide significantly shortens episode duration and time spent in a fib for vagal afibbers. Disopyramide would also appear to shorten both frequency and duration, but these observations did not reach statistical significance due to the small sample size. Sotalol and amiodarone did not appear to be effective for vagal afibbers and may actually increase the number of episodes, possibly due to their beta-blocking effect.

Efficacy of Drugs in Vagal LAF				
DRUG	# OF USERS	EPISODES(1)	DURATION(2) Hrs	AFIB BURDEN (3)
No drug	49	6	7	45
Flecainide	15	6	4	24
Disopyramide	9	2	3	16
Sotalol	6	19	8	48
Amiodarone	4	14	11	80
Combination	11	4	6	48

1. median number of episodes over a 6-month period
2. median duration of episodes in hours over a 6-month period
3. total time [hrs] spent in afib over a 6-month period

Conclusion

Considering that ablation therapy is now achieving success rates of 80-90% and results in a complete cure, it would probably not be too much to expect that an effective pharmaceutical drug properly prescribed should be able to keep an afibber in normal sinus rhythm for at least 6 months. Even if the drug was able to achieve this goal for just 50% of its users it might be worthwhile. According to this latest survey a total of 21 drug treated afibbers out of 125 (17%) had achieved the enviable goal of staying in sinus rhythm for 6 months.

Among afibbers not on drugs 12 out of 105 or 11% had achieved an afib-free 6-month period - hardly an impressive difference.

In conclusion, there is no evidence that pharmaceutical drugs, as currently prescribed, are generally effective in preventing or shortening afib episodes for the vast majority of afibbers. A notable exception is flecainide and disopyramide, which would appear to shorten episodes among vagal afibbers.

On-Demand therapy with antiarrhythmics

The fact that flecainide and disopyramide shorten episodes, but do not prevent them leads to the idea of the on-demand approach [20]. This approach involves taking 200 mg of flecainide or 300 mg of propafenone within 5 minutes of the onset of an episode rather than on a continuous, preventive basis. Best results are obtained if the tablets are crushed first and then swallowed with warm water. Italian researchers originally evaluated the on-demand approach in atrial tachycardia and found it safe and effective [21]. More recently a team of American and German researchers confirmed the safety and efficacy of this method for converting atrial fibrillation to normal sinus rhythm [22].

Twenty-six afibbers out of 138 respondents (19%) had tried the on-demand approach (1 adrenergic, 9 mixed and 16 vagal). Nineteen or 73% of the on-demand users had found the approach beneficial, 4 or 15% believed the approach worked sometimes while the remainder was not sure. Only 10% had found that the effectiveness decreased over time. The average conversion time was 5 hours for both mixed and vagal afibbers and never exceeded 36 hours.

The most commonly used on-demand drug was flecainide which was used by 62% in dosages between 100 and 400 mg with 200 mg being the most common dosage. Propafenone was used by 19% in dosages of 150 to 600 mg (average of 250 mg).

Surprisingly, there was no indication that the on-demand users on average actually experienced shorter episodes than experienced by afibbers who used no drugs or used drugs on a continuous preventive basis. This is a bit of a puzzle and can perhaps be explained by the possibility that afibbers who used to have very long episodes preferentially used the on-demand approach and that the approach just brought them back to a more "normal" level. I know this is the case for myself. I have experienced episodes as long as 223 hours, but have been able to shorten several of my more recent episodes to 2-4 hours and never longer than 36 hours. So if you have very long episodes the on-demand approach may well be worth trying. If your episodes, on the other hand, are relatively short (less than 6 hours) you may not gain much by using this approach. Most effective dosages would seem to be 200 mg of flecainide or 300 mg of propafenone perhaps preceded by 12.5 mg of atenolol or 80 mg of verapamil.

On-Demand therapy with beta and calcium channel blockers

There was not enough data to reach a conclusion as to whether taking a calcium channel blocker or a beta-blocker during an episode reduces duration or intensity or lowers the heart rate. However, there is ample anecdotal and medical evidence that doing so does indeed make an episode more tolerable.

Use of stroke prevention medications

A total of 297 respondents indicated their form of stroke prevention regimen. Aspirin and natural remedies (fish oil, vitamin E, and ginkgo biloba) tied in popularity at 49% each with warfarin coming in at 24%. Ten per cent of the respondents did not take any stroke prevention measures. Thirty-nine per cent of aspirin users also used natural approaches while only 24% of warfarin users also used natural remedies.

Use of Stroke Prevention Medications					
AFIB TYPE	#	NO PREVENTION	ASPIRIN	WARFARIN	NATURAL
Adrenergic	33	15%	39%	27%	55%
Mixed	91	12%	46%	23%	50%
Vagal	136	9%	57%	16%	47%
Paroxysmal	260	11%	51%	20%	49%
Permanent	37	5%	38%	54%	49%

Please note that percentages do not add up to 100% due to the fact that many afibbers combined stroke prevention regimens, particularly aspirin and natural approaches.

Only 25 respondents answered the question regarding the use of aspirin on-demand. Six out of these 25 (2 adrenergic, 1 mixed and 3 vagal) used the stroke prevention technique of taking an aspirin at the onset of an episode.

The median age (61 years) of warfarin users was significantly higher than that of both aspirin users (56 years) and natural remedy users (57 years). There was no significant difference in gender distribution between users of warfarin, aspirin and natural remedies.

Warfarin users had significantly longer episodes (median duration: 12 hours) than did non-users of warfarin (median duration: 5 hours). It is not possible to deduce whether this is because warfarin prolongs the episodes or because afibbers with long lasting episodes are more likely to use warfarin. There was no difference in episode duration among users and non-users of aspirin.

Heart Rhythm

Heart rhythm parameters

A total of 151 paroxysmal afibbers (19 adrenergic, 53 mixed and 79 vagal) provided full or partial data regarding their daily heart rhythm parameters. The participants rated their days as good or bad depending on whether they experienced a few or many ectopic beats (PACs or PVCs) on a particular day.

114

The average ratio of good to bad days was remarkably consistent overall at 23:7 (good:bad) for both adrenergic, mixed and vagal afibbers, but did vary considerably from individual to individual from 9:21 to 29:1 for adrenergic, from 3:27 to 29:1 for mixed, and from 5:25 to 29:1 for vagal. There was no gender difference in the number of good and bad days. The actual number of ectopic beats experienced in a day, based on 10-minute observations, showed quite a large variation.

Ectopic Beats/Day							
		GOOD DAY			BAD DAY		
AFIB TYPE	#	Mean	Median	Range	Mean	Median	Range
Adrenergic	11	177	0	0-864	1944	1440	0-7200
Mixed	36	194	0	0-2160	5570	936	0-4320
Vagal	48	110	0	0-2880	1164	468	0-7200
Paroxysmal	95	150	0	0-2880	2924	758	0-4320

The median number of ectopic beats per day over a 30-day period was 96 for adrenergic, 221 for mixed, 75 for vagal, and 133 for all paroxysmal afibbers combined.

The difference in ectopic beats per day was statistically significant when comparing mixed to vagal afibbers on a bad day and on an average day. No other differences between the various afib types or between male and female afibbers were statistically significant. However, there was clearly a significant difference between a good day and a bad day for all afibbers.

Forty-seven afibbers (3 adrenergic, 17 mixed and 27 vagal) had Holter monitor recordings which showed the distribution between PACs and PVCs during a 24-hour period.

Holter Monitor Recordings				
AFIB TYPE	RESPONDENTS	PACs	PVCs	BOTH
Adrenergic	3	1	1	1
Mixed	17	9	4	4
Vagal	27	20	5	2
Paroxysmal	47	30	10	7

PACs are clearly the predominant form of ectopics, particularly for vagal afibbers. There was no indication that the type of ectopic beats experienced was associated with the number of ectopics on a bad or average day.

One hundred and twenty-one afibbers (14 adrenergic, 43 mixed and 64 vagal) had observed the nature of their ectopic beats, i.e. whether they were single or came in runs of 2, 3 or more.

Nature of Ectopic Beats				
AFIB TYPE	RESPONDENTS	SINGLE	RUNS	BOTH
Adrenergic	14	5	7	2
Mixed	43	13	23	7
Vagal	64	24	33	7
Paroxysmal	121	42	63	16

Ectopic beats in runs were the predominant form for all afibbers and the most frequent number of beats in a run was 2-3 (experienced by 30 afibbers) followed by 3-4 or more (experienced by 9 afibbers). Seventy-one afibbers (67% of adrenergic, 79% of mixed and 67% of vagal) associated a run of ectopic beats with the initiation of an episode while 28 afibbers had observed no such association.

One hundred and eleven afibbers (10 adrenergic, 37 mixed and 64 vagal) had observed the frequency of their ectopic beats prior to an episode. Most (53%) had not observed any change, but 42% had noted an increase and 5% had noted a decrease.

Ninety-one afibbers responded to the question as to whether they had observed any change in frequency in ectopic beats with changes in position, stress, rest, etc.

Number of Respondents Experiencing Change in Ectopic Beat Frequency								
Afib Type	#	No Change*	With Stress	With Rest	With Exercise	With Time**	With Position	With Eating
Adrenergic	9	2	5	1	0	1	0	0
Mixed	31	7	8	1	1	7	6	1
Vagal	51	12	4	4	1	10	15	5
Paroxysmal	91	21	17	6	2	18	23	6

* during the day   **with time of day

A change in position was associated with an increase in ectopic beats by 25% of all afibbers (29% among vagal afibbers). An increase in ectopic beats was also significantly associated with time of day (20% of all afibbers) and exposure to stress (19% of all afibbers), but 23% of all afibbers reported that their ectopics were evenly spread throughout the day and not influenced by anything they were aware of.

The finding that almost 80% of all afibbers have noticed a connection between increased ectopy and an event involving a change in autonomic nervous system balance clearly underscores the important role of the ANS in the etiology of afib.

There was a significant association between episode frequency and the number of ectopic beats experienced in an average day ($r=0.23$, $p=0.03$). The association was particularly strong ($r=0.4815$, $p=0.02$) in afibbers who had been diagnosed on a Holter monitor as having predominantly PACs (premature atrial complexes). An association between PVC-type ectopic beats and episode frequency was not observed, possibly due to the small number of afibbers diagnosed with PVCs as the predominant ectopy (N=7) or because PVCs do not affect episode frequency. The finding that a higher number of PACs on an average day correlates with more frequent episodes is certainly not surprising, as PACs are believed to initiate the episodes. However, it does point out the importance of avoiding PAC-generating activities as much as possible.

Atrial flutter

The prevalence of atrial flutter was 25% among adrenergic afibbers, 28% among mixed, 18% among vagal, and 29% among permanent. The observed differences in prevalence were not statistically significant.

There were no differences in average age (55 years) or gender distribution (20% women) among afibbers with flutter and those without, nor were there any differences in afib episode frequency or duration. There was no difference in drug use between afibbers with flutter and those without; however, afibbers with flutter were significantly more likely to have hypoglycemia (idiopathic postprandial syndrome) then were those without flutter (39% versus 17%). It is tempting to speculate that an over-enthusiastic insulin response might play a role in atrial flutter and that those suffering from this condition could improve their situation by eating frequently, emphasizing low glycemic index foods, and ensuring protein in every meal and snack.

Thirty-five per cent of all those suffering from atrial flutter had undergone an ablation. The success rate was 62%; significantly lower than the oft-quoted number of 90%. A successful flutter ablation did not result in elimination of afib unless an AF ablation (left atrium) was performed at the same time.

Atrial Flutter Ablations				
AFIB TYPE	RESPONDENTS	"AFLUTTERERS"	ABLATIONS	SUCCESSES
Adrenergic	20	5	1	0
Mixed	51	14	6	4
Vagal	76	14	5	3
Paroxysmal	147	33	12	7
Permanent	14	4	1	1
TOTAL	161	37	13	8

REFERENCES

1. ACC/AHA/ESC Guidelines for the Management of Patients with Atrial Fibrillation: Executive Summary. Journal of the American College of Cardiology, Vol. 38, No. 4, 2001
2. Hypertension prevalence and the status of awareness, treatment, and control in the USA. Hypertension, Vol. 7, 1985, pp. 457-68
3. Nichols, GA, et al. Congestive heart failure in type 2 diabetes: prevalence, incidence, and risk factors. Diabetes Care, Vol. 24, September 2001, pp. 1614-19
4. Harrison's Principles of Internal Medicine, 12th edition, 1991, McGraw-Hill, NY, pp. 1977-85
5. Bots, Michiel, L., et al. Homocysteine and short-term risk of myocardial infarction and stroke in the elderly. Archives of Internal Medicine, Vol. 159, January 11, 1999, pp. 38-44
6. Bostom, Andrew G., et al. Nonfasting plasma total homocysteine levels and stroke incidence in elderly persons. Annals of Internal Medicine, Vol. 131, September 7, 1999, pp. 352-55

7. Roach, Gary W., et al. Adverse cerebral outcomes after coronary bypass surgery. New England Journal of Medicine, Vol. 335, December 19, 1996, pp. 1857-63

8. Falk, Rodney H. and Podrid, Philip J., editors. Atrial Fibrillation: Mechanisms and Management, 2nd edition, 1997, Lippincott-Raven, NY, pp. 277-98

9. Gage, Brian F., et al. Validation of clinical classification schemes for predicting stroke. Journal of the American Medical Association, Vol. 285, June 13, 2001, pp. 2864-70

10. Saoudi, Nadir, et al., editors. Atrial Flutter and Fibrillation, 1998, Futura Publishing, Armonk, NY, pp. 229-36

11. Kopecky, Stephen L., et al. The natural history of lone atrial fibrillation. New England Journal of Medicine, Vol. 317, No. 11, 1987, pp. 669-74

12. van Walraven, C., et al. A clinical prediction rule to identify patients with atrial fibrillation and a low risk for stroke while taking aspirin. Archives of Internal Medicine, Vol. 163, April 28, 2003, pp. 936-43

13. Merck Manual of Medical Information (home edition), Simon & Schuster, NY, 1997, p. 382

14. Transient Ischemic Attack
http://emedicine.com/EMERG/topic604.htm

15. Karjalainen, Jouko, et al. Lone atrial fibrillation in vigorously exercising middle aged men: case-control study. British Medical Journal, Vol. 316, June 13, 1998, pp. 1784-85

16. www.diabetes.org

17. Abdulla, AJ, et al. Leg cramps in the elderly: prevalence, drug and disease associations. International Journal of Clinical Practice, Vol. 53, No. 7, October/November 1999, pp. 494-96

18. Asthma Prevalence 2001
www.cdc.gov/mmwr/preview/mmwrhtml/mm5217a2.htm

19. Common Cold {Medline Plus]
www.nlm.nih.gov/medlineplus/ency/article /000678.htm.

20. Larsen, HR. Lone Atrial Fibrillation: Towards a Cure. International Health News, Victoria, Canada, 2003, p. 78

21. Alboni, P, et al. Efficacy and safety of out-of-hospital self-administered single-dose oral drug treatment in the management of infrequent, well-tolerated paroxysmal supraventricular tachycardia. Journal of the American College of Cardiology, Vol. 37, February 2001, pp. 548-53

22. Marrouche, NF, et al. Oral bolus of IC antiarrhythmic drugs for atrial fibrillation: outpatient versus inpatient administration. Journal of the American College of Cardiology, March 19, 2003, p. 98A

Candida and Migraines

By Hans R. Larsen [2004]

The **February 2004** survey, our first web-based survey, was designed to determine a possible association between LAF and migraine headaches and between LAF and the presence of *candida* overgrowth (yeast infection). A total of 65 lone afibbers without heart disease participated in the survey. Twenty-three per cent of respondents were women, a proportion similar to that observed in previous surveys. The average age of respondents was 55 years (range of 31 to 84 years). The average age at diagnosis was 49 years (range of 20 to 77 years) and the average number of years of having lived with afib was 6 years. There were no significant differences between men and women in regard to age or years of afib.

The majority (87%) of respondents had the paroxysmal (intermittent) kind of LAF; 5% had persistent LAF, and 8% the permanent variety. Of the paroxysmal afibbers, 13% had the adrenergic type, 45% the mixed, and 42% were vagal.

Episode **frequency** was distributed as follows:

Episodes in 6-month Period	%
None	7%
1-3	21%
4-6	12%
7-10	16%
11-20	16%
More than 20	28%

Episode **duration** was distributed as follows:

Average Episode Duration [hrs]	%
No episodes	7%
01-1 hrs	16%
1-2 hrs	7%
3-6 hrs	14%
7-12 hrs	22%
13-19 hrs	10%
20-29 hrs	3%
30-48 hrs	10%
More than 48 hrs	11%

Ablation procedures

Twelve respondents (18.5%) had undergone ablation therapy. Six of the procedures (50%) had been successful. This success rate is somewhat low, partly due to the fact that 2 of the so far unsuccessful ablations were performed quite recently. Of some concern is the finding that afibbers who had reported an unsuccessful ablation prior to 2003 were likely to be experiencing more and longer-lasting episodes than did afibbers who had not undergone ablation. These findings confirm observations from earlier surveys and clearly need further investigation.

Use of pharmaceutical drugs

Fifty-two per cent of all respondents were taking pharmaceutical drugs on a regular basis to manage their LAF, while 22% were using the on-demand approach (200 mg flecainide or 300 mg propafenone crushed and swallowed with warm water immediately at onset of an episode). There was no indication that drug use, regular or on-demand, had any effect on the average episode frequency or duration. There was also no indication that taking statin drugs or fish oils affected episode frequency or duration. However, there was a slight, statistically non-significant (p=0.06) trend for women to be more likely to take drugs and fish oils on a regular basis.

Migraines

Fourteen of 65 respondents had experienced a migraine headache in the past and eight were still experiencing them (1-3 in a 6-month period). Thus the current prevalence of migraines among the 65 respondents is 12.3%, not significantly different from the 10.3% experienced among the general US population. There was no correlation between the number of migraine episodes and the frequency and duration of afib episodes. Only one out of 11 had ever noticed an association between migraines and afib episodes. There was no indication that afib type (adrenergic, mixed, vagal, and permanent) was related to the prevalence of migraines. Thus it is unlikely that there is an association between migraine headaches and LAF.

Candida

Forty-one of 65 respondents had done the saliva test for *candida* overgrowth and 41% had tested positive, 49% negative, and 10% were unsure. Thirteen or 20% of the 65 respondents had been officially diagnosed with *candida* at one point or another and 10 (77%) of these were still battling the disorder when completing the survey. The most common location for *candida* overgrowth was the colon (46%) followed by the genital area (38%), and mouth (16%). Two respondents had overgrowth in more than one location. Women were more likely to have been diagnosed with *candida* than were men; however, there was no gender-related difference according to the saliva test. This could indicate that *candida* overgrowth is under-diagnosed in men.

Of the 13 respondents who had been diagnosed with *candida* 10 had taken the saliva test. Seven (70%) of these tested positive, 2 tested negative, and 1 was not sure. Of the 10 respondents currently battling *candida* 8 had taken the

120

saliva test and 7 (88%) tested positive. Thus it would appear that the saliva test is a reasonably accurate indication of the presence of *candida* overgrowth. It would also appear that *candida* is difficult to overcome on a permanent basis.

There was no statistically significant association between the presence of *candida* and episode frequency or duration. Two out of 10 respondents had however, observed an association between *candida* episodes and afib episodes.

In conclusion, there is no statistically significant association between migraine headaches and LAF nor between *candida* overgrowth and LAF.

2004 Ablation/Maze Survey

By Hans R. Larsen [2004]

The purpose of this survey was to evaluate and share information about the outcome of various catheterization and surgical approaches for eliminating afib. A total of 83 afibbers responded to the survey. The treatment modalities were distributed as follows:

- Radiofrequency (RF) ablation (left atrium)   63 respondents
- Cryoablation (left atrium)   2 respondents
- Maze procedure   10 respondents
- ICD implantation   4 respondents
- AV node ablation + pacemaker   2 respondents
- RF flutter ablation (right atrium)   2 respondents

RF Ablation of Left Atrium

Sixty-three respondents had undergone RF ablation of the left atrium. However, an additional 49 sets of data were available from previous LAF surveys giving a total of 112 responses for evaluation.

Demographics

The majority of the 112 respondents (77%) had the paroxysmal form of LAF, 15% were permanent, while the remaining 8% had persistent afib prior to their ablation. Among the paroxysmal afibbers 3 (3%) were adrenergic, 46 (54%) were mixed (random), 30 (35%) were vagal, and 7 (8%) were not sure about their type.

The average age of respondents was 56 years with a range of 33 to 84 years. The average age at diagnosis was 47 years with a range of 16 to 81 years. Thus, the average number of years that LAF had been present was 9 years with a range of 1 to 69 years. These numbers are not significantly different from the averages obtained by considering all the entries in our main database, so there is no reason to believe that respondents to the ablation survey were either younger or older than the general population of afibbers.

Thirty per cent of respondents were female, slightly higher than the proportion in our total database.

The average age at which the ablation was performed was 54 years with a range of 30 to 81 years.

Most respondents (98%) had no underlying heart disease, but 14% had been diagnosed with mitral valve prolapse (MVP).

Success Rating [See Definition of Terms]				
Parameter	Complete Success	Partial Success	Failure	Total*
# in group	55	15	37	107*
Total by group, %	51	14	35	100
Paroxysmal, %	54	12	34	100
Adrenergic, %	100	0	0	100
Mixed, %	40	14	46	100
Vagal, %	69	7	24	100
Not sure, %	57	29	14	100
Persistent, %	38	37	25	100
Adrenergic, %	0	100	0	100
Mixed, %	40	20	40	100
Vagal, %	50	50	0	100
Not sure,%	0	0	0	0
Permanent, %	47	6	47	100
Present age (mean), yrs	56	60	54	55
Age at diagnosis (mean), yrs	47	47	46	47
Age at ablation (mean), yrs	54	59	52	54
Age at ablation (range), yrs	30-70	48-81	30-75	30-81
Years of AF (mean)	8	13	10	9
Females, %	31	36	24	29
Underlying heart disease, %	0	7	5	3
Mitral valve prolapse, %	18	10	6	14
Success among women, %	55	16	29	100
Success among men, %	50	12	38	100
*5 cases of uncertain outcome omitted All ratings refer to most recent ablations				

None of the observed differences in Table 1 were statistically significant, although the difference between the success rate for paroxysmal vagal afibbers (69%) and that for mixed afibbers (40%) did come close to being so (p = 0.07).

The overall success rate of 51%, or 65% including afibbers still on drugs, is somewhat disappointing, but as we shall see further on, the success rate is highly dependent on when and where the procedure was performed.

There were 5 afibbers who had their ablation at age 70 years or older. Four (subjectively) considered their procedure a complete success, while one considered it a failure. Looking at the success rate using objective criteria shows that 2 afibbers were totally successful, 2 were partially successful, and 1 was a failure. Thus, based on this very small sample, ablations in elderly afibbers are not significantly less successful than those in younger ones.

There was a general trend for ablatees to judge the results of their ablation more favourably than would be the case if objective criteria were used. This indicates that any kind of improvement following an ablation is considered a blessing.

	Objective Judgment	Subjective Judgment
Complete success	49%	59%
Partial success	13%	13%
Failure	34%	25%
Uncertain	4%	3%
All 112 cases included		

Afib Severity Prior to Ablation 107 Paroxysmal Afibbers			
Parameter	Complete Success	Partial Success	Failure
# in group	55	15	37
# of episodes (1)	21	8	13
Episode duration, hrs (2)	8	3	6
Afib burden, hrs (3)	175	34	125
(1) Median # of episodes in 3 months prior to ablation (2) Median duration of episodes in hours (3) # of episodes x duration of episodes over a 3–month period			

The differences observed in Table 2 are not statistically significant, thus providing no indication that the severity of paroxysmal afib prior to ablation has any effect on the outcome.

Year of Ablation
Technological advances in mapping technology and ablation protocols, as well as skills progression along a fairly steep learning curve, have substantially improved the success rate for RF ablation over the years.

Success Rate by Year of 1st Ablation				
1st Procedure	# of Ablations	Complete Success, %	Partial Success, %	Failure, %
1997-2000	16	13	0	87
2001	12	9	33	58
2002	28	32	7	61
2003	37	65	8	27
2004	15	53	7	40
Overall	108	41	9	50

The prevalence of repeat ablations (touch-ups) was 22% overall and 46% considering only initially unsuccessful ablations. Considering only the outcome of the most recent ablations (touch-ups included) improves success rates further. The success rate for touch-up procedures was not impressive. Only 10 of 26 procedures (38%) were fully successful, 15% were partially successful, and 42% were failures. The fate of one touch-up procedure was uncertain.

Success Rate by Year of Final Ablation				
1st Procedure	# of Ablations	Complete Success, %	Partial Success, %	Failure, %
1997-2000	13	23	0	77
2001	9	11	44	45
2002	25	36	8	56
2003	39	80	10	10
2004	21	52	19	29
Overall	107	51	13	36
5 procedures were omitted because outcome was uncertain				

Five different procedures were used to perform the RF ablations.

Number of Procedures by Year						
Procedure	1997-2000	2001	2002	2003	2004	Total
Focal ablation	8 (62%)	2	6	5	2 (9%)	23
Pulmonary vein (PVA)	4	2	12	14	5	37
PVI	0	1	2	11	14 (60%)	28
Circumferential PVI	0	0	0	1	2	3
PVI + focal	0	2	5	7	0	14
Unspecified	1	2	-	3	0	6
Total	13	9	25	41	23	111

It is clear that the popularity of the various procedures has changed markedly over the years. The initial focal point procedure has gone from 62% in 1997-2000 to 9% in 2004, while the pulmonary vein isolation procedure (PVI) has gone from 0% in 1997-2000 to 60% in 2004. The circumferential PVI (Pappone method) is still relatively rare among the respondents to our survey.

The success rates of the various procedures are presented in the following table.

Success Rate of Procedures					
Procedure	Complete Success, %	Partial Success, %	Failure, %	Uncertain, %	Total, %
Focal ablation	22	13	61	4	100
PVA	50	11	36	3	100
PVI	66	14	17	3	100
Circumferential PVI	67	0	0	33	100
PVI + focal	57	14	29	0	100
Unspecified	33	17	33	17	100
Total	49	13	34	4	100

The success rate of purely focal ablation is clearly quite poor, while the success rate of pulmonary vein isolation (PVI) is substantially better at 66%. The difference is very significant in statistical terms (p = 0.003). Overall, based on our data, the PVI procedure is the best with a success + partial success rate of 80%. The circumferential PVI would also appear to have a reasonable success rate but, with only 3 afibbers so far having reported on this procedure, it is not possible to draw any conclusions.

Although the procedure used in the ablation is very important in determining the outcome, it is clear that the equipment, specific techniques, and the skill of the electrophysiologist play a major role as well.

Facilities and electrophysiologists

Although clearly arbitrary on my part, I believe the following facilities and electrophysiologists are among the top worldwide. I am sure Dr. Carlo Pappone's facility in Milan deserves inclusion as well, but I do not have any data from this facility. Also, I know that Dr. Richard Leather at the Royal Jubilee Hospital in Victoria, British Columbia has performed several hundred successful PVIs; however, only one afibber treated by Dr. Leather responded to the survey so I did not have enough data to "formally" include him among the top EPs. With those caveats here then are my top choices, in alphabetical order.

My Top Choices		
Facility	Electrophysiologist(s)	# of Ablations
Centinela Hospital, CA*	Dr. Nademanee	3
Cleveland Clinic, OH	Drs. Natale, Schweikert, Tchou, Saliba	28
Good Samaritan, Los Angeles	Dr. Bhandari	4
Good Samaritan, San Jose, CA	Dr. Coggins	2
Haut-Leveque, Bordeaux, FR	Drs. Haissaguerre, Jais	3
Johns Hopkins	Drs. Calkins, Berger	4
Marin General Hospital, CA	Dr. Natale	4
University of Pennsylvania	Dr. Callans	2
University of South Carolina	Dr. Wharton	3
Utah Valley Hospital	Dr. Hwang	2
*Pacific Rim Electrophysiology Research Institute		

These 10 facilities (Group A) performed 52% of the 106 ablations for which location and EP are known. A **comparison of their performance** with that of the remaining 48% (Group B) would thus be of interest.

Comparison of Baseline Demographics		
Parameter	Group A	Group B
# in group	55	51
Paroxysmal, %	79	76
Mixed(1), %	39	66
Vagal(1), %	46	25
Persistent, %	5	10
Permanent, %	16	14

Comparison of Baseline Demographics		
Parameter	Group A	Group B
Age at 1st ablation (range), yrs	33-81	30-75
Years of AF (mean)	7	7
Females, %	29	29
Underlying heart disease, %	4	2
(1) % of total paroxysmal and persistent		

Although there is no significant difference between the distribution of paroxysmal, persistent, and permanent afibbers among the two groups, there is a statistically significant (p = 0.02) difference between the percentage of mixed (39% versus 66%) and vagal afibbers (46% versus 25%) treated in the two groups. The success rate for vagal afibbers is generally higher than that for mixed afibbers. There were no differences in gender distribution and prevalence of underlying heart disease.

Comparison of Success Rates 2001-2004			
Parameter	Group A	Group B	Overall
# in sample	50	42	92*
After initial ablation			
Complete success, %	68	21	47
Partial success, %	12	10	11
Failure, %	20	64	40
Uncertain, %	0	5	2
After most recent ablation			
Complete success, %	76	29	55
Partial success, %	12	19	15
Failure, %	12	43	26
Uncertain, %	0	9	4
Touch-up rate (overall), %	10	38	23
Touch-up rate (successes), %	80	19	33
Touch-up rate (on failures), %	50	59	23
*omitting procedures performed during the period 1997-2000			

It is clear from the above table that the most important variables in the success of an RF ablation are the facilities and the expertise and skill of the electrophysiologist. The differences in success rates are dramatic, so dramatic in fact that I re-checked them twice. Essentially, while the complete success rate in Group A is 68% for the initial ablation and 76% with a touch-up, the corresponding numbers for Group B are 21% and 29%. Even including partial successes (no afib, but still on antiarrhythmics) the differences are still startling:

Group A – first ablation	80%
Group A – with touch-up	88%
Group B – first ablation	31%
Group B – with touch-up	48%

127

The conclusion is pretty inescapable – there are still a lot of EPs out there on the steep part of the learning curve. Unless you can have your ablation performed in a Group A center or equivalent, you are better off postponing your procedure for a couple of years.

Stenosis

Stenosis (narrowing of diameter) of the pulmonary veins can occur during ablation, particularly if the ablation is performed inside the veins (PVA). Stenosis is defined as a narrowing of one or more veins by at least 50%, while severe stenosis is defined as narrowing by 70% or more. It is important to check for stenosis about 3 months after the procedure, particularly in the case of PVA. This is usually done via a spiral CT scan.

Incidence of Stenosis			
	Group A	Group B	Combined
# in sample	55	51	106
All Procedures			
Stenosis check, %	44	25	35
Stenosis found(1), %	4	15	8
PVA Procedures			
Stenosis check, %	53	25	37
Stenosis found(1), %	0	40	15
(1) In patients checked			

It is clear that the practice of checking for stenosis is significantly less prevalent in Group B centers than in Group A and that the actual incidence of stenosis is substantially higher in Group B centers, particularly in the case of PVAs. At least one case of confirmed severe stenosis occurred in a Group B center.

Adverse Effects

Adverse effects related to the ablation procedure were reported by 8% of Group A ablatees and 19% of Group B ablatees (overall rate: 14%). The most common adverse effects were hematomas in the area of catheter insertion and bruising. More serious effects involved one case of severe damage to the mitral valve (necessitating replacement), development of atrial flutter (1 case), and penetration of the cardiac wall (tamponade) requiring open heart surgery (1 case). Forty per cent of the adverse events had resolved themselves at the time the survey was completed.

Recovery

For successful ablations the median time to recovery of normal sinus rhythm and no more afib episodes was 1 month (range 0-12 months). The median time to recovery of full physical capacity was 2 months (range 0-11 months with an outlier of 48 months). There was no correlation between age at ablation and time to recovery. About 20% of all successful ablatees reported experiencing a significant number of PACs and PVCs at the time they completed the survey. The corresponding percentage for unsuccessful ablatees was 46%.

The majority of successful ablatees (71%) no longer needed to avoid any triggers and 14% only needed to avoid some previous triggers. Fifteen per cent stated that it was too early to tell whether trigger avoidance was still necessary.

Blood Pressure
There was no significant difference in median blood pressure before the ablation (120/70) and after the ablation (118/72). Twenty-one out of 63 respondents (33%) reported using blood pressure lowering medications before the ablation, while 17 out of 63 (27%) reported using them after the procedure.

Prior to ablation 22 of 62 respondents (35%) were classified as being hypertensive, either because they had a blood pressure exceeding 140/90 or because they were on anti-hypertensive drugs. After ablation 17 out of 58 respondents (29%) were classified as being hypertensive. This difference was not statistically significant so there is no reason to suspect that blood pressure is affected by ablation.

Heart Rate
Many afibbers have noticed an increase in pulse (heart) rate after the ablation. For most, the rate returns to normal after a few months, but for others, it remains elevated. It is not clear what causes the elevation, but one possible explanation is that vagal nerve endings are damaged during the procedure, thus diminishing the "restraining" influence of the parasympathetic branch of the autonomic nervous system. Heart rate changes are detailed in Table 11.

Heart Rate Changes			
Direction of Change	Successful Group	Unsuccessful Group	Total Group
Up, %	53	32	45
Down, %	8	26	10
No change, %	39	42	42

The median difference in heart rate increase was somewhat lower in the successful group than in the unsuccessful one (11 bpm versus 20 bpm), but this difference was not statistically significant. The range in increase was quite wide, 4-52 bpm for the unsuccessful group and 2-25 bpm for the successful group.

Medication Usage Before and After Ablation

Medication Usage				
Parameter	Complete Success	Partial Success	Failure	Uncertain
# of respondents	31	12	14	3
Prior to procedure				
Use of antiarrhythmics	74 %	75 %	100 %	67 %
Use of blockers	74 %	67 %	86 %	67 %

After procedure				
Use of warfarin	100 %	67 %	100 %	67 %
Months used	3.5 %	1 %	8 %	2.5 %
Medication at Time of Survey				
Parameter	Complete Success	Partial Success	Failure	Uncertain
Use of antiarrhythmics	0 %	58 %	50 %	33 %
Use of blockers	0 %	58 %	36 %	67 %
Use of warfarin	12 %	25 %	71 %	67 %

Use of Statin Drugs

The use of statin drugs (Lipitor, atorvastatin) to control inflammation after the ablation was mainly confined to recent ablations carried out at the Cleveland Clinic. Group A centers used statin drugs in 47% of cases whereas Group B centers only used them in 17% of cases. Fourteen per cent of statin users experienced side effects, primarily muscle pain and weakness. Thirty-two per cent of statin takers were supplementing with coenzyme Q10 in order to counteract the long-term adverse effects of Lipitor.

Change in Afib Burden

A question uppermost in the minds of afibbers contemplating ablation is: "Will I be worse off if the ablation is unsuccessful?" Fourteen afibbers who had undergone an unsuccessful ablation supplied data regarding their afib severity for a 3-month period prior to the ablation and for a 3-month period after. Results are tabulated in Table 13 (medians used in all cases).

Change in Afib Burden			
Parameter	Before Ablation	After Ablation	Significance
# of episodes	44	5	P = 0.01
Duration of episodes, hrs	11	6	P = 0.15
Afib burden, hrs	600	28	P = 0.01
On antiarrhythmics	86 %	43 %	-
On beta-blockers(1)	79 %	36 %	-
(1) Or calcium channel blockers			

It is clear that even though the unsuccessful ablations did not eliminate afib completely, they did reduce the number of episodes and overall burden (number of episodes x duration) and also reduced the need for medication. In no case did an afibber end up with more or longer episodes after the ablation.

Satisfaction with Procedure

The majority (89%) of afibbers who had undergone a RF ablation would recommend it with 7% responding that it would depend on the circumstances, but that it should probably only be done as a last resort; 4% did not recommend the procedure. Even among afibbers having undergone an unsuccessful procedure 82% would still recommend it, while 18% would not.

Permanence of Procedures

The first ablation included in our survey performed in 1997 was not successful. The first ablation that is known to have been successful was done in February 2000 – almost 5 years ago. Another one done in May 2000 is also known to be successful to date. Several ablations done in 2001 are known to be "still holding". I am not aware of any initially successful ablations that have "stopped working", but my data in this area is quite limited. Nevertheless, at this point in time, I have no evidence to suggest that successful ablations eventually allow afib to resurface.

Conclusions

- Ablation outcome is not affected by afib severity prior to the procedure, nor by age at time of ablation. However, there is a trend for ablations involving vagal afibbers to have a greater likelihood of success than those involving mixed (random) afibbers.
- The overall average success rate of a first ablation has increased significantly over the years (from 13% in 1997-2000 to 53% in 2004).
- The success rates of different procedures vary significantly from 22% for focal ablation to 66% for pulmonary vein isolation (PVI).
- Stenosis (narrowing of pulmonary vein diameter) is a significant problem in facilities other than top-rated ones.
- The most important variable in determining the outcome of an ablation is the skills of the electrophysiologist and the facilities at his disposal. The average success rate (including touch-up) in a top-rated facility is 76% as compared to 29% in other facilities.
- Adverse effects, some quite serious, were reported by 8% of afibbers treated at top-rated facilities and by 19% of those treated at other facilities. Forty per cent of these effects resolved on their own.
- The median time to recovery of normal sinus rhythm and no more afib episodes was 1 month (range 0-12 months) for successful ablatees, while the median time to full physical recovery was 2 months (range 0-11 months with an outlier of 48 months). There was no correlation between age at ablation and time to recovery.
- About 20% of all successful ablatees reported experiencing a significant number of PACs and PVCs at the time they completed the survey. The corresponding percentage for unsuccessful ablatees was 46%.
- The majority of successful ablatees (71%) no longer needed to avoid any triggers and 14% only needed to avoid some previous triggers. Fifteen per cent stated that it was too early to tell whether trigger avoidance was still necessary.
- There is no indication that blood pressure is affected by RF ablation; however, 45% of ablatees noticed an increase in heart rate after the procedure.
- Use of antiarrhythmics and blockers decreased after an ablation whether successful or not.

- There is no indication that an unsuccessful ablation increases afib severity – actually, quite the opposite.
- The vast majority (89%) of ablatees would recommend RF ablation and, although data is very limited, there is no indication that afib resurfaced among afibbers who had undergone a successful ablation.

Cryoablation

Two male afibbers (ages 62 and 50 years) underwent cryoablation in March 2004 and April 2001 respectively. The March 2004 procedure was performed in Maastricht, The Netherlands (AZM) by Drs. Rodriguez and Timmermans and was 100% successful. Details about this particular procedure can be found in the November 2004 issue of The AFIB Report.

The procedure done in April 2001 was only partially successful and was followed by a touch-up RF ablation in January 2002, which was again only partially successful. The afibber involved is still experiencing episodes (12 episodes in the last 3 months lasting an average of 12 hours each); however, this frequency and duration is a substantial improvement over the near constant afib experienced prior to the ablations. This afibber is still taking antiarrhythmics and warfarin.

Thus, one out of two reported cryoablations was successful, the other partially successful. None of the ablatees were found to have any signs of stenosis. It is clear that much more data is required before I can draw any valid conclusions about the relative merit of cryoablation versus RF ablation, especially since cryoablation has been primarily done at European centers so far, and is just now beginning to become available in the United States.

Maze Procedure

The conventional maze procedure involves open-heart surgery, i.e. making a foot long incision through the sternum so that the ribs can be pushed aside and the heart exposed. The procedure is performed under general anesthesia and the use of cardiopulmonary bypass (heart/lung machine). The surgeon creates lesions (with a scalpel) on the heart wall so as to channel the electrical impulses across the atria from the SA node to the AV node and also creates lesions to prevent the chaotic electrical activity characterizing atrial fibrillation. The procedure has a high success rate, but does entail a much longer recovery time than do RF and cryoablations. The maze procedure is often done in conjunction with other open-heart surgery such as bypass operations, mitral valve repair, and valve replacement.

More recently, minimally invasive procedures have been developed in which the lesions are created with RF energy rather than with a scalpel. Doing the maze procedure this way avoids the necessity for a large incision to open up the rib cage and also eliminates the need for the use of the heart/lung machine.

Ten afibbers responding to the survey had undergone either the full maze or a minimally invasive procedure.

Demographics	
Parameter	% or Number
Paroxysmal, %	60 %
Persistent, %	20 %
Permanent, %	20 %
Present age (mean), yrs	58
Age at diagnosis (mean), yrs	43
Age at procedure (mean), yrs	55
Age at procedure (range), yrs	42-64
Years of AF (mean)	15
Years of AF (range)	2-52
Females, %	20 %
Underlying heart disease, %	0 %
Mitral valve prolapse, %	20 %

None of the above demographic parameters were significantly different from those observed for afibbers undergoing RF ablation, nor was the number of episodes, their average duration or the total afib burden prior to the procedure significantly different between the two groups.

Success rate

Seven (70%) of the maze procedures are known to have been fully successful. These procedures were performed between 1998 and 2001. One robotic maze procedure performed in March 2004 was not successful as the afibber is still experiencing episodes, although far fewer than before. The remaining two procedures were performed early in 2004 (January and March). The patients have experienced no episodes, but are still on antiarrhythmics and warfarin, so it is too early to tell whether the procedures were entirely successful or not.

The successful procedures were performed at the following facilities:

- Cleveland Clinic   Dr. Patrick McCarthy
- Mayo Clinic, Rochester   Dr. Dearani
- Ohio State University Hospital   Dr. James Cox
- OSF St. Francis Medical   Dr. Dale Geiss
- Texas Heart Institute   Dr. Ali Massumi

The success rate quoted for the maze procedure in the medical literature is 95-97%. Our very limited data would indicate a rate between 70 and 90%, most likely closer to 90%, and thus not significantly different from that obtainable with RF ablation performed at a top-rated facility.

Stenosis is unlikely to be a problem with the maze procedure and none was observed.

Recovery and adverse effects

Six out of the seven completely successful respondents regained consistent normal sinus rhythm immediately upon completion of the procedure, while one took a month to do so. One patient has been in consistent sinus rhythm since April 1998.

The time to full physical recovery was generally about 2 months, but one respondent reported a recovery time of 6 months and another a recovery time of 36 months. Only one of the 10 respondents still needed to avoid some triggers.

There were no serious side effects reported, but in one case the breastbone took longer than normal to heal because of a persistent cough.

There were no indications that blood pressure or heart rate were significantly changed due to the procedure.

Medication use

All respondents were taking antiarrhythmics and beta- or calcium channel blockers prior to the procedure. After the procedure only 3 out of 10 were doing so. None of the successful patients were on warfarin after the procedure.

Satisfaction with procedure

All respondents felt (subjectively) that the procedure had been a success and 9 out of 10 would recommend the procedure.

Implantable Pacemakers/Cardioverter-Defibrillators

Pacemakers have long been used to assist ailing hearts in maintaining a steady beat. The most common reason for implanting a pacemaker is because the heart's own pacemaker (the sino-atrial node) has become too slow because of heart disease, age or the use of heart medications. Pacemakers are also used to provide a regular electrical impulse directly to the ventricles in case the AV (atrioventricular node) is blocked. A pacemaker can only increase the heart rate; it cannot slow it down.

The pacemaker consists of a small metal housing containing a battery and a small computer and is connected to one or two leads (wires) that are threaded through a vein beneath the collar bone and positioned in the heart using an x-ray monitor. The pacemaker itself is placed in a pocket beneath the skin just below the collarbone. The entire installation procedure takes about an hour or two and is performed under local anaesthesia.

From its original application as a means of supporting ailing hearts, the pacemaker has now emerged as a viable means of preventing cardiac arrhythmias. Their first application was in the prevention and termination of potentially fatal ventricular arrhythmias, but they are now also used in the prevention of atrial fibrillation. Some later models also have the capability of terminating fibrillation episodes by rapid bursts of pacing or by delivering an internal shock to the heart at much lower energy levels than what is required for the conventional external cardioversion procedure. These new devices are called implantable cardioverter-defibrillators or ICDs and are highly sophisticated and expensive electronic devices.

A typical, modern ICD acts as a miniature Holter monitor, has electronic circuitry that will provide precisely-timed impulses to the atria, thus preventing afib from beginning, and if an episode does start has the capability to terminate it. The ICD works in two ways to prevent arrhythmia. It continuously senses the heart beat and if it drops below a certain rate transmits electrical impulses to one or more electrodes implanted in the heart and connected to the ICD. This speeds up the heart beat and prevents bradycardia (dangerously slow heart beat) and the subsequent compensatory atrial fibrillation. This approach would work particularly well for vagal afibbers whose episodes are almost always preceded by bradycardia.

The ICD also continuously senses the heart rhythm and quickly notices the occurrence of PACs (premature atrial complexes) that often are a prelude to an afib episode, particularly among mixed and adrenergic afibbers. When the ICD senses PACs it speeds up the heart rhythm in a step-wise fashion until the PACs no longer appear. It then slowly reduces the heart rate to its original level and leaves the heart to do its own pacing again.

Modern ICDs are programmable just by holding a special wand in front of them, and the built-in Holter monitor, which can store lengthy heart beat records, can be read in the same way. They are indeed highly sophisticated devices and, as such, take extremely competent cardiologists to install and program.

Four survey respondents had had a programmable pacemaker installed in order to control their afib. Two reported complete control of episodes for 6 months or more and a much improved quality of life. Attaining this desirable state was, however, only achieved after considerable experimentation with the settings of the pacemaker, and, in one case, partial ablation of the AV node was required.

An excellent description of one afibber's journey to successfully ridding himself of afib is given in the April 2004 issue of The AFIB Report. One afibber with an ICD was able to remain afib-free with the aid of 2 x 100 mg/day of flecainide and one was still experiencing very brief episodes about every month or so. The improvement in the latter patient's condition only came about after the ICD was adjusted to provide only atrial pacing rather than dual pacing (both atria and ventricles).

Although it is impossible to draw any valid conclusions from just 4 responses, I see no evidence that an implantable pacemaker would be a better option for lone afibbers than a PVI carried out at a top-rated facility. Of course, in cases where access to such a facility is not available, the implantation of an antiarrhythmia pacemaker would certainly be an option, particularly if supplements, lifestyle change, and medications have not worked.

Pacemaker Implantation with AV Node Ablation

Another approach to eliminating the effects of the fibrillation of the atria on ventricular performance is to isolate the AV node (the ventricular beat controller) from any extraneous impulses and feed it its "marching orders" from an implanted pacemaker. This procedure is considered a last resort only and is (or should be) reserved for afibbers with no other options. The procedure has five major drawbacks.

- It is irreversible.
- It does nothing to stop the fibrillation of the atria, which, in itself, can be quite uncomfortable. It also necessitates continued anticoagulation (warfarin) therapy for life.
- It makes the patient entirely dependent on the pacemaker. If it malfunctions or the batteries run out, the patient may die.
- It does nothing to remedy the fatigue and reduced exercise capacity caused by the fibrillation of the atria.
- It actually worsens the prognosis since it tends to convert paroxysmal afib to the persistent or permanent type.

The procedure itself is relatively safe and a Swedish study reported that recipients of the procedure reported an improvement in their quality of life.

Two survey respondents (one 76-year-old female and one 51-year-old male) reported that they had undergone AV node ablation and pacemaker implantation in February 2004 and October 2000 respectively. The procedure performed in February 2004 (permanent female afibber) was deemed successful by the recipient. She no longer experiences noticeable afib, is not taking antiarrhythmics or beta-blockers, and does not need to avoid any triggers. She is, however, still on warfarin. She would only recommend the procedure if medication does not work.

The procedure performed in October 2000 was not successful and was later followed by an open-heart maze procedure. This procedure was successful in eliminating afib, but the patient is still on antiarrhythmics and beta- or calcium channel blockers. He has been taken off warfarin.

The results of only two procedures clearly do not provide adequate information as to the viability of AV node ablation and pacemaker implantation. However, I see no evidence that would contradict current medical opinion that this procedure should only be used as a very last resort.

Flutter Ablation

Most cases of atrial flutter are associated with a conduction abnormality in the lower right atrium and can be successfully treated with a relatively simple ablation procedure that does not include penetrating the septum separating the right and left atrium. Both atrial flutter and atrial fibrillation may be at least partially due to an enlarged atrium and the two conditions can coexist in the same patient and one may convert to the other.

Two survey respondents (a 57-year-old male vagal afibber and a 61-year-old male mixed afibber) had experienced both afib and atrial flutter prior to their flutter ablations in May 2004 and March 2001 respectively. The ablations successfully eliminated flutter episodes, but afib episodes still occur unless controlled by medication.

This concludes the evaluation of the responses obtained in our 8th LAF survey covering surgical and catheterization approaches to dealing with afib. Radiofrequency ablation is clearly the most popular option and has an excellent success rate if performed by a highly skilled EP at a top-rated facility. The success rate for the maze procedure is also excellent. Insufficient data is available to gauge the success rate of cryoablation and pacemaker implantation with and without AV node ablation.

Pharmaceutical and Alternative Protocols

By Hans R. Larsen [2004]

The purpose of this survey was to gather information about and share the various approaches used by fellow afibbers to successfully manage their condition by the use of pharmaceutical drugs, supplements, dietary changes, or other protocols.

It is important to bear in mind when interpreting the results of this survey that only fibbers who had been **successful** in controlling their condition were invited to participate. There are many, many of us who have tried numerous approaches without success, but hopefully, these survey results will give us ideas for new approaches to try.

Profile of respondents

A total of 116 respondents provided data for this part of the survey. The majority (81%) were men. The average (mean) age of the respondents was 57 years (median: 57, range: 27-79). The mean age at diagnosis was 49 years (median: 51, range: 18-77). The number of years that the respondents had experienced afib varied between 1 and 41 years with a mean of 7 years and a median of 5 years. Only 8 respondents (7%) had been diagnosed with underlying heart disease, while 7 (6.2%) had been diagnosed with mitral valve prolapse. The majority (92%) had received a medical diagnosis of paroxysmal, persistent or permanent AF.

The majority (84%) of respondents had paroxysmal LAF with 37% having the vagal variety, 33% being mixed, 7% being adrenergic, and 7% unknown. Among the 10% who had persistent afib 3% had the vagal variety, 4% mixed, 0% adrenergic, and unknown 3%. Three percent were in permanent afib and the status for the remaining 3% was unknown. The types of interventions can be divided into three categories:

A. Pharmaceutical drugs as sole remedy (27 respondents)
B. Alternative methods as sole remedy (41 respondents)
C. Pharmaceutical drugs + alternative methods (50 respondents)

A. Pharmaceutical Drugs Only

Twenty-seven of the 116 survey respondents (23%) in this part of the survey had relied solely on the use of pharmaceutical drugs to manage their afib. The majority of respondents (78%) were men. The average (mean) age of the respondents was 56 years (median: 59, range: 27-74). The mean age at diagnosis was 51 years (median: 52, range: 26-68). The number of years that the respondents had experienced afib varied between 1 and 13 years with a mean of 5 years and a median of 4 years. Only one respondent had been diagnosed with underlying heart disease, while 3 had been diagnosed with mitral valve prolapse. The majority (89%) had received a medical diagnosis of paroxysmal, persistent or permanent atrial fibrillation.

The majority (92%) of respondents had paroxysmal LAF with 37% having the vagal variety, 37% being mixed, 7% being adrenergic, and 11% unknown. All afibbers with persistent afib had the mixed variety and there were no permanent afibbers who had successfully managed their condition with pharmaceutical drugs.

Fifteen respondents (56%) had experienced side effects from their drug regimen with the most common being:

- Fatigue or dizziness (4 out of 27 or 15%)
- Exercise intolerance (4 out of 27 or 15%)

Other reported side effects were shortness of breath, reduction in heart rate, skin flushing, and weight gain. One respondent on amiodarone had experienced the beginning of hyperthyroidism, while another reported increased sun sensitivity.

Nine respondents (33%) reported additional benefits from their drug regimen such as mental relief from not having to fear another episode, weight loss, and a reduction in PVCs.

Eleven respondents (40%) no longer needed to avoid their previous episode triggers such as exercise, alcohol, caffeine, MSG, cold drinks, large meals, etc. Five (19%) still needed to avoid their known triggers, 6 (22%) still needed to avoid some triggers, but not as many as before their drug regimen and the remaining 5 (19%) were not sure whether they still had to avoid triggers.

The majority (89%) would recommend their protocol to other afibbers, but 30% were still contemplating an ablation, while 41% were uncertain whether they would have one or not. Only 29% were quite certain they would not undergo an ablation. The sources of information used in arriving at the successful drug regimen are given below.

Cardiologist	67%
Electrophysiologist	37%
Afibbers.org Bulletin Board	11%
Lone Atrial Fibrillation: Towards a Cure	7%
Personal Research on the Internet	7%
The AFIB Report	4%
Primary physician (GP)	4%
Other sources	4%

Please note that percentages do not add up to 100% because many respondents reported having used more than one information source.

Not surprisingly, the majority of afibbers relying solely on pharmaceutical drugs to control their condition had obtained their information from a cardiologist or electrophysiologist.

Effectiveness of drug protocols

Flecainide (Tambocor) was, by far, the most widely prescribed drug among the 27 respondents. It was used either alone or in combination with beta- or calcium channel blockers by 13 afibbers or 48% of the group. Sotalol was used by 5 afibbers or 19%, while amiodarone and propafenone were each used by 2 respondents. The remaining 5 respondents used beta-blockers (2), a calcium channel blocker (diltiazem), disopyramide or digoxin.

It is of interest that, out of these 7 drugs, only flecainide and propafenone are actually labelled (approved) for use in the treatment of paroxysmal atrial fibrillation.

A total of 19 afibbers in the group had submitted sufficient data for detailed analysis and fulfilled the criteria of having spent at least 50% less time in afib (number of episodes x average duration) in the 3 months after their protocol became effective as compared to the 3 months prior to embarking on their protocol.

Episodes over 3 months	Before protocol	With protocol
Episode frequency [number]		
Mean	17	2
Median	8	0
Range	2 – 87	0 - 19
Episode duration [hours]		
Mean	17	4
Median	8	4
Range	2 – 94	0 – 18
Total hours spent in afib during 3 months		
Mean	264	11
Median	75	1
Range	6 – 1800	0 - 149

The 19 afibbers had been on their program for an average of 18 months (4-156 months) and the time before it became effective varied from 1 day to 3 months.

The percentage reduction in time spent in afib over a 3-month period varied from 60 to 100% with 8 (42%) of respondents reporting no episodes at all since their program became effective. The average (mean) reduction in time spent in afib among all the 19 afibbers was 94% (median 99%).

The reduction in episode frequency and duration reported by the 19 afibbers is substantial; however, it must be kept in mind that this is a very small sample indeed. There is certainly no guarantee that similar results would be obtained in the general afib population.

Eleven or 58% of the group of 19 were using flecainide either alone or in combination with a beta-blocker or calcium channel blocker; 3 were using sotalol, 2 propafenone, and 1 each amiodarone, Toprol XL (metoprolol), or diltiazem.

Flecainide (Tambocor) was used as sole remedy by 3 afibbers with the mixed variety and by 2 with vagal afib. It was used in combination with a beta-blocker (atenolol, metoprolol or bisoprolol) by 3 mixed and 2 vagal, and in combination with diltiazem by 1 mixed afibber. The dosage when used as a sole remedy ranged from 3x50 mg/day to 2x100 mg/day and the dosage when used in combination ranged from 1x50 mg/day to 2x100 mg/day. The most common concomitant dosage of metoprolol and atenolol was 25 mg/day with that for bisoprolol and diltiazem being 5 mg/day and 240 mg/day respectively.

Only 1 out of 5 (20%) reported negative side effects when using flecainide alone, while 5 out of 6 (83%) reported adverse effects when using combinations. This likely indicates that it is primarily the beta- or calcium channel blocker that is responsible for the side effects.

The average (median) percent reduction in time spent in afib for the 11 flecainide users was 99% and 5 of them had experienced no episodes at all since beginning their therapy. It is encouraging to note that 5 out of 11 (45%) flecainide users no longer needed to avoid the common afib triggers. Also of note is the finding that 2 persistent afibbers had benefited substantially from using flecainide with one having experienced no episodes at all since beginning therapy and one now experiencing episodes lasting only about 5 hours.

From this very small sample it would appear that flecainide, when it works, works very well indeed. Because peak plasma levels of the drug are reached about 3 hours after ingestion, it is best to take flecainide in divided doses throughout the day. A dosage of 50 mg taken every 8 hours or 50 mg taken every 12 hours would likely be a good starting regimen. A further refinement may be to make sure that one of the daily doses is taken about 3 hours before the most vulnerable period. So if bedtime (10-11 pm) is the "danger zone" then a dose should be taken around 7-8 pm. The absorption of flecainide is not affected by food or antacids.

Sotalol (Betapace) was used as the sole remedy by 1 mixed and 1 adrenergic afibber (daily dose of 2x80 mg). One vagal afibber reported good results with a combination of sotalol and irbesartan (Avapro). Irbesartan is an angiotensin II receptor blocker and has, on its own, been found to help maintain sinus rhythm for extended periods when combined with amiodarone. German researchers have found that lone afibbers have more angiotensin II receptors in the left atrium than do non-afibbers, so blocking these receptors could be important.

The two afibbers who used sotalol on its own both reported significant side effects (skin flushing and exercise intolerance), but had seen a 100% improvement in their condition. They had been taking sotalol for 3 and 5 years respectively and during that period had only experienced one episode between them. Two of the 3 sotalol users still needed to avoid the usual triggers to some degree and one was not sure whether avoidance was still required.

From this extremely small sample it would seem that sotalol can be of considerable benefit in selected individuals. Unfortunately, there is some evidence that there may not be too many of these individuals among lone afibbers. An earlier LAF survey found that not a single one of 38 respondents had found sotalol to be beneficial and 76% had experienced significant side effects.

Propafenone (Rythmol) was used as the sole remedy by 1 vagal afibber and in combination with verapamil (120 mg/day) by a mixed afibber. The daily dosage of propafenone was 3x150 mg/day in both cases. Neither of the 2 respondents had experienced any episodes since starting therapy (8 and 33 months respectively), nor felt any side effects, and they no longer had to avoid the usual triggers. The earlier LAF survey found that 7 out of 19 respondents had found propafenone to be beneficial and 47% had experienced significant side effects.

Peak plasma levels of propafenone are reached 1-2 hours after ingestion and the elimination half-life of the drug varies between 4 and 10 hours. Thus taking this drug in divided doses is even more important than in the case of flecainide. A dosage of 150 mg taken every 8 hours is the standard starting regimen, but I suspect some afibbers may need 4x150 mg/day to see a beneficial effect. Again, it may be possible to optimize the regimen by ensuring that a dose is taken a couple of hours prior to the most vulnerable period. Propafenone is better absorbed if taken with food.

Amiodarone (Cordarone) was used in combination with 5 mg bisoprolol by 1 mixed afibber. The daily dose was 200 mg. This respondent reported a 99% improvement (from 24 6-hour episodes in the 3-month period preceding therapy to two 4-hour episodes in the 18 months of therapy). However, a thyroid problem was developing. Amiodarone is absorbed very slowly and eliminated even more slowly. It can take 8 months or more to reduce plasma levels by 50%. Amiodarone is absorbed quicker and more fully if taken with food.

Toprol XL (slow-release metoprolol) had benefited 1 adrenergic afibber by reducing the number of episodes from 3 to 1 in the 3-month period before and after therapy initiation. Occasional dizziness was reported as a side effect and some triggers still had to be avoided. Obviously, a sample of one predicts nothing about the effectiveness of metoprolol. The earlier survey found that 2 out of 5 adrenergic and 4 out of 5 mixed afibbers had obtained benefits from using this beta-blocker, but 71% reported side effects such as fatigue, slow heart rate and low blood pressure.

Diltiazem (Cardizem) in one daily dose of 240 mg was used by 1 vagal afibber to obtain a reduction in afib frequency from 2 episodes per 3 months to 2 episodes per year. No side effects were reported and the usual trigger factors did not need to be avoided. Again, a sample of one is not enough on which to draw a valid conclusion. The earlier survey found that none out of 8 paroxysmal afibbers had found diltiazem useful in preventing episodes.

Profiles of 8 afibbers who had completely eliminated their episodes solely through the use of pharmaceutical drugs are presented below.

Female - 56 years of age with 4 years of paroxysmal, mixed LAF
Drug protocol: 2x100 mg/day of flecainide for 9 months
Number of episodes in 3 months prior to protocol: 50
Average duration of episodes prior to protocol: 36 hours
Number of episodes since beginning protocol: 0
Still need to avoid triggers: No

Supplements: None reported   Dietary changes: None reported
Other preventive measures: None reported
Side effects of protocol: Exercise intolerance

Male - 37 years of age with 9 years of paroxysmal, vagal LAF
Drug protocol: 100 mg/day of flecainide for 36 months
Number of episodes in 3 months prior to protocol: 3
Average duration of episodes prior to protocol: 2 hours
Number of episodes since beginning protocol: 0
Still need to avoid triggers: No

Supplements: None reported   Dietary changes: None reported
Other preventive measures: None reported
Side effects of protocol: None

Comment: Was able to reduce dosage from 2x100 mg /day

Male - 61 years of age with 4 years of paroxysmal, mixed LAF
Drug protocol: 50 mg/day flecainide + 25 mg/day metoprolol for 23 months
Number of episodes in 3 months prior to protocol: 25
Average duration of episodes prior to protocol: 3 hours
Number of episodes since beginning protocol: 0
Still need to avoid triggers: Don't know [have not tried alcohol and caffeine]

Supplements: None reported   Dietary changes: None reported
Other preventive measures: None reported
Side effects of protocol: None

Female - 57 years of age with 1 year of paroxysmal, mixed LAF
Drug protocol: 2 x 50 mg flecainide + 25 mg/day metoprolol for 8 months
Number of episodes in 3 months prior to protocol: 3
Average duration of episodes prior to protocol: 5 hours
Number of episodes since beginning protocol: 0
Still need to avoid triggers: Yes, but much less so

Supplements: None reported   Dietary changes: None reported
Other preventive measures: None reported
Side effects of protocol: Tiredness, shortness of breath upon exertion

---

Male - 67 years of age with 2 years of paroxysmal, vagal LAF
Drug protocol: 2 x 100 mg flecainide + 2 x 25 mg/day atenelol for 4 months
Number of episodes in 3 months prior to protocol: 20
Average duration of episodes prior to protocol: 2 hours
Number of episodes since beginning protocol: 0
Still need to avoid triggers: No

Supplements: None reported   Dietary changes: None reported
Other preventive measures: None reported
Side effects of protocol: Tiredness, lack of sex drive

Female - 54 years of age with 6 years of paroxysmal, vagal LAF
Drug protocol: 3 x 150 mg/day of propafenone for 33 months
Number of episodes in 3 months prior to protocol: 5
Average duration of episodes prior to protocol: 10 hours
Number of episodes since beginning protocol: 0
Still need to avoid triggers: No

Supplements: None reported   Dietary changes: None reported
Other preventive measures: None reported
Side effects of protocol: None

Male - 53 years of age with 2 years of paroxysmal, mixed LAF
Drug protocol: 3x150 mg propafenone + 120 mg/day verapamil for 8 months
Number of episodes in 3 months prior to protocol: 6
Average duration of episodes prior to protocol: 4 hours
Number of episodes since beginning protocol: 0
Still need to avoid triggers: No

Supplements: None reported   Dietary changes: None reported
Other preventive measures: None reported
Side effects of protocol: None

Male - 62 years of age with 4 years of paroxysmal, mixed LAF
Drug protocol: 2 x 80 mg/day of Sotalol for 34 months
Number of episodes in 3 months prior to protocol: 4
Average duration of episodes prior to protocol: 4 hours
Number of episodes since beginning protocol: 0
Still need to avoid triggers: Yes, but much less so

Supplements: None reported   Dietary changes: None reported
Other preventive measures: None reported
Side effects of protocol: Exercise intolerance, reduced heart rate

It is clear that a well-designed drug protocol can, on its own, be highly effective in reducing afib severity in a select group of afibbers. Flecainide (Tambocor) would appear to be the most successful antiarrhythmic and may be effective in a dose as low as 50 mg/day on its own or combined with a small amount of beta-blocker. Although flecainide has the potential for very serious adverse effects, a trial may be worthwhile in afibbers with sound hearts, especially those having the mixed or vagal variety of AF.

B. Alternative Therapies

Forty-one of the 116 survey respondents (35%) had relied solely on the use of alternative therapies rather than pharmaceutical drugs to manage their afib. The majority (83%) were men. The average (mean) age of the group as a whole was 56 years (median 57 years, range 36-73). The mean age at diagnosis was 47 years (median 51 years, range 18-71). The number of years the respondents had experienced afib varied between 1 and 41 years with a mean of 9 years and a median of 6 years. Four respondents (10%) had been diagnosed with underlying heart disease, while one (3%) had been diagnosed with mitral valve prolapse. The majority (88%) had received a medical diagnosis of paroxysmal, persistent or permanent atrial fibrillation. The distribution of the various types of afib follows:

Type of AF	# of Respondents	% of Respondents
Paroxsysmal	**36**	88%
- Adrenergic	2	5%
- Mixed	15	37%
- Vagal	16	39%
- Unknown	3	7%
Persistent	**2**	5%
- Adrenergic	0	0%
- Mixed	0	0%
- Vagal	1	2%
- Unknown	1	2%
Permanent	**2**	5%
Unknown	1	2%
TOTAL	**41**	**100%**

Six respondents (15%) had experienced minor "**side effects**" such as:
- missing a glass of wine or beer;
- limited food choices;
- bowel problems (detoxification);
- cutback on strenuous exercise;
- high cost of supplements.

The 15% who experienced minor side effects from the alternative protocols compares to 56% who experienced significant side effects from the pharmaceutical drug protocols. This is clearly a very significant difference.

Thirty respondents (73%) reported additional benefits from their regimen. This is substantially lower than the 33% who reported additional benefits from their drug regimen. Among the **benefits reported** were:

Able to discontinue antiarrhythmics	41%
More energy	27%
Weight loss	20%
Improved mental outlook	17%
Improved general health	13%
Improved digestion	13%
Less stress and anxiety	10%
Better sleep	7%
Clearer thinking	7%
Less noticeable heart beat	7%
Lower blood pressure	3%
Clearer skin	3%
Please note percentages do not add up to 100% because some respondents reported more than one benefit.	

It is clear that the protocols used by this group had very substantial overall benefits above and beyond the control of afib severity.

Only 4 out of 41 respondents (10%) no longer needed to avoid their previous episode triggers such as exercise, alcohol, caffeine, MSG, cold drinks, large meals, etc. This percentage is clearly significantly lower than the 40% reported by the pharmaceuticals group. Thus, it is clear that the alternative approach to afib management requires continued vigilance to a greater extent than does a pure drug protocol. Ten respondents (25%) still needed to avoid some triggers, but not as many as before. Twenty-two (53%) had observed no improvement as far as trigger avoidance is concerned, while the remaining 5 (12%) were not sure whether they still had to avoid triggers.

The majority of respondents (90%) would recommend their program to other afibbers and only 5% were contemplating an ablation as compared to 30% in the pharmaceuticals group. Twelve respondents (29%) were not sure whether they would have an ablation (41% in the drug group), and 27 (66%) were quite certain that they would not undergo an ablation. The desire to have an ablation

146

is probably largely related to how serious an impact afib has on one's life. Thus, it would seem that the impact of afib is less pronounced among afibbers using alternative means than among those using antiarrhythmics – or perhaps users of pharmaceutical drugs are more comfortable with surgical interventions.

The sources of information used in arriving at the successful regimen were as follows:

Cardiologist	22%
Electrophysiologist	5%
Afibbers.org Bulletin Board	44%
Other bulletin boards	12%
Lone Atrial Fibrillation: Towards a Cure	46%
Personal Research on the Internet	46%
The AFIB Report	32%
Primary physician (GP)	7%
Naturopath	0%
Other health care practitioner	7%
Other sources	34%

Please note that percentages do not add up to 100% because many respondents reported having used more than one information source.

It is clear that afibbers who relied on alternative therapies for managing their afib were much less likely to have obtained their information from a cardiologist or electrophysiologist than were those relying on pharmaceutical drugs. The main information sources for afibbers using alternative management were the book *Lone Atrial Fibrillation: Towards a Cure*, personal research on the Internet, the affibers.org Bulletin Board, and The AFIB Report.

Protocols Used in Management

The protocols used by this group of 41 afibbers to control their afib fall into 5 broad categories:

- Supplementation – used by 73% of respondents
- Dietary changes – used by 41% of respondents
- Trigger avoidance – used by 39% of respondents
- Stress reduction and other methods – used by 41% of respondents
- Elimination of GERD – used by 7% of respondents

Among supplement users, magnesium was by far the most popular and was used by 54% of respondents, fish oils were used by 34%, vitamin E by 27%, coenzyme Q10 by 24%, vitamin C by 20%, potassium, including low-sodium V8 juice by 17%, and a daily multivitamin by 20%.

The Paleo diet was used by 12% of respondents and the Zone diet and the Mediterranean diet by one respondent each. Other dietary changes included elimination of dairy products (22%) and grains (20%), and an increase in the consumption of fruits and vegetables (20%).

Eliminating caffeine had been found beneficial by 20% of respondents, eliminating alcohol by 17%, eating smaller meals by 12%, and eliminating MSG, aspartame and glutamate from their diet had benefited 12% of respondents. Three respondents had reduced their afib severity very significantly by taking steps to eliminate their GERD (gastroesophageal reflux disease).

The stress reduction methods used by the group were many and varied and included breathing exercises (used by 15%), cognitive thinking, meditation, and smelling or ingesting valerian root. Two afibbers had found relief by having an ICD (implantable cardioverter defibrillator) installed or reprogrammed, and one had reduced episode frequency by 98% by having jaw bone cavitations removed.

Effectiveness of Protocols

A total of 23 afibbers in the group had sufficient data for detailed analysis and fulfilled the criteria of having spent at least 50% less time in afib (number of episodes x average duration) in the 3 months after their program became effective as compared to the 3 months prior to embarking on their program.

The 23 afibbers had been on their program for an average of 18 months (4-62 months) and the time before it became effective varied from 1 day to 12 months with a median of 2 months. Afib severity parameters for a 3-month period before and for a 3-month period after the program became effective are presented below:

Episodes over 3 months	Before protocol	With protocol
Episode frequency [number]		
Mean	18	1
Median	5	0.3
Range	1 - 90	0 - 6
Episode duration [hours]		
Mean	30	4
Median	14	1.5
Range	1 – 237	0 – 18
Total hours spent in afib during 3 months		
Mean	381	5
Median	56	1
Range	4 – 2160	0 - 45

The average (median) reduction in time spent in afib by the group of 23 was an impressive 98%.

A comparison between the above data and the corresponding data for the 19 afibbers using drugs shows that the total hours [median] spent in afib over a 3-month period prior to beginning the successful protocol were similar [75 hours for pharmaceuticals vs. 56 hours for alternative protocols]. The total time spent in afib in a 3-month period after the protocol became effective were identical [1 hour] indicating that an alternative protocol can be just as effective as a drug-based protocol. The alternative protocols, of course, has the added advantage of many other beneficial effects and no serious side effects. Nevertheless, a sample of 23 is small indeed and there is obviously no guarantee that a program based on alternative protocols would work as well in the general afib population.

The protocols used by the select group of 23 afibbers with complete data paralleled those used by the entire group of 41 afibbers, except that the 3 respondents who had found improvement by controlling their GERD were all in the select group. The percentage of afibbers using the various supplements did not differ between the select and total group. The percentage of afibbers having found improvement through dietary changes was somewhat higher in the select group (56%) than among the remaining 18 afibbers (33%). There were no differences between the select group and the remaining group as far as the use of stress reduction and other methods are concerned nor in the percentage having found trigger elimination beneficial.

Ten afibbers (24%) in the group of 41 had completely eliminated their afib episodes for at least a 3-month period and two had seen a 99.9% improvement. Their profiles are presented below:

Female - 62 years of age with 4 years of paroxysmal, vagal LAF
Number of episodes in 3 months prior to protocol: 4
Average duration of episodes prior to protocol: 1 hour
Months on protocol: 7
Number of episodes since beginning protocol: 0
Still need to avoid triggers: Not sure

Supplements [Daily]: Magnesium (800 mg), potassium (1800 mg as low-sodium V8 juice), fish oil (6 g), coenzyme Q10 (60 mg), taurine (4 g), vitamin E (1200 IU), vitamin C (6 g), B-complex, (50 mg), arginine (4 g), garlic (2500 mg), vitamin B-12 (1000 mcg), multivitamin

Dietary changes: Paleo diet, elimination of wheat
Stress reduction protocol: None reported
Triggers avoided: None specified
Other preventive measures: None reported
Other benefits of protocol: Improvement in general well-being
Adverse effects of protocol: None

Female - 44 years of age with 22 years of permanent LAF
Number of episodes in 3 months prior to protocol: permanent
Average duration of episodes prior to protocol: permanent
Months on protocol: 36
Number of episodes since beginning protocol: 3
Still need to avoid triggers: Yes

Supplements: None reported

Dietary changes: Whole fresh foods [approaching Paleo diet], elimination of grains and dairy, at least 10 servings/day of fruit and vegetables
Stress reduction protocol: Cognitive thinking
Triggers avoided: Glutamates, MSG, and all other food additives
Other preventive measures: 1.5-2 L/day of mineral water, green tea

Other benefits of protocol: Clear skin, loss of cellulite, greater energy, clearer thinking, no anxiety, loss of stomach fat, "glad to be alive"
Adverse effects of protocol: None

Comment: 100% commitment is required for this program to work

---

Male - 42 years of age with 18 years of paroxysmal, mixed LAF
Number of episodes in 3 months prior to protocol: 1
Average duration of episodes prior to protocol: 72 hours
Months on protocol: 5
Number of episodes since beginning protocol: 0
Still need to avoid triggers: Yes

Supplements: magnesium

Dietary changes: Increased intake of raw natural foods and vegetable juices
Stress reduction protocol: None reported
Triggers avoided: Caffeine

Other preventive measures: None reported
Other benefits of protocol: None reported
Adverse effects of protocol: None reported

Comment: Cutting out all caffeine and supplementing with magnesium worked for me

Male - 51 years of age with 3 years of paroxysmal, vagal LAF
Number of episodes in 3 months prior to protocol: 5
Average duration of episodes prior to protocol: 12 hours
Months on protocol: 26
Number of episodes since beginning protocol: 0
Still need to avoid triggers: Yes, but much less so

Supplements: Magnesium orotate and chelate [280 mg/day], potassium [100 mg/day]

Dietary changes: None reported
Stress reduction protocol: None reported
Triggers avoided: None specified
Other preventive measures: None reported

Other benefits of protocol: Was able to discontinue flecainide
Adverse effects of protocol: None reported

Male - 59 years of age with 1 year of paroxysmal, mixed LAF
Number of episodes in 3 months prior to protocol: 3
Average duration of episodes prior to protocol: 18 hours
Months on protocol: 3
Number of episodes since beginning protocol: 0
Still need to avoid triggers: Yes, but much less so

Supplements: Magnesium, coenzyme Q10 [50 mg/day], fish oil [10 ml/day]
Dietary changes: None reported

Stress reduction protocol: Diaphragmatic breathing
Triggers avoided: None specified
Other preventive measures: None reported

Other benefits of protocol: More relaxed and happily detached with positive attitude
Adverse effects of protocol: None reported

Male - 51 years of age with 2 years of permanent LAF
Number of episodes in 3 months prior to protocol: Permanent
Average duration of episodes prior to protocol: Permanent
Months on protocol: 18
Number of episodes since beginning protocol: 0
Still need to avoid triggers: Yes

Supplements: Coenzyme Q10 [50 mg/day]

Dietary changes: No dairy, no big meals at night, drink lots of water
Stress reduction protocol: Reduced work-related stress
Triggers avoided: Coffee [used to drink 15 cups a day]
Other preventive measures: Discontinued all medications

Other benefits of protocol: None reported
Adverse effects of protocol: None reported

Comment: Was successfully cardioverted 18 months ago

Male - 55 years of age with 3 years of paroxysmal, vagal LAF
Number of episodes in 3 months prior to protocol: 4
Average duration of episodes prior to protocol: 12 hours
Months on protocol: 7
Number of episodes since beginning protocol: 0
Still need to avoid triggers: Yes

Supplements: Magnesium glycinate [200 mg/day]

Dietary changes: Lots of fresh fruit daily [at least one banana]
Stress reduction protocol: None reported
Triggers avoided: Alcohol
Other preventive measures: Avoid sleeping on left side

Other benefits of protocol: None reported
Adverse effects of protocol: Miss a glass of red wine with dinner

Comment: Cutting out alcohol [red wine] was what worked for me

Male - 53 years of age with 5 years of paroxysmal, vagal LAF
Number of episodes in 3 months prior to protocol: 2
Average duration of episodes prior to protocol: 18 hours
Months on protocol: 4
Number of episodes since beginning protocol: 0
Still need to avoid triggers: Yes, but much less so

Supplements: Magnesium glycinate [1500 mg/day], vitamin B6

Dietary changes: None reported
Stress reduction protocol: None reported
Triggers avoided: None specified
Other preventive measures: Discontinuing beta-blockers

Other benefits of protocol: Elimination of heartburn
Adverse effects of protocol: None reported

Comment: Increase in magnesium intake worked for me

Male – 36 years of age with 16 years of paroxysmal, vagal LAF
Number of episodes in 3 months prior to protocol: 2
Average duration of episodes prior to protocol: 7 hours
Months on protocol: 5
Number of episodes since beginning protocol: 0
Still need to avoid triggers: Don't know yet

Supplements: 1.2 gram/day of pharmaceutical grade fish oil

Dietary changes: Changed to Zone Diet
Stress reduction protocol: None reported
Triggers avoided: None specified
Other preventive measures: Discontinuing propafenone

Other benefits of protocol: Increased energy and concentration
Adverse effects of protocol: None reported

Comment: Your book lead me to the Zone Diet and I've never felt better

Male - 67 years of age with 4 years of paroxysmal, mixed LAF
Number of episodes in 3 months prior to protocol: 8
Average duration of episodes prior to protocol: 237 hours
Months on protocol: 6
Number of episodes since beginning protocol: 2 [at 6 hours each]
Still need to avoid triggers: Yes

Supplements [daily]: B complex (100 mg), B12 (1 mg), vit C (3 g), vit E (800 IU),
1 multi-vitamin/mineral, chromium (200 mg), mag glycinate (300 mg), mag
taurate (250 mg), mag citrate (100 mg), selenium (200 mcg), fish oil (5 g
providing 1080 mg EPA and 720 DHA), lycopene (10 mg), coenzyme Q10 (200
mg), alpha lipoic acid (400 mg), acetyl-l-carnitine (1.5 g), l-carnitine (1 g), taurine
(1 g), saw palmetto (320 mg), digestive enzymes (1.5 g), milk-free acidophilus (80
g)

Dietary changes: No dairy, low glycemic index Mediterranean diet, organic
apples, no coffee or beer
Stress reduction protocol: Meditation
Triggers avoided: Wine, getting out of bed quickly
Other preventive measures: Discontinued taking flecainide, reduced water
intake to 2.5 L/day, stopped eating daily tuna fish sandwich

Other benefits of protocol: General health benefits
Adverse effects of protocol: Cost of supplements, limited variation in diet
Comment: Main elements of my success were supplementing with
acidophilus and taurine, reducing water consumption, discontinuing
flecainide, and reducing mercury level (hair analysis) from 9.3 to 0.9 ppm
by discontinuing to eat tuna sandwiches daily

Male - 38 years of age with 4 years of paroxysmal, vagal LAF
Number of episodes in 3 months prior to protocol: 4
Average duration of episodes prior to protocol: 3 hours
Months on protocol: 23
Number of episodes since beginning protocol: 4 [lasting 10 minutes or less]
Still need to avoid triggers: Yes

Supplements: None reported
Dietary changes: Reduced carbohydrates and added protein to every meal
Stress reduction protocol: None reported
Triggers avoided: None specified
Other preventive measures: Drinking plenty of water

Other benefits of protocol: Better sleep, overall feeling of well-being
Adverse effects of protocol: None reported
Comment: I believe my program lead to better insulin response and
elimination of dehydration

Male - 38 years of age with 2 years of paroxysmal LAF
Number of episodes in 3 months prior to protocol: 2
Average duration of episodes prior to protocol: 14 hours
Months on protocol: 14
Number of episodes since beginning protocol: 0
Still need to avoid triggers: Yes, but much less so

Supplements: low sodium V8 (2 glasses/day), MoloCure Aloe Vera (9 caps/day), Coromega fish oil (1 pouch/day)

Dietary changes: 1 cup blueberries daily
Stress reduction protocol: None reported
Triggers avoided: None specified
Other preventive measures: None reported

Other benefits of protocol: None reported
Adverse effects of protocol: None reported
Comment: I believe my program has reduced my GERD (specifically the aloe vera), reduced systemic inflammation, and increased potassium stores

It is clear that a well-designed non-drug program can be just as effective as a program based on antiarrhythmics and beta- or calcium channel blockers. The big challenge is to find the protocol that is just right. This clearly can involve a great deal of experimentation and can be costly as well, particularly if supplements and fresh, organic food are part of the program. A successful program can be as simple as eliminating triggers such as alcohol or caffeine, wheat and dairy or just increasing the intake of magnesium and potassium. However, in many cases fundamental dietary changes, a vast arsenal of supplements, and faithful adherence to stress reduction protocols are required to achieve the afib-free nirvana.

The alternative protocols adopted by the respondents to this survey clearly have no serious side effects and many highly desirable benefits over and above the elimination of afib or, at least, a substantial reduction in episode severity. Will they work for everyone? Probably not – we are all an experiment of one it seems, but certainly the afibbers whose programs have been covered here have shown the way and provided many ideas for the rest of us to try.

C. Pharmaceutical Drugs and Alternative Therapies

Fifty of the 118 survey respondents (42%) had relied on a combination of alternative protocols and pharmaceutical drugs to manage their afib [Note: two afibbers joined the survey after the results of the use of pharmaceutical drugs and alternative protocols had been published thus increasing the total survey population to 118]. The majority (78%) were men. The average (mean) age was 57 years (median 57, range 39-79) for the entire group. The mean age at diagnosis was 50 years (median 51, range 19-77). The number of years the

155

respondents had experienced afib varied between a few months and 36 years with a mean of 7 years and a median of 4 years. Three respondents (6%) had been diagnosed with underlying heart disease and 5 (10%) had been diagnosed with mitral valve prolapse. The majority (92%) had received a medical diagnosis of paroxysmal, persistent or permanent atrial fibrillation.

Type of AF	# of Respondents	% of Respondents
Paroxsysmal	**43**	86%
- Adrenergic	4	8%
- Mixed	17	37%
- Vagal	20	40%
- Unknown	2	4%
Persistent	**5**	10%
- Adrenergic	0	0%
- Mixed	2	4%
- Vagal	1	2%
- Unknown	2	4%
Permanent	**2**	4%
Unknown	0	0%
TOTAL	**50**	**100%**

Twenty-one (42%) had experienced side effects from their protocol with the most common being:

- **Fatigue** was experienced by 8 respondents and was associated with flecainide (Tambocor), metoprolol (Toprol), and propafenone (Rythmol).
- **Dizziness** was experienced by 3 respondents and was associated with flecainide, metoprolol and disopyramide (Norpace).
- **Constipation** was experienced by 2 respondents and was associated with flecainide and amiodarone (Cordarone).

Other side effects experienced by one respondent each included dry mouth, exercise intolerance, decrease in urinary stream, acid reflux, chest and joint pain, eye floaters, headaches, and gas and belching.

The frequency of **side effects** was thus slightly less than for the drugs-only group (56%), but higher than that experienced by the alternative protocol group (15%).

Thirty-four (68%) had noticed additional **benefits** from their regimen. Five respondents reported reduction in their stress level and greater peace of mind. Four of these were taking flecainide (2 with supplements), while one was taking valsartan (Diovan), an angiotensin II blocker. Two had undertaken a program of meditation or stress management. Three respondents reported disappearance of their gastroesophageal reflux disorder (GERD). One of these was taking omeprazole (Losec).

Three respondents reported a greater energy level. All were taking numerous supplements as well as the drugs flecainide, propafenone (on demand) or dofetilide (Tikosyn).

Other reported benefits were better exercise tolerance, normalized blood pressure, weight loss, fewer ectopic beats, better sleep, and less cramping when running.

Eleven respondents (22%) no longer needed to avoid their previous triggers such as exercise, alcohol, caffeine, MSG, cold drinks, large meals, etc. Sixteen (32%) still needed to avoid their known triggers, 20 (40%) still needed to avoid some triggers, but not as many as before they began their protocol, and the remaining 3 (6%) were not sure whether they still had to avoid triggers.

Most of the afibbers who had used a combined drug and alternative protocol to manage their afib would seem to have combined information obtained from their cardiologist with that learned from the afibbers.org Bulletin Board, the *Lone Atrial Fibrillation: Towards a Cure* book and The AFIB Report.

Cardiologist	46%
Electrophysiologist	10%
Afibbers.org Bulletin Board	44%
Other bulletin boards	4%
Lone Atrial Fibrillation: Towards a Cure	44%
Personal Research on the Internet	36%
The AFIB Report	42%
Primary physician (GP)	18%
Naturopath	6%
Other health care practitioner	4%
Other sources	24%

Please note that percentages do not add up to 100% because many respondents reported having used more than one information source.

The majority (86%) would recommend their program to other afibbers, but 24% were still contemplating an ablation, while 32% were uncertain whether they would have one or not. The majority (44%) was quite sure they would not undergo an ablation.

The percentage of afibbers in this group who would not contemplate an ablation (44%) compares to 29% in the drugs only group and 66% in the alternative protocol only group.

Protocols Used in Management

All afibbers included in this group used one or more pharmaceutical drugs to manage their afib. In addition, they used one or more of the following modalities:

- Supplementation – used by 76% of respondents
- Trigger avoidance – used by 18% of respondents
- Dietary changes – used by 16% of respondents
- Stress reduction – used by 20% of respondents
- Elimination of GERD – used by 6% of respondents
- Other methods – used by 10% of respondents

Pharmaceutical Drugs

Forty-six of the 50 respondents were using antiarrhythmics, beta-blockers or calcium channel blockers as part of their afib management program. One had achieved control through the use of omeprazole (Losec) to manage GERD, one was using valsartan (Diovan), an angiotensin II receptor blocker, and two respondents were managing their afib with tranquilizers or antidepressants. It is clear that flecainide is the most prescribed antiarrhythmic and that monotherapy (using just one drug) is still the most widely used treatment.

Pharmaceutical Drug Protocols

Drug	Brand Name	Sole Drug	w/Blocker	w/Other
Flecainide	Tambocor	26%	13%	2%
Propafenone	Rythmol	13%	-	-
Disopyramide	Norpace	4%	4%	-
Sotalol	Betapace	7%	-	-
Digoxin	Lanoxin	4%	-	-
Amiodarone	Cordarone	-	-	2%
Dofetilide	Tikosyn	-	2%	-
Metoprolol	Toprol	13%	-	2%
Atenolol	Tenormin	2%	2%	-
Nadolol	Corgard	2%	-	-
NOTE: Two of the flecainide users and one propafenone user were taking their drugs on demand only.				

Supplement Protocols

Supplement	Daily Dosage	Used By
Magnesium	100-1000 mg	89%
Potassium	100-1200 mg	42%
Fish oil	500-6000 mg	33%
Coenzyme Q10	10-300 mg	33%
Vitamin C	250-2000 mg	31%
Multivitamin	-	31%
Vitamin E	250-800 mg	22%
B vitamins	-	22%
L-carnitine	500-1000 mg	19%
Calcium	300-1000 mg	17%
Selenium	100 mcg	17%
Zinc	20-25 mg	11%
Taurine	500 mg	8%
Three respondents used low sodium V8 juice as their potassium source		

158

Thirty-eight out of 50 (76%) respondents were using one or more supplements in their afib management protocol.

Magnesium is clearly the most popular supplement followed by potassium, fish oil and coenzyme Q10. Most of the 38 supplement users (55%) used just 1 or 2 daily supplements, but 22% used 7 or 8 and 5% used 9 or more daily supplements.

Trigger Avoidance
Nine out of the 50 (18%) respondents had used conscious trigger avoidance as an important component in their afib management program. The majority (67%) had found it beneficial to strictly avoid caffeine in all its forms. Others (56%) had found that avoiding alcohol was important. Three afibbers (33%) had found relief from avoiding glutamates, MSG, and aspartame (NutraSweet), while one had noted benefits from sharply reducing sugar consumption. It is interesting that one afibber had found relief from cutting out salt, while another had found that a low-salt diet resulted in more episodes.

Dietary Changes
Eight out of 50 (16%) respondents had found dietary changes to be effective. The most popular measure was to discover a suitable diet program and stick with it. The Paleo, Atkins, Zone, and Dean Ornish diets had been used successfully by at least one respondent. Avoidance of grains and gluten was cited as beneficial by 50% of the afibbers who reported dietary changes with avoiding dairy products and eating lots of bananas and nuts being other reported measures.

Stress management
Ten respondents (20%) reported that they had found stress management highly beneficial in controlling their afib. Several respondents used more than one method with the following being the most popular:

- Meditation – practiced by 50%
- Breathing exercises – practiced by 30%

Acupuncture, yoga, Tai Chi, brisk exercise, and forgiveness were other stress management techniques practiced by one respondent each.

GERD Elimination
One respondent had used omeprazole (Losec) to control GERD, and 2 had been able to eliminate it by cutting out grains, especially wheat in their diet.

Other Protocols
One respondent had found relief by having all dental amalgam fillings and dissimilar metals in the mouth removed. One had found psychoanalysis useful, and 3 had found weight loss beneficial. One afibber who had been in permanent afib eliminated episodes through an estrogen/testosterone balancing program.

Effectiveness of Protocols

A total of 36 afibbers in the group had sufficient data for detailed analysis and fulfilled the criteria of having spent at least 50% less time in afib (number of episodes x average duration) in the 3 months after their protocol became effective as compared to the 3 months prior to embarking on their protocol.

Afib severity parameters for a 3-month period before starting protocol and for a 3-month period after the protocol became effective are presented below:

Episodes over 3 months	Before protocol	With protocol
Episode frequency [number]		
Mean	12	1.4
Median	6	0.3
Range	1 - 90	0 - 18
Episode duration [hours]		
Mean	15	11
Median	8.5	1.5
Range	1-96	0 – 168
Total hours spent in afib during 3 month period		
Mean	172	11
Median	75	1
Range	1 – 2160	0 - 106

The average (median) reduction in time spent in afib by the group of 36 was 99%.

The 36 afibbers had been on their protocol for an average of 19 months (2-60 months) and the time before it became effective varied from 1 day to 36 months with a median of 1 month. The 36 afibbers had been afib-free or at least vastly improved for anywhere from 3 months to 5 years with an average (median) of 13 months. Profiles of 10 typical respondents follow:

Male - 55 years of age with 3 years of paroxysmal, vagal LAF
Number of episodes in 3 months prior to protocol: 2
Average duration of episodes prior to protocol: 12 hours
Months on protocol: 30
Number of episodes since beginning protocol: 0
Still need to avoid triggers: Yes

Pharmaceutical drugs: flecainide
Supplements: None reported

Dietary changes: Lost 25 pounds
Stress reduction protocol: Reduced exposure to stress
Triggers avoided: alcohol
Other preventive measures: None reported

Other benefits of protocol: Happier, less worry, better overall health
Adverse effects of protocol: None reported

Male – 48 years of age with 7 years of paroxysmal, mixed LAF
Number of episodes in 3 months prior to protocol: 1
Average duration of episodes prior to protocol: 2 hours
Months on protocol: 16
Number of episodes since beginning protocol: 0
Still need to avoid triggers: Yes, but much less so

Pharmaceutical drugs: omeprazole [Losec] 20 mg/day
Supplements: Magnesium 250 mg/day

Dietary changes: Cut out all sugar
Stress reduction protocol: None reported
Triggers avoided: Stress
Other preventive measures: Controlling GERD with medication

Other benefits of protocol: More energy, no depression
Adverse effects of protocol: None reported
Comment: Eliminating GERD eliminated afib

Male - 58 years of age with 5 years of paroxysmal, mixed LAF
Number of episodes in 3 months prior to protocol: 7
Average duration of episodes prior to protocol: 4 hours
Months on protocol: 36
Number of episodes since beginning protocol: 0
Still need to avoid triggers: Yes, but much less so

Pharmaceutical drugs: flecainide [2x100 mg/day]
Supplements: Magnesium 400 mg/day, coenzyme Q10 125 mg/day, N-acetylcarnitine 2x50 mg/day

Dietary changes: None reported
Stress reduction protocol: None reported
Triggers avoided: None reported
Other preventive measures: None reported

Other benefits of protocol: None reported
Adverse effects of protocol: Fatigue

Comment: Flecainide use resulted in my improvement

Male - 62 years of age with 4 years of paroxysmal, vagal LAF
Number of episodes in 3 months prior to protocol: 12
Average duration of episodes prior to protocol: 9 hours
Months on protocol: 23
Number of episodes since beginning protocol: 0
Still need to avoid triggers: No

Pharmaceutical drugs: disopyramide [Norpace]
Supplements: None reported

Dietary changes: Cut out cereals
Stress reduction protocol: None reported
Triggers avoided: None specified
Other preventive measures: None reported

Other benefits of protocol: GERD and indigestion gone
Adverse effects of protocol: None reported

Comment: Would recommend this protocol to vagal afibbers

Male – 66 years of age with 26 years of paroxysmal, vagal LAF
Number of episodes in 3 months prior to protocol: 3
Average duration of episodes prior to protocol: 3 hours
Months on protocol: 6
Number of episodes since beginning protocol: 0
Still need to avoid triggers: Yes, but much less so

Pharmaceutical drugs: flecainide [2x100 mg/day]
Supplements: None reported

Dietary changes: None reported
Stress reduction protocol: None reported
Triggers avoided: Alcohol, aspartame, caffeine
Other preventive measures: None reported

Other benefits of protocol: None reported
Adverse effects of protocol: Fatigue, dizziness, constipation, dry mouth and eyes

Comment: Took 2 months before flecainide worked

Male - 68 years of age with 18 years of paroxysmal, vagal LAF
Number of episodes in 3 months prior to protocol: 6
Average duration of episodes prior to protocol: 12 hours
Months on protocol: 40
Number of episodes since beginning protocol: 1
Still need to avoid triggers: Yes, but much less so

Pharmaceutical drugs: flecainide [150 mg/day slow-release]
Supplements: Magnesium, fish oil, coenzyme Q10, vitamin C, vitamin E, selenium, multivitamin

Dietary changes: changed to Zone diet
Stress reduction protocol: Meditation, yoga
Triggers avoided: None reported
Other preventive measures: Total amalgam removal and detoxification

Other benefits of protocol: Better overall health
Adverse effects of protocol: None reported

Comment: Eliminating dental amalgams had an immediate, beneficial effect

---

Male - 57 years of age with 3 years of paroxysmal LAF
Number of episodes in 3 months prior to protocol: 12
Average duration of episodes prior to protocol: 2 hours
Months on protocol: 30
Number of episodes since beginning protocol: 2
Still need to avoid triggers: Yes, but much less so

Pharmaceutical drugs: flecainide [3x100 mg/day], metoprolol [25 mg/day]
Supplements: None reported

Dietary changes: Peppermint tea at meals
Stress reduction protocol: None reported
Triggers avoided: Caffeine and alcohol
Other preventive measures: Regular exercise program

Other benefits of protocol: None reported
Adverse effects of protocol: Tiredness

Comment: I still experience a few PACs after a big meal

Afib burden before and with successful protocol

	Pharmaceuticals	Alternatives	Combination
# of respondents	19	23	36
Frequency before	8	5	6
Frequency with	0	0.3	0.3
Reduction	8 [100%]	4.7 [94%]	5.7 [95%]
Duration before	8 hrs	14 hrs	8.5 hrs
Duration with	4 hrs	1.5 hrs	1.5 hrs
Reduction	4 hrs [50%]	12.5 hrs [89%]	7 hrs [82%]
Afib burden before	75 hrs	56 hrs	75 hrs
Afib burden after	1 hr	1 hr	1 hr
Reduction	74 hrs [99%]	55 hrs [98%]	74 hrs [99%]

Before: A 3 month period before starting successful protocol
With: A 3 month period while on successful protocol
Episode frequency, duration and afib burden [hours spent in afib over a 3 month period] are averages [medians]

These numbers show that it is possible to significantly reduce afib burden with pharmaceutical drugs, alternative therapies or combinations thereof. However, considering that participation in the LAF-7 survey was limited to afibbers who felt they had control of their afib, the overall proportion of afibbers who have completely eliminated their afib with pharmaceutical drugs, alternative protocols or both is likely to still be disappointingly small.

LAF vs AF – Shape Matters

By Patrick Chambers, MD [2006]

SIZE MATTERS! That has been the banner proclamation for Godzilla and mainstream medicine, when it comes to atrial fibrillation (AF) risk. However, the results of this survey suggest that shape trumps size and is the primary determinant of the risk of **lone** atrial fibrillation (LAF).

Before proceeding Hans and I would like to thank all of you that took the time out of your busy schedules to complete yet another survey. And I would personally like to thank Hans for allowing me the opportunity to exploit his wonderful resource, all of you. I believe you will find the objective data uncovered by the survey titillating and hope your reaction to the ensuing discussion of that data to be likewise.

What is lone atrial fibrillation?

Lone atrial fibrillation (LAF) is AF in the absence of structural heart disease (enlarged heart, rheumatic heart disease, coronary artery disease, valvular heart disease, congenital heart disease, etc.). Mitral valve prolapse, frequently encountered in the general population, is not generally considered to represent structural heart disease. Hypertension, which causes the heart to enlarge, is the biggest risk factor for AF in the U.S, according to the American Heart Association (AHA). Some studies on LAF include those with hypertension, while others do not.

Due to the increase in cardiovascular disease with age, once 65 is attained the "lone" is often dropped. Furthermore, aging results in progressive LENGTHENING of the atrial effective refractory period (AERP). NOTE: AERP is the rest period following the contraction of the heart muscle. The cell does not respond to stimulation during this period [1,2,3]. Parasympathetic and sympathetic stimulation can both trigger LAF, because they both cause SHORTENING of the AERP. This is why onset of true LAF after age 65 is most unlikely and why the mechanisms for LAF v. AF may differ [1].

What percent of AF is LAF? The answer to this question depends on what you consider to be organic heart disease and how hard you look for that disease. According to one study, "AF is associated with organic heart disease in 70% to 80% of such patients. AF can occur in the absence of detectable organic heart disease, so-called "lone AF," in about 30% of cases" [4]. "In material based on hospital observations, 35% of all fibrillation was described as being of paroxysmal type" [5]. "About 50% of the patients with paroxysmal AF are lone. This proportion falls to <20% in patients with persistent or permanent forms" [6]. So, these two studies also translate to about 30% of AF being LAF. In other studies a more conservative figure is given. According to the AHA, only 5 to 15 percent of patients with AF have no apparent heart disease or identifiable contributing factor [7].

Because only about 5-30% of AF is lone, most studies on AF make no distinction. Instead AF categorization is limited to paroxysmal (spontaneously terminating and less than 48 hours duration for some v. less than seven days for others), persistent (medically or electrically cardiovertible) or permanent (not cardiovertible).

Could AF and LAF be two different diseases requiring different treatments? Previously differentiation between the two rested on an expensive battery of tests, e.g., EKG, chest radiograph, treadmill test, 24 Holter test, and perfusion scan ... Perhaps there is an easier way. Cardiac structural disease may be reflected in body structure, which is much more readily measured. Hence, this survey was undertaken in an attempt to explore this possibility. Hopefully the results of this survey will underscore the legitimacy and utility of this approach.

Anthropometric analysis

Anthropometry is the measurement and study of the human body and its parts and capacities. The anthropometric data from this survey suggest that LAF and AF are most definitely distinct afflictions and that shape not size is the critical parameter. The survey reveals that, whereas pear body shape (gynoid) is good and apple body shape (android) is bad, when it comes to cardiovascular disease risk, the opposite applies for LAF. Furthermore, age at onset/diagnosis, blood pressure and possibly specific lab data may provide further delineation.

	LAF Patients		Normal Population	
Demographics	Men	Women	Men	Women
Respondents (77) by gender, %	79.2	20.8	-	-
Mean present age, yrs.	58.9	63.6	-	-
Mean age at diagnosis/onset, yrs.	49.8	53.7	-	-
Means years of AF	9.1	9.9	-	-
Mean height, inches[8]	71.4	66.6	69.2	63.8
Mean body mass index (BMI)[8]	26.2	24.9	27.8	28.1
Mean waist/hip ratio (WHR)[9,10]	0.91	0.77	0.95	0.88
Mean waist/height ratio (WTR)[12]	0.51	0.47	0.53	0.55
Mean waist circumference (WC)[11]	36.6	31.2	38.8	36.3
Mean blood pressure mm Hg	121/74			

Statistical analysis of the differences of the **means** between LAF patients {afibbers] and the normal population on all of the above anthropometric measurements range from significant, i.e., p=. 01, (male WTR) to very significant, p < .001, (female BMI and height) to extremely significant, p < .0001, (everything else).

After elimination of several respondents for probable structural heart disease a total of 77 respondents were included in the survey. This included 61 men and 16 women, a 4:1 ratio. Average present age is 59 for males and 64 for females, while the average age at onset/diagnosis is 50 for males and 54 for females (overall mean of 51). Curiously the latter is 50 for all vagal afibbers. There are many anthropometric measures of cardiovascular disease risk, BMI, WHR, WTR and WC [13]. So, data to calculate them all was requested. Afibbers are taller with males and females both being about two to three inches taller than their average counterparts (LAF averages are 71.5" and 66.3" respectively).

Regarding BMI, the average male weighed in at 26.2 kg/m2 (includes one BMI over 38), while for the average female BMI is 24.9. The frequency distribution curve for BMI is bell shaped. While BMI is the oft quoted barometer for assessing overweight and obesity, there has been much recently written on waist to hip ratio (WHR) [9,10]. For male afibbers this is .91 and for females it is .77 with an overall average of .88, well under the North American average WHR of .90. However, the latest data indicates that the waist to tallness ratio (WTR) is the most sensitive and specific standard for measuring obesity and related cardiovascular disease risk with limits of .55 for men and .53 for women [12]. WTR for the afibbers participating in this survey is .51 for males and .47 for females.

Afibbers are not hypertensive with an average BP of 121/74. Much of the rest of the data was difficult to assimilate, but there was one other noteworthy result. Only seven afibbers have undergone intracellular mineral analysis, but all seven are either below normal or very near the lower limit of normal for intracellular magnesium. The normal range is 33.9-41.9 mEq/L, and that of afibbers ranged from 30.0-35.0 mEq/L. All of the height, weight, BMI, age, gender and BP results conform to those determined by the 2003 General Survey.

After analyzing the data from this survey, a pattern began to emerge and additional data from earlier surveys proved relevant. The 2001 General Survey revealed that 25% of all respondents (50) had hypoglycemia (idiopathic postprandial syndrome) and another 24% had symptoms of hypoglycemia, yet no one had diabetes. The 2003 General Survey reported the prevalence of diabetes to be 0.6% amongst afibbers (vs. 6% for the U.S. population). The prevalence of hypoglycemia amongst 140 afibbers with vagal or mixed type was reported to be 27% and the prevalence among 24 afibbers with adrenergic type was reported to be 42%.

So, what does this all mean? And what is the link between LAF and hypoglycemia? Hypoglycemia is generally due to either increased insulin sensitivity (decreased blood insulin and glucose levels) or increased insulin. It appears that LAF is highly correlated with increased insulin sensitivity and that this may be directly reflected in body shape. The following elaborates on this hypothesis.

Obesity and LAF

The risk of AF increases by 4% for every unit increase in BMI [14]. Since body size is related to heart size and larger atria more easily accommodate AF, the medical literature has linked this increased AF risk directly to increased heart size. This is why AF is often seen in syndrome X (metabolic syndrome) and in the tall, or so it has been reported [15,16]. But this is clearly not the case for afibbers, where increasing BMI over 26 kg/m2 is associated with decreasing LAF risk. Furthermore, the above weight and waist data reflect measurements taken on average eight years after onset/diagnosis. And, of course, these figures tend to go south as we age. In addition progression of episodes over this nine-year period may have restricted any pre-existing exercise regimen. This would negatively impact ensuing weight and waist measurements. And finally delineation of LAF from AF can sometimes be quite difficult. Undoubtedly some of the latter may have been inadvertently included in this survey, compromising their anthropometric distinction.

Gender, age, blood pressure and AF/LAF

The 4:1 male to female ratio is difficult to explain. However, this survey does contain a clue. The mean age at onset/diagnosis of vagal afibbers in females is a year less than that of male vagal afibbers. Whatever protective hormone may be at work in females appears to be effective predominantly against the adrenergic component. Age at onset/diagnosis of vagal/mixed/adrenergic types of LAF is 50.3/49.7/49.0 in males and 48.8/58.6/ in females. No female reported pure adrenergic type LAF.

Data from the Framingham Heart Study have established that the prevalence of atrial fibrillation rises with increasing age -- occurring in less than 0.5% of 25- to 35-year-olds, about 1.5% of people up to 60 years of age, and increasing to 9% in people aged over 75 years [17]. This is in contrast to the pattern for LAF where the frequency distribution curve for age at onset/diagnosis is bell shaped with a mean of about 50.6 years.

Hypertension is the biggest risk factor for AF. The relationship between insulin level and systolic/diastolic blood pressure persists after adjustment for body mass index, WHR, norepinephrine, age, smoking, physical activity level, and antihypertensive medication use [18]. Mean blood pressure amongst afibbers is 121/74 mm Hg; ie. well below the range for hypertension.

Hypoglycemia and AF/LAF

In one canine study the AERP was shortest under hypoglycemia in the left atrium and longest under hyperglycemia in the right atrium [19]. Other research indicates that ACTH mediates this through sympathoadrenal stimulation and catecholamine stimulated hypokalemia [20]. Hypoglycemia is a potent stimulant of ACTH secretion [21,22]. Hypokalemia is clearly aggravated by the additional action of increased ACTH driven aldosterone secretion.

According to the Merck Manual on Potassium Metabolism, "Numerous factors affect the movement of potassium between the intracellular and extracellular fluid compartments. Among the most important is circulating insulin level. In the presence of insulin, potassium moves into cells, thus lowering plasma potassium concentration.... Stimulation of the sympathetic nervous system also affects transcellular potassium movement. Beta-agonists, especially selective beta$_2$-agonists, promote cellular uptake of potassium.... High-circulating aldosterone levels lead to increased potassium secretion and kaliuresis" [23]. Insulin, catecholamines (adrenaline) and aldosterone all work to lower blood potassium.

Height and insulin sensitivity

Although endurance athletes are typically of average height, tall males also seem to be at increased risk for LAF (Bill Bradley, Akeem Olajuwon and recently 6'4" Mario Lemieux). Since insulin and glucose both inhibit growth hormone (GH) [24], those with increased insulin sensitivity (lower blood insulin and glucose levels) should be taller.

Tallness is a function of growth hormone (GH) secretion during the developmental stage. Growth hormone exerts its effect through insulin-like growth factor 1 (IGF-1), produced by the liver. "Tall height and high BMI at 7 yr. were associated with low IGF-1 in adulthood but only in those subjects whose current BMI was below median. On further analysis these interactive effects were particularly strong for height in childhood and adult lean BMI (lean body mass/height^2). Serum IGF-I was positively correlated with fasting glucose, fibrinogen concentrations and blood pressure" [25]. Hence tallness appears to be associated with insulin/IGF-1 sensitivity. As an aside, increased IGF-1 levels have been directly linked with increased cancers of breast, colon, prostate, lung and ovary. Obese men and women demonstrated significantly more deaths due to these cancers, as well as cancers of the esophagus, liver, gallbladder, pancreas, kidney, endometrium, non-Hodgkins lymphoma and multiple myeloma than normal weight controls. The heaviest men were 52% more likely to die of cancer than thin/normal weight men; and the most obese women were 62% more likely to die than thin/normal weight women [26]. LAF seems a small price to pay for extra protection against heart disease AND numerous cancers.

Body fat distribution and insulin sensitivity

Lower-body obesity in women has been associated with hypoglycemia and a high level of beneficial high-density lipoprotein (HDL). Insulin sensitivity is highest in those with moderate lower-body overweight (11.2), intermediate in controls (6.1) and lowest in those with upper-body obesity (2.6) [27]. Body fat distribution is a more relevant determinant of insulin resistance than obesity. Compared to the normal female, female afibbers appear to carry relatively more of their weight in their hips (WHR=.77). Perhaps female afibbers of normal weight are also relatively insulin sensitive compared to non-LAF females of normal weight.

Thigh fat may contribute to lipoprotein profiles that predict lower risk of cardiovascular disease [28,29]. However, a few afibbers appear to prefer weight lifting to aerobic endeavors. This may not be as beneficial to lipoprotein profile, as demonstrated by one study on HDL levels in professional football players [30]. Weight gain aggravates insulin sensitivity and weight loss improves it [31]. HDL is a surrogate for insulin sensitivity.

Autonomic tone and insulin sensitivity

Our stomachs often remind us when we're hungry. This is because insulin induced hypoglycemia stimulates efferent vagal signals to the stomach. However, a recent study has shown that no simultaneous signals are sent to the heart [32]. Therefore, any role that insulin induced hypoglycemia might play in triggering LAF appears to be more related to subsequent electrolyte imbalance. On the other hand, insulin sensitivity clearly regulates cardiac autonomic tone [33]. These studies suggest that the role of parasympathetic tone in the possible genesis of LAF precedes hypoglycemia [33,34].

There appears to be a substance yet to be isolated, produced in the liver and released by parasympathetic signals that sensitizes tissue to insulin. It is called hepatic insulin sensitizing substance (HISS) [35]. The HISS hypothesis has been proposed as a new paradigm for diabetes and obesity by Canadian pharmacologist Wayne Lautt [36]. Could this be the missing link connecting parasympathetic tone and insulin sensitivity in afibbers?

Exercise and insulin sensitivity/autonomic tone

"The proportion of sportsmen among patients with lone atrial fibrillation is much higher than that reported in the general population of Catalonia: 63% vs. 15%" [57]. The prevalence of lone atrial fibrillation in master orienteers was at least six-fold higher than in controls [58].

Physical fitness has also been shown to increase HDL and insulin sensitivity [37,38,39]. In fact HDL (or HDL/TG (triglyceride)) can be taken as a measure of insulin sensitivity [40]. Heart rate recovery after exercise is also related to HDL and can also be taken as a reflection of insulin sensitivity [41], further underscoring the link between cardiac autonomic tone and insulin resistance/sensitivity [42]. On the other hand obese patients have increased sympathetic activity and a withdrawal of vagal activity [43], and these autonomic disturbances improve after weight loss [44,45].

Obesity and inflammation

Not only is body shape/size intimately tied to hypertension, insulin sensitivity, lipoprotein profile, and autonomic tone but also to inflammation [46]. Commonly used tests for detecting inflammation, e.g., high-sensitivity C-reactive protein (hs-CRP), serum amyloid A (SAA), white blood cell (WBC) count, fibrinogen, are much more frequently elevated in the obese [46,47,48]. These inflammatory markers decrease with weight loss. It has been suggested that a WBC in the upper range of normal is yet another manifestation of the insulin resistance syndrome (syndrome X, metabolic syndrome) along with hypertension, increased cholesterol and increased triglycerides [49]. Afibbers may have a white blood cell count at the lower limit of normal.

Inflammation and LAF

Although fibrosis and inflammation have been described in LAF and reactive oxygen species (ROS) generated by endurance sports has been suggested as causative, perhaps LAF precedes the inflammation, unlike in pathologic AF. After all, exercise and HDL are both anti-inflammatory [50] and AF by itself can produce a measurable increase in left atrial ROS [51]. Indirect support for this view may be found in Canadian and Spanish meta-analyses [52,53]. Angiotensin converting enzyme inhibitors (ACEIs) and angiotensin receptor blockers (ARBs) prevent recurrent and new onset AF in those with structural heart disease, but such findings have not been demonstrated for LAF with or without mild hypertension

Left atrial angiotensin II type 1 receptors (AT1s), but not AT2s are increased in afibbers [54]. On the other hand, pathologic AF is associated with decreased atrial AT1s and increased AT2s [55]. Furthermore, the decrease in AT1s is greater in permanent than paroxysmal atrial fibrillation. Why do the left atrial AT1s differ between LAF and AF? Angiotensin II/aldosterone are prominent players in cardiac remodeling and fibrosis. Therefore, increased left atrial AT1s in LAF should portend greater damage, yet ACEIs and ARBs confer no benefit. Recent research suggests a possible solution to this dilemma. Increased left atrial ATIs in LAF may be no more than a marker for mechanical stress and angiotensin II may not actually be involved [56].

LAF/AF both causes inflammation, whereas perhaps only AF may actually be caused by inflammation. The anthropometric data also support this interpretation.

Alcohol, glutamate, coffee and LAF

Alcohol has been well described as a trigger for LAF episodes (holiday heart syndrome). Alcohol-induced hypoglycemia often occurs during the fasting state. Hypoglycemia may result from alcoholic inhibition of gluconeogenesis (creation of glucose by the liver) [59,60] in combination with glycogen (storage form of glucose) depletion. "Light to moderate alcohol intake is associated with enhanced insulin sensitivity and this improvement in sensitivity results in higher HDL cholesterol levels" [61]. Furthermore, the acute effect of a moderate dose of alcohol on the heart is vagotonic [62].

In the 2003 General Survey approximately 21% of 166 LAFers associated glutamate intake with initiation of episodes. L-glutamate appears to play a direct role in insulin release, although the precise mechanism remains elusive [63,64].

Although caffeine has been widely reported to increase insulin resistance (small, short-term studies), long-term coffee consumption decreases insulin resistance. Two recent reports, one epidemiologic study and one meta-analysis, have confirmed this [65], even after adjustment for age, body mass index, and other risk factors [66]. Could coffee aggravate LAF by increasing insulin sensitivity?

Potassium and adrenergic LAF

The risk of AF can be quantified by the equation: wavelength (WL)=AERP x conduction velocity (CV). According to Moe's wavelet theory, the circumference of each wavelet is > WL and six or more wavelets appear to be required to sustain AF [67,68,69]. Both atrial dilatation and smaller wavelets provide this sustenance. Therefore, since shorter WL=>smaller wavelets, shorter WL translates to greater risk of AF. Because adrenergic LAF (ALAF) or stress triggered LAF is associated with sympathetic tone, which causes relatively less AERP shortening (v. vagal tone) and increases CV, then ALAF requires additional arrhythmogenic input. Electrophysiologic studies show that increased dispersion may provide this arrhythmogenic shortfall [70]. Perhaps this is mediated by hypoglycemia. Hypoglycemia not only shortens AERP but also increases dispersion (heterogeneity) and both are potentiated by hypokalemia. The fact that 42% of adrenergic afibbers and only 24% of vagal afibbers are hypoglycemic supports this greater role for hypoglycemia in adrenergic afibbers.

The Na-K ATPase pump maintains intracellular potassium in the face of a 30:1 gradient with the extracellular space. The lower the blood potassium levels, the more this pump is challenged and the greater the leakage of potassium from within cells. This "conductance" of potassium forces faster repolarization and hence shortens the refractory period. Therefore, insulin-induced hypoglycemia and its ultimate impact on blood potassium appear to work in tandem with

174

autonomic tone to shorten the AERP. Additional research has shown that low blood glucose increases dispersion of this refractoriness and that this is prevented by the administration of potassium [71]. Blood potassium may be lower in adrenergic than in vagal afibbers, because ACTH is not only driven by hypoglycemia but also by stress. This stress mediated ACTH release leads to increased catecholamine and aldosterone secretion. An inability to maintain intracellular potassium in the face of a growing gradient may be at the heart of LAF. In adrenergic LAF the gradient may be greater but of shorter duration, whereas in vagal LAF the opposite may occur (less gradient but longer duration).

Potassium and vagal LAF

In vagally mediated AF (VMAF) it may not be the magnitude of the gradient that is critical but its duration, i.e., an extended period of lower range blood potassium. As Hans speculated on p. 63 of *Lone Atrial Fibrillation: Towards A Cure*, the flat or blunted glucose tolerance test curves associated with increased vagal tone may be implicated in LAF. These flat or blunted curves indicate extended periods during which blood glucose is in the lower range of normal. Frank hypokalemia or hypomagnesemia may not even be required for VMAF.

The prominence of nighttime episodes in VMAF may be due not only to increased nighttime vagal tone but also to the midnight diurnal nadir of blood potassium. "Plasma potassium values exhibit a circadian rhythm (average peak-to-trough difference 0.60 mmol/L, with lowest values at night) and also decrease postprandially because of insulin released in response to an ingested carbohydrate load" [72]. Slow leakage of intracellular potassium can also cause muscle cramps and twitching. Twenty one percent of 166 afibbers in the 2003 General Survey complained of leg cramps, especially at night.

Magnesium and LAF

Intracellular potassium is difficult to maintain in the face of low intracellular magnesium. Magnesium is necessary for proper functioning of the Na-K ATP requiring pump that performs this function. The fact that magnesium was either low or at the very lower limit of normal in seven of seven afibbers undergoing intracellular mineral analysis supports emphasis of its exalted status in preventing LAF episodes. However, the sampling is quite small and no sweeping conclusions can be drawn. Furthermore, this pump is inhibited by digoxin and may explain why digoxin is problematic for afibbers, especially vagal ones [73,74].

According to magnesium expert Mildred Seelig, "Stress causes secretion of epinephrine (adrenaline) and corticosteroids (aldosterone) and results in magnesium loss in animals and in humans. The types of stresses that can increase magnesium needs can be physical (exhausting or competitive exercise, extremes of temperature, and accidental or surgical trauma), or psychological (anger, fear, anxiety, overwork and crowding)" [75,76]. To this list insulin induced hypoglycemia (idiopathic postprandial hypoglycemia) might be specifically added.

Magnesium also impacts cholesterol. According to her book *The Magnesium Factor*, magnesium inhibits HMG-CoA reductase, the rate-limiting step in cholesterol synthesis, thereby working to lower total cholesterol. Furthermore, the insulin to glucagon ratio also influences cholesterol metabolism by either stimulating (high ratio) or inhibiting (low ratio) the activity of this same enzyme [77]. Insulin sensitivity should result in a lower ratio and lower total cholesterol.

Summary

In summary, body fat distribution is inextricably entwined with insulin sensitivity/resistance, lipoprotein profiles, autonomic tone and inflammation. The anthropometric data of this survey indicate afibbers to be quite distinct in their body shape. LAF (physiologic AF) appears to be the opposite of diabetes, and HDL cholesterol, total cholesterol, triglycerides, BP, WTR, WHR and age at onset/diagnosis may help to differentiate it from pathologic AF. Elevated total cholesterol in the face of normal BMI and WTR may indicate low intracellular magnesium, especially amongst vagal afibbers and especially if accompanied by nighttime muscle cramps and/or fasciculations (muscle twitching). Further delineation of the utility of these lab tests in differentiating LAF from AF awaits a future LAF survey. Low blood glucose and potassium appear to conspire in creating an arrhythmogenic substrate. Low blood potassium may represent the final common pathway for both vagally mediated and adrenergic forms of LAF. LAF may represent physiologic AF primarily mediated by low potassium, whereas AF associated with structural heart disease is pathologic AF and predominantly characterized by visceral obesity, cardiac fibrosis and other age related changes.

REFERENCES

1. "Relation Of Age And Sex To Atrial Electrophysiological Properties In Patients With No History Of Atrial Fibrillation", Sakabe et al., Pacing Clin Electrophysiol, 2003 May; 26(5): 1238-44
2. "Electrophysiologic And Electroanatomic Changes In The Human Atrium Associated With Age", P.M. Kistler et al., J Am Coll Cardiol. 2004 Jul 7, 44(1): 109-16
3. "Age-Related Changes in Human Left and Right Atrial Conduction", Kojodjojo et al., J Cardiovasc Electrophysiol, Vol. 17, pp. 1-8, February 2006
4. "Epidemiology and Classification of Atrial Fibrillation", S. Levy, J Cardiovasc Electrophysiol, 1998, Aug; 9(8 Suppl): S78-82

5. "Arrhythmia-Provoking Factors And Symptoms At The Onset Of Paroxysmal Atrial Fibrillation: A Study Based On Interviews With 100 Patients Seeking Hospital Assistance", Hansson et al., BMC Cardiovascular Disorders 2004, 4:13

6. "Pathophysiology and Prevention of Atrial Fibrillation", Allessie et al., Circulation. 2001; 103:769

7. American Heart association http://www.americanheartassociation.com/downloadable/heart/1075_russo.pdf

8. "Mean Body Weight, Height, and Body Mass Index, United States 1960–2002", Ogden et al., Advance Data from Vital and Health Statistics, number 347, Oct 27, 2004.

9. "Waist-to-Hip Ratio vs. BMI May Be More Accurate Predictor of CV Risk", Yusuf et al., Lancet. 2005; 366:1589-1591, 1640-1649

10. "Abdominal Obesity Identified as Independent Risk Factor for Stroke", Seung-Han Suk, Northern Manhattan Stroke Study, International Stroke Conference, Columbia-Presbyterian Medical Center in New York, reported on Feb. 8, 2002.

11. "Trends in Waist Circumference among U.S. Adults", Ford et al., Obes Res. 2003 Oct 11(10) 1223-31.

12. "Waist to Tallness Ratio Effective Indicator of Obesity, CVD, 87th Annual Meeting of the Endocrine Society, June 4-7, 2005, San Diego, http://www.diabeticmctoday.com/HtmlPages/DMC0905/DMC1005Conference.html

13. "Use of Anthropometric Measurements in Assessing Risk for Coronary Heart Disease: A Useful Tool in Worksite Health Screening?" Oshaug et al., Int Arch Occup Environ Health, 1995, 67 (6): 359-66.

14. "Obesity and the Risk of New-Onset Atrial Fibrillation", Thomas J. Wang et al., JAMA, vol. 292, No. 20, 11/24/04

15. "Irregular Heartbeats Linked to Tallness", American Heart Association Scientific Sessions 2004, New Orleans, Nov. 7-10, 2004. News release, American Heart Association.

16. "Is Obesity A Risk Factor For Atrial Fibrillation?", Gianluca Iacobellis, Nature Clinical Practice Cardiovascular Medicine (2005) 2, 134-135.

17. "Safety of Antiarrhythmic Agents: The Final Frontier in Treating Atrial Fibrillation", John Camm, 2000 Medscape Portals, Inc

18. http://www.medscape.com/viewarticle/420862

19. "Influence Of Insulin, Sympathetic Nervous System Activity, And Obesity On Blood Pressure: The Normative Aging Study", Ward et al., J Hypertens 1996 Mar; 14(3): 301-8

20. "Susceptibility Of The Right And Left Canine Atria To Fibrillation In Hyperglycemia And Hypoglycemia", P.E. Vardas et al., J Electrocardiol 1993 Apr, 26(2): 147-53.

21. "Mechanisms of Abnormal Cardiac Repolarization During Insulin-Induced Hypoglycemia", Robinson et al., Diabetes 52:1469-1474, 2003.

22. "Aldosterone Response To Hypoglycemia: Evidence Of ACTH Mediation", Hata et al., Journal of Clinical Endocrinology & Metabolism, Vol. 43, 173-177, Copyright © 1976 by Endocrine Society

23. "Hormonal Responses To Insulin-Induced Hypoglycemia In Man", Watabe et al., Journal of Clinical Endocrinology & Metabolism, Vol. 65, 1187-1191, Copyright © 1987 by Endocrine Society

24. http://www.merck.com/mrkshared/mmanual/section2/chapter12/12c.jsp

25. "Insulin Suppresses Growth Hormone Secretion By Rat Pituitary Cells", Melmed et al., J Clin Invest, 1984 May; 73(5): 1425-33

26. "Serum Insulin-Like Growth Factor (IGF)-I And IGF-Binding Protein-1 In Elderly People: Relationships With Cardiovascular Risk Factors, Body Composition, Size At Birth, And Childhood Growth", Kajantie et al., J Clin Endocrinol Metab 2003 Mar; 88(3): 1059-65

27. "Overweight, Obesity, And Mortality From Cancer In A Prospectively Studied Cohort Of U.S. Adults", Calle et al., NEJM, 2003 Apr 24;348(17):1625-38.

28. "Insulin Sensitivity Measured With The Minimal Model Is Higher In Moderately Overweight Women With Predominantly Lower Body Fat", Raynaud et al., Horm Metab Res, 1999 Jul; 31(7): 415-7

29. "Contributions Of Regional Adipose Tissue Depots To Plasma Lipoprotein Concentrations In Overweight Men And Women: Possible Protective Effects Of Thigh Fat", R.B. Terry et al., Metabolism, 1991 July, 40(7): 733-40.

30. Plasma High-Density Lipoprotein Cholesterol: Association with Measurements of Body Mass. The Lipid Research Clinics Program Prevalence Study", Glueck et al., Circulation, 1980 Nov; 62(4 Pt 2): IV-62-9

31. "Analysis of Lipoproteins and Body Mass Index in Professional Football Players", Garry et al., Preventive Cardiology, 02/28/2002. http://www.medscape.com/viewarticle/424725

32. "Insulin Sensitivity Among Obese Children and Adolescents, According to Degree of Weight Loss", Reinehr et al., Pediatrics Vol. 114 No. 6 December 2004, pp. 1569-1573

33. "Insulin-Induced Hypoglycemia Stimulates Gastric Vagal Activity and Motor Function without Increasing Cardiac Vagal Activity", Hjelland et al., Digestion 2005, 72:43-48.

34. "Insulin Sensitivity Regulates Autonomic Control of Heart Rate Variation Independent of Body Weight in Normal Subjects", Bergholm et al., Journal of Clinical Endocrinology & Metabolism Vol. 86, No. 3 1403-1409, Copyright © 2001 by The Endocrine Society

35. "Does the Autonomic Nervous System Play A Role in the Development of Insulin Resistance? A Study On Heart Rate Variability In First-Degree Relatives Of Type 2 Diabetes Patients And Control Subjects", Lindmark et al., Diabet. Med. 20, 399-405 (May, 2003)

36. "Meal-Induced Peripheral Insulin Sensitization Is Regulated By Hepatic Parasympathetic Nerves", Lautt et al., 083P University of Cambridge, Summer Meeting July 2005

37. "A New Paradigm For Diabetes And Obesity: The Hepatic Insulin Sensitizing Substance (HISS) Hypothesis", Journal of Pharmacological Sciences, 2004; 95(1): 9-17).

38. "The Acute Versus The Chronic Response To Exercise", Thompson et al., Medicine & Science in Sports & Exercise. 33(6) Supplement S438-S445, June 2001.

39. "Exercise And Insulin Sensitivity: A Review", L. B. Borghouts et al., Int. J Sports Med, 2000 Jan, 21(1): 1-12.

40. "Physical Activity, Insulin Sensitivity, And The Lipoprotein Profile In Young Adults: The Beaver County Study", RP Donahue et al., American Journal of Epidemiology, Vol. 127, Issue 1 95-103, Copyright © 1988 by Oxford University Press

41. "Association of Triglyceride–to–HDL Cholesterol Ratio With Heart Rate Recovery", Shishehbor et al., Diabetes Care 27:936-941, 2004

42. "Heart Rate Recovery after Exercise Is Related to the Insulin Resistance Syndrome and Heart Rate Variability in Elderly Men", Lind et al., Am Heart J. 2002 Oct; 144 (4): 580-2.

43. "Dysregulation of the Autonomic Nervous System Can Be a Link between Visceral Adiposity and Insulin Resistance", Lindmark et al., Obesity Research 13:717-728 (2005)

44. "Heart Rate Variability and Obesity Indices: Emphasis on the Response to Noise and Standing", Kim et al., Journal of the American Board of Family Practice, 18:97-103 (2005).

45. "Heart Rate Variability In Obesity And The Effect Of Weight Loss", Karason et al., Am J Cardiol 1999 Apr 15; 83(8): 1242-7

46. "Cardiac Parasympathetic Activity Is Increased by Weight Loss in Healthy Obese Women", Rissanen et al., Obesity Research 9:637-643 (2001)

47. "Elevated C-Reactive Protein Levels in Overweight and Obese Adults", Visser et al., JAMA. 1999;282:2131-2135

48. "Echocardiographic and Hemodynamic Data in Obese Patients", H. Schunkert, Heart Metab. 2002; 17:14–19

49. "Coagulation, Fibrinolysis And Haemorheology In Premenopausal Obese Women With Different Body Fat Distribution", G. Avellone et al., Thromb Res 1994 Aug 1; 75(3): 223-31,

50. "The White Blood Cell Count: Its Relationship To Plasma Insulin And Other Cardiovascular Risk Factors In Healthy Male Individuals", Targher et al., Journal of Internal Medicine, Volume 239 (5): 435 (May 1996)

51. "Body Mass Index, but Not Physical Activity, Is Associated with C-Reactive Protein", E. Rawson et al., Medicine & Science in Sports & Exercise. 35(7): 1160-1166, July 2003

52. "Atrial Fibrillation Increases Production Of Superoxide By The Left Atrium And Left Atrial Appendage: Role Of The NADPH And Xanthine Oxidases", Dudley et al., Circulation. 2005 Aug 30, 112(9): 1266-73.

53. "The Role of Angiotensin Receptor Blockers and/or Angiotensin Converting Enzyme Inhibitors in the Prevention of Atrial Fibrillation in Patients with Cardiovascular Diseases", Madrid et al., Pacing Clin Electrophysiol 27(10): 1405-1410, 2004.

54. "Prevention of atrial fibrillation with angiotensin-converting enzyme inhibitors and angiotensin receptor blockers: a meta-analysis", Healey et al., J Am Coll Cardiol, 2005 Jun 7; 45(11): 1832-9.

55. "Expression Of Angiotensin II Receptors In Human Left And Right Atrial Tissue In Atrial Fibrillation With And Without Underlying Mitral Valve Disease", Boldt et al., J Am Coll Cardiol. 2003 Nov 19; 42(10): 1785-92.

56. "Regulation of Angiotensin II Receptor Subtypes During Atrial Fibrillation in Humans", Goette et al., (Circulation. 2000; 101:2678.)

57. "Mechanical Stress Activates Angiotensin II Type 1 Receptor Without The Involvement Of Angiotensin II", Zou et al., Nature Cell Biology 6, 499 - 506 (2004)

58. "Long-Lasting Sport Practice and Lone Atrial Fibrillation", Mont et al., Eur Heart J. 2002 Mar, 23 (6): 431-3.

59. 'Lone Atrial Fibrillation In Vigorously Exercising Middle Aged Men: Case-Control Study", Karjalainen et al., BMJ 1998; 316:1784-1785 (13 June)

60. "The Inhibition Of Gluconeogenesis Following Alcohol In Humans", Siler et al., Am J Physiol Endocrinol Metab 275: E897-E907, 1998

61. "Role Of Gluconeogenesis In Sustaining Glucose Production During Hypoglycemia Caused By Continuous Insulin Infusion In Conscious Dogs", Frizzell et al., Diabetes, Vol. 37, Issue 6 749-759, Copyright © 1988 by American Diabetes Association

62. "Alcohol and Insulin Sensitivity", van de Wiel, Neth J Med, 1998 Mar: 52(3): 91-4.

63. "Vagal Mediation of the Effect of Alcohol on Heart Rate", Newlin et al., Alcohol Clin Exp Res, 1990 Jun; 14(3): 421-4

64. "Glutamate Inhibits Protein Phosphatases And Promotes Insulin Exocytosis In Pancreatic Beta-Cells", Lehtihet et al., Biochem Biophys Res Commun. 2005 Mar 11, 328(2): 601-7.

65. "Glutamate Stimulates Insulin Secretion And Improves Glucose Tolerance In Rats", Bertrand et al., AJP - Endocrinology and Metabolism, Vol. 269, Issue 3 E551-E556.

66. "Coffee Consumption And Risk Of Type 2 Diabetes: A Systematic Review", Van Damm et al., JAMA. 2005 Jul 6; 294(1): 97-104.

67. "Coffee Consumption and Risk for Type 2 Diabetes Mellitus", Salazar-Martinez et al., Ann Intern Med. 2004: 140:1-8.

68. "Evolution of Curative Therapies For Atrial Fibrillation", Khasnis et al., Indian Pacing Electrophysiol. J. 2004; 4(1): 10-25

69. "Principles and Applications of Bioelectric and Biomagnetic Fields" by Jaakko Malmivio and Robert Plonsey, Chapter 24, Cardiac Defibrillation in Bioelectromagnetism, Oxford University Press, 1995.

70. "Wavelength And Vulnerability To Atrial Fibrillation: Insights From A Computer Model Of Human Atria", Jacquemet et al., Europace 2005 7(s2): S83-S92

71. "Differing Sympathetic And Vagal Effects On Atrial Fibrillation In Dogs: Role Of Refractoriness Heterogeneity", Liu et al., American Journal of Physiology - Heart and Circulatory Physiology, Vol. 273, Issue 2 805-H816 (1997) "Mechanisms of Abnormal Cardiac Repolarization During Insulin-Induced Hypoglycemia", Robinson et al., Diabetes 52:1469-1474, 2003.

72. "The Diurnal Rhythm Of Plasma Potassium: Relationship To Diuretic Therapy", Solomon et al., J Cardiovasc Pharmacol, 1991 May, 17(5): 854-9.

73. "Digoxin And Membrane Sodium Potassium ATPase Inhibition In Cardiovascular Disease", Kumar et al., Indian Heart J. 2000 May-Jun; 52(3): 315-8

74. "Effects Of Digoxin On Acute, Atrial Fibrillation-Induced Changes In Atrial Refractoriness", Sticherling et al., Circulation, 2000 Nov 14; 102(20): 2503-8

75. "Consequences of Magnesium Deficiency on the Enhancement of Stress Reactions; Preventive and Therapeutic Implications (A Review)", Seelig, Journal of the American College of Nutrition, Vol. 13, No. 5, 429-446 (1994)

76. "Magnesium Requirements in Human Nutrition," Mildred S. Seelig, Contemporary Nutrition, January, 1982, Vol. 7 No. 1

77. "Relationship of Nutrition to Blood Glucose Control", Arline McDonald http://www.feinberg.northwestern.edu/nutrition/tools-resources/sbm-files/SBM-BloodGlucose2001.doc

Non-Ablation/Surgery Interventions

By Hans R. Larsen [2007]

The findings and conclusions of this survey are based on responses from 224 afibbers who had attempted to reduce or eliminate their afib burden through means other than ablation or surgical procedures, and who had been on their program for at least 6 months. More than half the respondents believed they had found a way to materially reduce or completely eliminate their afib episodes. The successful protocols used to eliminate afib were evenly split between the use of pharmaceutical drugs and the use of alternative approaches such as trigger avoidance, supplementation, dietary changes, stress management, and elimination of underlying conditions such as GERD (gastroesophageal reflux disease), sleep apnea and hypoglycemia.

The survey cannot accurately predict what proportion of the total afib population will be able to materially reduce or eliminate their afib through means other than ablation or surgery. Nevertheless, it is likely that a substantial proportion of those who give it a sincere try will be able to substantially improve their condition.

The survey was conducted in September/October 2007 and received a total of 248 responses (189 males and 59 females). The purpose of the survey was two-fold:

- To determine the proportion of afibbers who have been successful in managing their afib through means other than ablation or surgical procedures.
- To obtain and share information about successful protocols.

Baseline Characteristics			
Variable	Male	Female	Total
Gender distribution, %	76	24	100
Median age, yrs*	59	60	60
Age range, yrs*	26-78	34-80	26-80
Median age at 1st episode, yrs	50	51	50
Age range at 1st episode, yrs	10-75	7-75	7-75
Median no. of years of AF	7	6	7
LAF confirmed by diagnosis, %	86	92	87
Underlying heart disease, %	3.7	1.6	3.2
Median weight, lbs/kg	183/83	147/66.7	175/79.5
Median height, ft/meters	5'11"/1.80	5'5"/1.65	5'10"/1.78
Median BMI	25.2	23.6	25.1
Median birth weight, kg	3.620	3.365	3.410
Median resting heart rate, bpm	60	68	60
Median blood pressure	120/75	117/70	120/75

Variable	Male	Female	Total
Blood type O, %	42	39	41
Blood type A, %	37	41	38
Blood type B, %	15	10	13
Blood type AB, %	6	10	7
*at time of completing survey			

Success in managing afib was defined as a 50% reduction in afib burden over the most recent 6-month period as compared to a 6-month period prior to starting on the protocol that ultimately proved successful.

There were no significant differences in the base characteristics between males and females except for the expected differences in weight and height, which were highly significant ($p < 0.0001$). The difference in BMI was also significant, but somewhat less so ($p = 0.04$), as was the difference in birth weight ($p = 0.03$). The difference in resting heart rate, 60 bpm vs. 68 bpm, was very significant at $p < 0.0001$.

Afib type
A total of 218 respondents had provided detailed information about their type of afib prior to starting their quest to reduce or eliminate their afib burden.

Type of Afib			
	Male, %	Female, %	Total, %
Adrenergic	7	6	6
Mixed	32	34	33
Vagal	51	46	50
Total paroxysmal	90	86	89
Persistent	5	2	5
Permanent	5	12	6
TOTAL	100	100	100

Type of afib did not correlate with age at diagnosis, blood type, height, or presence of heart disease. However, a correlation was observed between afib type and weight and BMI with mixed afibbers having a lower weight and BMI than persistent afibbers. Birth weight was significantly higher for permanent afibbers than for mixed and vagal afibbers.

Afib burden
A total of 190 paroxysmal afibbers had provided data about their episode frequency and duration over a 6-month period prior to beginning their quest to eliminate or reduce their afib burden.

Mixed afibbers experienced significantly more episodes over the 6-month period than did vagal afibbers ($p = 0.0002$). Adrenergic afibbers had the highest overall burden of afib and this was significantly higher than the burden experienced by vagal afibbers ($p = 0.03$).

183

Afib Burden				
	#	Median # of Episodes	Median Duration, hrs	Median Burden, hrs
Adrenergic	12	7	12	164
Mixed	63	15	6	96
Vagal	93	7	6	48
Not known	22	12	5	79
Total paroxysmal	190	10	6	84

Paroxysmal afib burden prior to program implementation did not correlate with age at diagnosis, years of afib, weight, height, BMI, birth weight, resting heart rate, blood type, or presence of heart disease.

Intervention Program Results

A total of 248 respondents participated in the survey. Of these, 6 (2.4%) had made no attempt to reduce their afib burden by means other than ablation and surgical procedures. Eighteen respondents (7%) had been on their intervention program for less than 6 months leaving 224 respondents for further evaluation. These respondents had been on their program for a median of 36 months.

In answer to the question, "Did you ultimately find a program that was successful in materially reducing or eliminating your afib burden?" 144 respondents (64%) answered "YES" and 80 (36%) answered "NO". A total of 29 NO-responders went on to have an ablation/maze procedure, of which, 19 (66%) were deemed to be successful. Five of the NO responders stated that their intervention program had been partially successful, but they decided to undergo an ablation or maze procedure anyway.

Seven YES responders had undergone an unsuccessful ablation/maze procedure, but had ultimately found a non-ablation, non-surgical approach to manage or eliminate their afib. Another YES responder had managed their afib successfully with drugs, but decided to have an ablation (successful) to be able to discontinue the drugs. Finally, one YES responder had found a successful protocol, but had undergone a maze procedure in connection with open-heart surgery for other heart-related problems.

Among the respondents who had not tried to reduce their afib burden with means other than ablation/surgery, two had undergone a successful ablation, and finally, among afibbers who had been on their protocol for less than 6 months, five had undergone an ablation, of which, two were successful.
Overall, 45 of the 248 respondents (18%) had undergone an ablation/maze procedure with 25 or 56% being successful.

Characteristics of YES and NO responders

Baseline characteristics of the 224 afibbers who had tried to manage or eliminate their afib for 6 months or longer are presented below.

Baseline Characteristics of Respondents		
Variable	YES Responders	NO Responders
# in sample	144	80
Female, %	22.2	22.5
Male, %	77.8	77.5
Median age, yrs*	60	59
Age range, yrs*	26-80	35-77
Median age at 1st episode, yrs	51	50
Age range at 1st episode, yrs	7-75	10-71
Median no. of years of AF	6	8
LAF confirmed by diagnosis, %	85	93
Underlying heart disease, %	3.5	3.8
Median weight, kg	79.5	80.2
Median height, meters	1.78	1.80
Median BMI	25.1	24.9
Median birth weight, kg	3.410	3.475
Median resting heart rate, bpm	60	60
Median blood pressure	120/75	120/75
Blood type O, %	39	45
Blood type A, %	41	33
Blood type B, %	12	17
Blood type AB, %	8	5
*at time of completing survey		

There were no statistically significant differences in baseline characteristics.

Afib type

The types of afib encountered in the two groups prior to beginning the intervention protocol are shown below.

Afib Type		
Responders	YES	NO
Adrenergic, %	9	3
Mixed, %	27	45
Vagal, %	56	38
Total paroxysmal, %	92	86
Persistent, %	6	1
Permanent, %	2	13
TOTAL, %	100	100
Not sure, #	16	9

The difference in percentage of mixed and vagal afibbers (27% vs 45% and 56% vs 38%) between the YES and NO responders was statistically significant (p= 0.03). This difference would indicate that vagal afib is comparatively easier to manage than is mixed afib.

Afib burden

Ninety-six YES responders and 42 NO responders had provided data to allow a comparison of the paroxysmal afib burden experienced prior to the start of the intervention protocol.

Afib Burden*		
	YES Responders	NO Responders
Median # of episodes	11	8
Median duration, hrs.	6	8
Median burden, hrs.	90	78
*during 6-month period prior to beginning intervention program		

There was no significant difference in afib burden prior to program implementation when comparing YES responders to NO responders indicating that initial afib burden, as such, is not a determinant of ultimate success in reducing or eliminating afib.

A summary of the percentage of YES and NO responders who had used different modalities in their quest to relieve or eliminate their afib burden is presented below. Please note that percentages do not add up to 100 since most respondents had tried more than one modality.

Main Components of Intervention Programs			
Modalities	YES Responders	NO Responders	Total
Trigger avoidance, %	86	93	88
Dietary changes, %	51	63	55
Supplementation, %	81	91	84
Drug therapy, %	79	78	79
Other therapies, %	51	61	55
Disease treatment, %	35	39	37
Ablation/maze, %	6	36	17
Total in group, #	144	80	224

Most (85%) of NO respondents had tried more than one modality with 46% trying four or more, 21% trying three, and 18% trying two. Among YES respondents 78% had tried more than one modality with 37% trying four or more, 20% trying three, and 22% trying two. Thus, there was no indication that NO responders had been less persistent in their search for a protocol that worked. Of course, it is not possible to conclude anything about the diligence with which the various options were pursued in the two groups.

Program Details

A total of 124 YES responders (86%) and 74 NO responders (93%) had attempted to reduce or eliminate their afib through trigger avoidance. The percentage of afibbers who had practiced avoidance of some common triggers is shown below.

Trigger Avoidance, %			
Triggers	YES Responders	NO Responders	Total
MSG	32	39	34
Aspartame	36	43	38
Alcohol	52	64	56
Caffeine	64	74	67
Tyramine-containing foods	5	11	7
High glycemic index foods	22	24	22
Cold drinks	17	36	24
Heavy evening meals	38	50	42
Dehydration	33	54	40
Stress	32	38	34
Physical overexertion	40	34	38
Sleeping on left side	35	60	44
Other	21	18	20
Total in group, #	144	80	224

Among other triggers avoided wheat, gluten, sugars, bending over, and lack of sleep figured prominently. Caffeine was clearly the most common trigger factor avoided followed by alcohol (especially red wine), sleeping on the left side, heavy evening meals, dehydration, physical overexertion, and aspartame and other food additives.

Among YES responders 36% believed that trigger avoidance on its own had reduced their afib burden by at least 50% over the most recent 6-month period after beginning the protocol. Another 14% believed it had made little or no difference, and 50% believed that trigger avoidance, in combination with other measures, had resulted in at least a 50% reduction in afib burden. Among NO responders 24% felt that trigger avoidance had improved their condition somewhat, but not by 50% or more.

Over half of all respondents (58%) who had embarked on trigger avoidance had noted other benefits.

Additional Benefits of Trigger Avoidance	
Better overall health	10%
Weight loss	9%
Improved mood, less anxiety, calmer	6%
Fewer ectopic beats	5%
Better sleep	4%
Better digestion, less bloating	4%
More energy (less tired)	3%
Fewer colds and infections	2%
Percentages are based on the total group of 198 respondents who practiced trigger avoidance.	

Dietary changes

A total of 74 YES responders (51%) and 50 NO responders (63%) had attempted to reduce or eliminate their afib through diet changes. The percentage of those who had tried various approaches is shown below.

Dietary Changes, %			
Triggers	YES Responders	NO Responders	Total
Eliminated gluten	11	16	13
Eliminated wheat	13	15	14
Eliminated/reduced dairy	9	21	13
Changed to Paleo diet	8	11	9
Changed to Zone diet	5	6	5
Changed to Atkins diet	1	1	1
Reduced sugar intake	4	6	5
Increased veggies/fruits	0	6	2
Eat smaller portions	3	1	3
Other	26	13	21
Total in group, #	144	80	224

Among the YES responders 30% believed that dietary changes had reduced their afib burden by at least 50% over the most recent 6-month period after beginning the protocol. Another 15% believed it had made little or no difference, and 55% believed that dietary changes, in combination with other measures, had resulted in at least a 50% reduction in afib burden.

Eliminating wheat, eliminating gluten, or switching to the Paleo diet or Zone diet all has one thing in common – the elimination of wheat. Thus, it would be of interest to determine if the baseline characteristics of those afibbers who benefited from wheat elimination are different from those who did not. Twenty-seven respondents had observed no benefit from wheat elimination (including 10 who had switched to the Paleo diet), while 26 respondents had observed a benefit (including 10 who had switched to the Paleo diet). The percentage of vagal afibbers in the successful group was substantially higher than in the unsuccessful group (62% vs. 29%, $p = 0.04$). The percentage of females in the

188

successful group was also substantially higher than in the unsuccessful group (50% vs. 19%, p = 0.04). This same ratio also applied to the Paleo diet on its own.

In other words, women (especially vagal afibbers) who try the Paleo diet or wheat elimination are far more likely to be successful than are men. The reason could well be that most women still do the meal preparation and may be more inclined to be strict in their adherence to the diet if they have afib themselves than if it is the husband's problem. Also, men are probably more inclined to ignore the possible benefits of strict adherence and be less diligent.

The fact that vagal afibbers experienced more success with wheat elimination supports the contention that vagal afib is easier to manage than are the mixed, adrenergic, and permanent types. Of course, the possible influence of genetic differences between the sexes cannot be ruled out, but it seems unlikely to be a major cause in the difference in success with wheat elimination.

Any adverse effects from diet changes were minor with the need for adjustment of fiber content being the most significant. Fifty-nine per cent of respondents who had embarked on diet changes felt that their changes had made a significant overall positive impact on their health and wellbeing, quite apart from any effects on their afib.

Other Benefits of Dietary Changes	
Weight loss	23%
Better overall health	10%
Improved digestion	10%
More energy	8%
Less anxiety and depression	2%
Percentages are based on the total group of 124 respondents who had made diet changes.	

Use of Supplements
A total of 117 Yes responders (81%) and 73 NO responders (91%) had attempted to reduce or eliminate their afib burden through supplementation with vitamins, minerals, and herbs. The percentage of those who had tried various supplements and the percentage of those who had found them beneficial are given below.

The average number of supplements tried by each respondent was 7. The most popular one was fish oil, which had been tried by 71% of all respondents. Only 25% of YES responders, and 7% of NO responders had found it beneficial as far as reducing their afib burden was concerned. Fish oil supplementation, of course, has many other benefits independent of any effect on afib, most notably, stroke prevention. The second-most popular supplement was magnesium glycinate, which had been tried by 65% of all respondents and found beneficial by 71% of YES responders and 17% of NO responders. Coenzyme Q10 had been tried by 60% of all responders and found beneficial by 18%, while potassium had been tried by 55% and found beneficial by 17%. Taurine had been tried by 43% of all respondents and found beneficial by 51% of YES responders.

Supplements Used by Respondents						
	YES Responders		NO Responders		Combined	
Supplement	Tried, %	Benefit, %	Tried, %	Benefit, %	Tried, %	Benefit, %
Fish oil	68	25	74	7	71	18
Magnesium glycinate	62	71	71	17	65	48
Coenzyme Q10	60	24	60	9	60	18
Potassium	52	21	60	11	55	17
Vitamin C	44	10	56	5	49	8
Vitamin E	44	15	42	6	44	12
B-vitamins	43	18	45	6	44	13
Multivitamin	40	6	42	6	41	6
Taurine	38	51	49	8	43	32
Low-sodium V8 juice	25	34	23	12	24	26
L-carnitine	20	17	29	5	23	11
Zinc	20	4	18	0	19	3
Magnesium oxide	19	41	30	9	23	25
Calcium	18	5	27	0	22	2
Selenium	17	5	19	0	18	3
Probiotics	15	24	26	5	19	14
Digestive enzymes	10	33	19	7	14	19
L-arginine	9	9	15	9	12	9
Sea salt	9	9	16	0	12	4
Melatonin	5	0	8	0	6	0
Waller water	3	25	11	13	6	17
Ribose	3	100	1	0	2	75
Magnesium infusions	2	50	8	0	4	13
PAC-tamer drink	1	0	3	0	2	0
One or two respondents had found the following supplements beneficial – celery juice, hawthorn, niacin, flax oil, and a lysine/proline combination.						

Other supplements which had been found beneficial by 50% or more of the YES responders who had tried them include magnesium infusions and ribose; however, as only 3 and 2 respondents had tried them nothing can be concluded about their effectiveness in a larger population, particularly since 6 NO responders had tried infusions and none had found them beneficial. Nevertheless, the ribose results look promising and it is to be hoped that this supplement will receive a more thorough evaluation. Somewhat surprisingly, 19% of YES responders had tried magnesium oxide supplements and 41% had found them beneficial (vs. only 9% among NO responders). This may indicate a placebo effect, or that magnesium oxide is better absorbed than reported in the medical literature. Low-sodium V8 juice, probiotics, digestive enzymes, and Waller water had been found beneficial by 34%, 24%, 33%, and 25% respectively of the YES responders who had tried them.

Among the YES responders 25% believed that supplementation had reduced their afib burden by at least 50% over the most recent 6-month period after starting their protocol. Another 22% believed it had made little or no difference, and the remaining 53% believed that supplementation, in combination with other measures, had resulted in at least a 50% reduction in afib burden. In contrast, 82% of NO responders felt that supplementation had been of no benefit. The remaining 18% felt that they had achieved some benefit, but not enough to reduce their afib burden by 50%. It is of interest that 92% of those claiming some benefit had been supplementing with magnesium. Among YES responders who claimed that supplementation had helped, 56% had been supplementing with magnesium glycinate.

Comparing baseline characteristics of those who had benefited from magnesium glycinate supplementation and those who had not revealed that those who had benefited had experienced afib for only 3 years vs. 7 years for those who had not benefited ($p=0.04$). This could perhaps indicate that magnesium supplementation is more likely to be successful if started early in one's afib career. There was a strong correlation between having made successful dietary changes and supplementing with magnesium glycinate ($p = 0.04$) and a trend for blood type O to be more common among those who had not benefited from magnesium supplementation ($p=0.06$). Finally, it is worth noting that about 50% of those supplementing with magnesium glycinate also supplemented with potassium and taurine.

Seventeen percent of the 190 respondents had noted adverse effects from taking supplements. The most prevalent of these are listed in Table 13.

Adverse Effects of Supplementation	
Loose stools and diarrhea*	5%
Upset stomach, bloating	2%
Niacin flush	1%
Carnitine and Q10 causing afib	1%
*mostly from magnesium supplementation.	

Among other less frequent adverse effects (mentioned by one respondent each) were an increased frequency of afib or ectopics caused by B-vitamin, potassium, zinc, l-arginine and magnesium.

Thirty-nine percent of 190 respondents had noted further beneficial effects of their supplementation program

Additional Benefits of Supplementation	
Increased energy	8%
Better overall health	6%
Fewer ectopic beats	6%
Less severe symptoms	3%
Cholesterol reduction	3%
Improved digestion	3%
Elimination of leg cramps	2%
Reduction of blood pressure	2%

Other benefits mentioned by one or two respondents included improved mood, better weight control, fewer colds/flus, softer skin (vitamin C), and the heart feeling calmer.

Use of pharmaceutical drugs

A total of 114 YES responders (79%) and 62 NO responders (78%) had attempted to reduce or eliminate their afib burden through the use of prescription drugs (antiarrhythmics, beta-blockers or calcium channel blockers). The percentage of those who had tried various drugs and the percentage who had found them beneficial in reducing their afib burden are given below.

Use of Pharmaceutical Drugs						
	YES Responders		NO Responders		Combined	
Drug	Tried, %	Benefit, %	Tried, %	Benefit, %	Tried, %	Benefit, %
Beta-blocker	49	45	55	21	51	36
Flecainide	38	74	39	33	38	60
Sotalol	20	43	24	13	22	32
Calcium channel blocker	20	35	34	19	25	27
Propafenone	17	47	21	15	18	34
Digoxin	14	13	16	10	15	12
On-demand flecainide	13	53	10	33	12	48
ACE inhibitors	12	36	6	0	10	28
Amiodarone	9	70	11	57	10	65
Proton pump inhibitor	8	67	6	25	7	54
Tranquilizers	7	50	11	43	9	47
Disopyramide	6	43	0	0	4	43
Rythmol SR	6	29	10	33	7	31
On-demand propafenone	5	50	5	0	5	33
Angiotensin II blocker	4	60	5	0	5	38
Antidepressants	4	25	5	0	4	14
Dofetilide	3	67	5	33	3	50
On-demand beta-blocker	3	0	10	17	5	11
Aldosterone blockers	1	100	2	0	1	50
Procainamide	1	0	2	0	1	0

The average number of drugs tried by each respondent was 2.5 and there was no indication that NO responders had tried fewer drugs than had YES responders. The most popular drugs were beta-blockers, which had been tried by 51% of all respondents and found beneficial by 36% (Yes responders 45%, NO responders 21%). The second-most popular drug was flecainide (Tambocor), which had been tried by 38% and found beneficial by 60% (74% among YES responders and 33% among NO responders). In third place came calcium channel blockers, which had been tried by 25% and found beneficial by 27% (35% among YES responders and 19% among NO responders). Sotalol (Betapace) had been tried by 22% of all respondents and 32% of them had found this drug beneficial (43% of YES responders and 13% of NO responders). Amiodarone had been tried by 10% of all respondents and had been found beneficial by 65% (70% of YES responders and 57% of NO responders). Although only tried by 7% of responders, proton pump inhibitors (omeprazole, etc) had been found effective by 54%. Finally, 6 respondents had tried dofetilide (Tikosyn) with half of those finding it beneficial.

Beta-blockers and propafenone (Rythmol) were the most effective drugs for adrenergic afibbers; for mixed it was dofetilide (Tikosyn), propafenone, amiodarone, and flecainide that were the most effective, while for vagal afibbers amiodarone, flecainide, and calcium-channel blockers were most effective. The most effective drug overall was amiodarone, while the least effective was digoxin (Lanoxin). Somewhat surprisingly, 30% of vagal afibbers who had tried beta-blockers on a continuous basis had found them effective. NOTE: Half of them were taking the beta-blocker in combination with flecainide or amiodarone.

One respondent had eliminated his afib by correcting a low serum potassium level (3.2 mEq/l) with 50 mg/day of the aldosterone blocker, eplerenone, plus 2000 mg/day of potassium. He also took 50 mg of flecainide before bedtime. This protocol brought his potassium level up to 4.2 mEq/l.

Among the YES responders 56% believed that the use of prescription drugs had reduced their afib burden by at least 50% over the most recent 6-month period after beginning their protocol. Another 19% believed it had made no difference, and the remaining 25% believed that the use of drugs, in combination with other measures, had resulted in at least a 50% reduction in afib burden.
Thirty-five percent of the 176 respondents had noticed adverse effects from their medications. The most prevalent of these are listed below.

Flecainide users (34%) were the most likely to report adverse events followed by amiodarone (29%) and sotalol (26%) users.

Adverse Effects of Drugs	
Tiredness, fatigue	15%
Hypotension (Low blood pressure)	3%
Sexual dysfunction	2%
Constipation	2%
Increased ectopics	2%
Thyroid problems*	1%
Headaches	1%
Dizziness/lightheadedness	1%
Sleeping problems	1%
*associated with amiodarone	

Eleven percent of the 176 respondents had noted further benefits from their medications.

Additional Benefits of Drugs	
Reduction of blood pressure	4%
Fewer ectopics beats	2%
Lower heart rate	2%
Fewer migraine attacks	1%
Decrease in GERD symptoms	1%
Calmer	1%

Use of alternative therapies

A total of 74 YES responders (51%) and 49 NO responders (61%) had attempted to reduce or eliminate their afib burden through the use of stress management or other alternative therapies. The percentage of those who had tried various protocols and the percentage who had found them beneficial in reducing their afib burden are given in Table 18.

Use of Alternative Therapies						
	YES Responders		NO Responders		Combined	
Therapy	Tried, %	Benefit, %	Tried, %	Benefit, %	Tried, %	Benefit, %
Relaxation therapy*	39	52	43	10	41	34
Breathing exercises	38	57	47	17	41	39
Acupuncture	15	18	18	0	16	10
Chiropractic	5	25	4	0	5	17
	YES Responders		NO Responders		Combined	
Chinese herbals	7	40	12	0	9	18
Meditation	32	42	27	23	30	35
Yoga	20	60	16	38	19	52
Qi gong	5	75	6	33	6	57
Tai chi	5	50	6	0	6	29
Cognitive thinking	12	67	8	0	11	46
Amalgam removal	14	50	6	0	11	38
*mostly adrenergic afibbers who benefited						

Relaxation therapy had been tried by 41% of respondents and found beneficial by 34% (mostly adrenergic afibbers). Breathing exercises had also been tried by 41% and found beneficial by 39%. Meditation had been tried by 30% and found beneficial by 35%. The most effective therapy was Qi Gong, which had been tried by 6% of respondents and found beneficial by 57%. Yoga and cognitive thinking therapy were also found effective at 52% and 46% success rates respectively.

Among the YES responders 19% believed that the use of stress management and other alternative therapies had reduced their afib burden by at least 50% over the most recent 6-month period after beginning their protocol. Another 28% believed it had made no difference, and the remaining 53% felt that the use of alternative therapies, in combination with other measures, had resulted in at least a 50% reduction in afib burden.

Only 2 respondents (2%) reported adverse effects of their alternative therapy program and both were related to vigorous exercise. In contrast, 26% of respondents who had tried alternative therapies reported additional benefits over and above the effect on afib burden. The most prevalent of these benefits were an increased sense of mental and physical wellbeing (7%), feeling calmer and more relaxed (7%), more flexible due to yoga training (3%), and more energy (2%).

Treatment of underlying disease

A total of 52 YES responders (36%) and 30 NO responders (38%) had attempted to reduce or eliminate their afib burden by dealing with underlying disease conditions.

Elimination of Diseases						
	YES Responders		NO Responders		Combined	
Disease	Tried, %	Benefit, %	Tried, %	Benefit, %	Tried, %	Benefit, %
GERD	42	41	43	0	43	26
Digestive problems	33	53	47	0	38	29
Food allergies	12	50	13	0	12	30
	YES Responders		NO Responders		Combined	
Sleep apnea	21	27	13	0	18	20
Hyperthyroidism	2	100	3	0	2	50
Hypothyroidism	10	20	10	0	10	13
Hypoglycemia	10	20	3	0	7	17
Other conditions treated were constipation, tooth abscesses, hypokalemia (1 each)						

GERD (gastroesophageal reflux disease) and digestive problems affected a total of 36 or 44% of the 82 respondents. Half of them (22%) had reduced their afib burden by effectively dealing with these conditions. Sleep apnea affected

18% of respondents and was dealt with successfully in 20% of cases. Food allergies were reported by 12% and effectively treated by 30%.

Somewhat surprisingly, only about 10% of GERD patients had used proton pump inhibitors (Nexium, Prilosec) in treating their problem. The remaining had used diet (58%) or probiotics and digestive enzymes (33%) to help alleviate GERD. Sleep apnea sufferers were generally overweight or obese and most had used a CPAP machine to alleviate their problem.

Among the YES responders 35% believed that dealing with underlying disease conditions had reduced their afib burden by at least 50% over the most recent 6-month period after starting their regimen. Another 21% believed it had made no difference, and the remaining 44% felt that dealing with underlying conditions, in combination with other measures, had resulted in at least a 50% reduction in afib burden. In contrast, 83% of NO Responders felt that attempting to deal with their underlying conditions had made no difference.

An impressive 63% of the 82 respondents who had dealt with underlying disease conditions in an attempt to reduce their afib burden had observed additional benefits, the most common of which are summarized below.

Additional Benefits from Treatment of Underlying Disease Conditions	
Improved digestion and bowel function	17%
No more acid reflux (heartburn)	17%
Better sleep	16%
Overall better health and wellbeing	6%
More energy	4%
No more fluctuations in blood sugar	4%
Weight loss	4%

Shortening episodes

A total of 110 respondents (49% - YES and NO respondents combined) had found one or more ways of shortening their episodes. The number and percentage of those who had found effective protocols are presented below.

Means of Shortening Episodes		
Effective Protocol	#	%
On-demand flecainide	27	25
Light exercise	26	24
Resting	23	21
Vigorous exercise	19	17
On-demand beta-blocker	17	15
Tranquilizers	11	10
On-demand propafenone	11	10
Hydrotherapy	9	8

Effective Protocol	#	%
Meditation	8	7
Valsalva maneuver	7	6
Increased supplements*	7	6
On-demand calcium channel blocker	5	5
Acupuncture/acupressure	3	3
Increase regular medication	3	3
Drink lots of water	3	3
Standing up (when resting at onset)	2	2
Coughing	2	2
Sleeping in cool room	2	2
Warm bath	1	1
*especially magnesium, taurine and potassium		

Twenty-five percent of the 110 respondents had found the on-demand (pill-in-pocket) approach with flecainide to be effective in hastening conversion to normal sinus rhythm. This approach was equally effective for mixed and vagal afibbers, but significantly more effective for YES responders than for NO responders.

Twenty-four percent had found light exercise to be effective, 23% had benefited from resting (equal benefit for all afib types), 19% from vigorous exercise, 17% from on-demand beta-blockers, and 11% from tranquilizers. The most effective therapies for women were hydrotherapy, meditation, tranquilizers and resting, while the most effective therapy for men was vigorous exercise. NOTE: 80% of respondents who had found vigorous exercise beneficial were male, vagal afibbers.

Preventing ectopics

Sixty-eight respondents (33%) had found one or more means of preventing ectopics (premature beats, PVCs, PACs), 21% did not experience ectopics, and the remaining 46% had not found a way of preventing ectopics.

Prevention of Ectopics		
Effective Protocol	#	%
Supplementation with magnesium*	30	44
Supplementation with potassium*	29	43
Low-sodium V8 juice	18	26
Supplementation with taurine*	16	24
Beta-blocker	10	15
Tranquilizers	7	10
Additional supplements**	7	10
Additional antiarrhythmics	4	6
PAC-tamer drink	1	1
*mostly in combination (magnesium/potassium/taurine) **specifically potassium and coenzyme Q10		

197

By far the most effective way of preventing ectopics is by supplementing with magnesium and/or potassium, preferably in combination with taurine. Forty-four percent of all respondents had found this approach to be effective, while 26% had found drinking low-sodium (high potassium) V8 juice to be effective in preventing ectopics. Beta-blockers and tranquilizers were also found to be somewhat effective. In my own experience the most effective way of preventing or eliminating ectopics is by drinking (over a 10-minute period) 8 ounces of lukewarm water containing the following:

- 1 pouch of *Emergen-C*
- 1 teaspoon of magnesium citrate (*Natural Calm*)
- 1 teaspoon of potassium gluconate
- 1000 mg of taurine (may be taken separately in capsule form)

This drink will provide, besides 1000 mg of vitamin C, 740 mg of elemental potassium and 265 mg of elemental magnesium in a highly absorbable form.

Other suggestions for preventing ectopics include avoiding trigger factors such as caffeine, sugar, and sleeping on the left side.

Overall results of intervention protocols

One hundred and forty-four respondents (64% of the total) answered YES to the question, "Did you ultimately find a program that was successful in materially reducing or eliminating your afib burden?" The average time these respondents had been on their successful program varied from 6 to 120 months with a median of 22 months. Ninety-one YES responders had kept track of the number of episodes and duration during their time on the program as well as before they started.

Overall Results		
Burden over 6 months	Before Protocol	After Implementation
# of episodes	10	0.8
Average duration, hrs.	6	1
Afib burden, hrs.	72	2
Permanent AF is counted as 24 hours/day for 180 days, ie. 4320 hours over 6 months.		

The differences in the two columns were all statistically extremely significant. Perhaps even more impressive is the fact that almost a third of respondents had experienced no episodes at all since implementing their protocol. Nevertheless, 45 of the respondents still needed to avoid triggers, while 30% did not. The remaining 25% still needed to avoid triggers, but much less so.

Ninety-five percent of respondents would recommend their program to fellow afibbers, but 5% would not, primarily because their programs involved the use of amiodarone or drastic measures such as early retirement.

Overall, 157 respondents who had not undergone ablation and had been on their program for 6 months or longer had kept records of their afib burden prior to implementing their program and for the most recent 6 months while on the program. These respondents can be assigned to 4 different groups:

- Worsened or no improvement   40 respondents
- Less than 50% improvement   11 respondents
- Better than 50%, but not eliminated   57 respondents
- No episodes in most recent 6 months   42 respondents

In addition, 7 persistent afibbers either completely eliminated their afib (4 respondents) or became paroxysmal. Thus, out of the group of 157 respondents with complete data, 68% had reduced their afib burden by 50% or more, and 29% had experienced no episodes in the most recent 6 months.

It clearly would be of interest to determine the relevant differences between the group of 46 respondents (Group A) who managed to completely eliminate their afib for at least a 6-month period (including former persistent afibbers) and the group of 40 respondents (Group B) whose condition worsened or remained the same. To do so is the purpose of the following section.

Comparison between Groups A and B

In this section the baseline characteristics and actions taken will be compared for a group of 46 afibbers (Group A) who experienced no afib episodes over the latest 6-month period and a group of 40 afibbers whose condition worsened or remained the same (Group B).

Comparison of Baseline Characteristics		
Variable	Group A	Group B
Female, %	24	33
Male, %	76	67
Median age at completion, yrs	60	58
Age range at completion, yrs	33-77	40-77
Median age at 1st episode, yrs	50	52
Age range at 1st episode, yrs	16-69	20-71
Median no. of years of AF	7	7.5
LAF confirmed by diagnosis, %	89	93
Underlying heart disease, %	4.8	2.5
Median weight, kg	81.6	78.8
Median height, meters	1.78	1.80

Comparison of Baseline Characteristics		
Variable	Group A	Group B
Median body mass index (BMI)	25.8	25.0
Median birth weight, kg	**3.280**	**3.700**
Median resting heart rate, bpm	60	62
Median blood pressure	120/75	120/73
Months on program	36	48
Blood type O, %	39	47
Blood type A, %	42	30
Blood type B, %	14	17
Blood type AB, %	5	6
Adrenergic	10	3
Mixed	24	42
Vagal	63	45
Paroxysmal	98	90
Permanent	2	10
Total	100	100

There were no statistically significant differences in baseline characteristics between the two groups except for median birth weight which was almost a pound (420 grams) higher in Group B.

The afib burden 6 months prior to beginning the protocols and for the most recent 6-month period are shown below.

Afib Burden				
	Before Intervention		After Intervention	
Afib Burden	Group A	Group B	Group A	Group B
Median # of episodes	4	6	0	24
Median duration hrs.	6	8	0	12
Median burden hrs.	33	56	0	208

There was no statistically significant difference between the pre-intervention afib burden of Groups A and B. However, the difference in pre- and post-intervention burden was highly significant for both groups with Group B getting much worse and Group A eliminating afib altogether, at least for a 6-month period.

Intervention modalities

A summary of the percentage of Group A and B members who had used different modalities in their quest to relieve or eliminate their afib burden is presented below. Please note that percentages do not add up to 100 since most respondents had tried more than one modality.

There was no indication that members of Group B had tried fewer interventions than had those of Group A – quite the contrary. Most surprising was the finding that only 41% of those in Group A had made dietary changes as compared to

70% in Group B (p=0.02). Trigger sensitivity was not significantly different between the two groups, except that those in Group B had found sleeping on the left side to be more detrimental than had those in Group A (53% vs 28%, p= 0.05).

Main Components of Intervention Program		
Component	Group A, %	Group B, %
Trigger avoidance	85	93
Dietary changes	41	70
Supplementation	70	90
Drug therapy	72	75
Other therapies	54	63
Disease treatment	41	36

Dietary changes

Seventy percent of Group B and 41% of group A had tried changing their diet. The percentage of those having tried different approaches and their rate of success is presented below.

Dietary Interventions				
	Group A		Group B	
Intervention	% Tried	% Success*	% Tried	% Success*
Elimination of gluten	13	33	20	0
Elimination of wheat	13	33	18	0
Reduced dairy	11	60	20	0
Changed to Paleo diet	9	75	5	0
*% of those who had tried the intervention and believed it had reduced their AF burden by 50% or more				

There clearly was a substantial difference in the degree of success experienced in the two groups. Group B had no luck at all, while Group A found that diet changes had reduced their afib burden by 50% or more in from 33 to 75% of cases. The major difference between the two groups was that there were no mixed afibbers in Group A, while the proportion of mixed afibbers in Group B was 55%. It was also noted that 75% of Group A members who had found diet changes beneficial were women.

Supplements

Ninety percent of Group B and 70% of Group A had tried supplementation.

The most beneficial supplement was magnesium glycinate (chelated magnesium), which had been tried by 55% of all 86 responders and found beneficial by 38%. Thirty-nine percent of Group A had tried magnesium glycinate and two-thirds had found this supplement beneficial. Potassium and taurine were also found to be effective with 24% and 22% of those having tried them finding them beneficial (54% and 67% respectively in Group A). Fish oil was the most popular supplement, but only 14% (23% in Group A) had found it beneficial as far as afib was concerned.

Supplement Interventions						
	Group A (N=46)		Group B (N=40)		Combined	
Supplement	Tried, %	Benefit, %	Tried, %	Benefit, %	Tried, %	Benefit, %
Magnesium glycinate	39	67	81	21	55	38
Magnesium infusions	2	100	6	0	3	33
Potassium	28	54	58	5	40	24
Taurine	20	67	50	0	31	22
Magnesium oxide	20	44	28	0	22	21
Low-sodium V8 juice	7	67	22	0	13	18
Digestive enzymes	13	33	14	0	13	18
Coenzyme Q10	37	24	67	13	48	17
Fish oil	48	23	75	7	57	14
Probiotics	11	0	28	0	17	0

It is not surprising that magnesium turned out to be highly beneficial. Magnesium has proven antiarrhythmic properties and magnesium sulfate injections have been found to shorten episode duration. It is also worth noting that 80% of the US adult population (excluding those who supplement) do not get the recommended daily allowance of 420 mg/day for men and 320 mg/day for women from their diet.[1] Furthermore, there is also evidence that magnesium intake is inversely proportional to the level of the inflammatory marker C-reactive protein.[1] This all adds up to the conclusion that magnesium is likely the most effective supplement for lone afibbers. It also points to the possibility that the massive extent of magnesium deficiency in the USA, and likely in Canada and Western Europe as well, may be at least partly responsible for the afib epidemic.

In the experience of many afibbers a combination of magnesium, potassium, and taurine is even more effective than magnesium alone. A commonly used combination is:

- 3 x 100-200 mg/day of elemental magnesium from magnesium glycinate
- 3 teaspoons/day of potassium gluconate powder providing 3 x 540 mg/day of elemental potassium
- 3 x 1000 mg/day of taurine

When the above combination is first started it is a good idea to begin just with magnesium and taurine as there is evidence that it is difficult to remedy a low potassium level without first ensuring an adequate level of magnesium. Also, it is advisable to gradually increase magnesium over a couple of weeks (3x100 mg/day to 3x200 mg/day) so as to avoid any stomach upset. The above supplements are best taken in juice or in a protein shake. NOTE: *Natural Calm* magnesium citrate can also be used, but needs to be started slowly to avoid loose stools.

Coenzyme Q10 had been tried by 48% of all respondents and found beneficial by 17% (24% in Group A). However, some afibbers have found that coenzyme Q10 is too excitatory and worsens their condition. Experimentation is definitely required here.

Pharmaceutical drugs
Seventy-five percent of Group B and 72% of Group A had tried pharmaceutical drugs. NOTE: Only drugs which had been tried by at least 5% of the total group, are included here.

Pharmaceutical Interventions						
	Group A		Group B		Combined	
Drug	Tried, %	Benefit, %	Tried, %	Benefit, %	Tried, %	Benefit, %
Amiodarone	7	100	3	100	5	100
Tranquilizers	7	33	8	100	7	67
Proton pump inhibitors	11	60	3	0	7	50
Flecainide	28	69	25	20	27	48
Beta-blocker	37	41	38	40	37	41
Calcium channel blocker	17	38	23	33	20	35
Sotalol	22	40	20	25	21	33
ACE inhibitors	11	40	8	0	9	25
Propafenone	13	33	8	0	10	22
Digoxin	13	17	13	0	13	9

Amiodarone, although only tried by 4 afibbers, had a 100% success rate, but was accompanied by a 50% rate of adverse effects involving thyroid problems. Tranquilizers (Ativan, Xanax, Valium) were found quite effective for mixed afibbers and proton pump inhibitors (PPI) were effective for those with GERD or digestive problems. Flecainide had been tried by 27% of the total group of 86 respondents and had been found effective by 48%. Beta-blockers had been tried by 37% and had been found effective by 41%; however, 84% of those who had found beta-blockers successful were taking antiarrhythmics as well. Sotalol had been tried by 21% and found effective by 33%. There was no indication that sotalol was any less effective for vagal afibbers than for mixed.

Alternative therapies
Seventy-five percent of Group B and 54% of Group A had tried to reduce their afib burden with the use of alternative therapies.

Alternative Protocols						
	Group A		Group B		Combined	
Alternative Therapy	Tried, %	Benefit, %	Tried, %	Benefit, %	Tried, %	Benefit, %
Breathing exercises	26	58	28	18	27	39
Relaxation therapy	17	38	33	31	24	33
Meditation	20	44	25	30	22	37
Yoga	9	75	10	25	9	50
Acupuncture	7	0	13	0	9	0
Amalgam removal.	7	67	3	0	5	50
Cognitive thinking	2	0	8	0	5	0
Qi gong	2	100	3	100	2	100
Chiropractic	2	0	3	0	2	0
Tai chi	2	0	3	0	2	0

Breathing exercise was the most popular protocol; it had been tried by 27% of the total group and found beneficial by 39%. Relaxation therapy had been tried by 24% and found beneficial by 33%, while meditation had been tried by 22% and found beneficial by 37%. Yoga had been found beneficial by half of the 9% of the group who had tried it. Two afibbers had tried Qi Gong and both had found it beneficial.

Treatment of underlying disease

A total of 18 Group A members (39%) and 14 Group B members (35%) had attempted to reduce or eliminate their afib burden by dealing with underlying disease conditions.

Elimination of Underlying Conditions						
	Group A		Group B		Combined	
Condition	Tried, %	Benefit, %	Tried, %	Benefit, %	Tried, %	Benefit, %
Sleep apnea	9	75	5	0	7	50
GERD	20	33	15	17	17	27
Digestive problems	11	60	18	0	14	25
Food allergies	9	50	10	0	9	25
Hypoglycemia	9	25	3	0	6	20
Hypothyroidism	4	0	3	0	3	0

Treatment of sleep apnea (with a CPAP machine) was the most effective of the disease elimination protocols with an overall success rate of 50% (75% in Group A). The most common disease condition was GERD (gastroesophageal reflux disease), which 17% of the 32 afibbers had attempted to eliminate with a 27% success rate as far as reduction or elimination of afib is concerned. Fourteen percent had tried to eliminate digestive problems and 25% (60% in Group A) had been able to eliminate or reduce (by 50% or more) their afib burden by doing so.

Preventing ectopics
Thirty percent of Group A did not experience ectopics, while only 17% of Group B were free of this annoyance. One third of Group A had found an effective means of dealing with ectopics, while only 15% of Group B had done so. The most effective way of preventing ectopics was through supplementation with potassium (including low-sodium V8 juice) which 60% of Group A had found beneficial. Forty percent had found magnesium supplementation beneficial either on its own or in combination with potassium, and 20% (all vagal) had found the use of tranquilizers to be beneficial for ectopics.

Trigger avoidance
Forty-five percent of Group A no longer had to avoid triggers, while 28% still had to do so, but to a lesser extent.

Review of successful protocols
The main modalities used by Group A were almost evenly split between the use of pharmaceutical drugs and the use of other approaches. Ultimately, 22 Group A respondents (no afib episodes in the last 6 months) had managed to achieve their afib-free status through the use of antiarrhythmic drugs (mostly flecainide). Fourteen had relied solely on drugs, while 4 had combined drugs, supplements (mostly magnesium), and alternative protocols. Four had combined antiarrhythmics with trigger avoidance, dietary changes, and elimination of GERD.

The remaining 24 respondents had managed to remain afib-free for at least 6 months through the use of protocols not involving pharmaceutical drugs. Trigger avoidance had been successfully practiced by 14 Group A members, but was usually accompanied by other protocols such as supplementation (10 respondents), dietary changes (4 respondents), and stress management and other alternative therapies (6 respondents). Diet changes had been made by 9 respondents, 8 of whom had also used supplementation (mostly magnesium) and 3 had also used other alternative methods. One respondent had managed to become afib-free through dietary changes alone. Seventeen (71%) of the 24 respondents had used supplementation with 3 relying on supplementation alone. It is interesting that no mixed afibbers had been successful in using dietary changes to eliminate their afib burden. The most successful – based on this albeit very small sample – were female, vagal afibbers who switched to a paleo diet.

Conclusions

A total of 248 afibbers (189 males and 59 females) participated in the 2007 LAF Survey. The majority (89%) had paroxysmal afib with 50% having the vagal type and 33% the mixed. Mixed afibbers experienced significantly more episodes than did vagal ones, but adrenergic afibbers carried the highest overall afib burden (# of episodes x average duration) prior to the implementation of their programs.

A total of 224 respondents had attempted to reduce or eliminate their afib using means other than ablation or surgical procedures and had been on their program for 6 months or longer (36 months on average).

In answer to the question, "Did you ultimately find a program that was successful in materially reducing or eliminating your afib burden?" 144 respondents (64%) answered "YES" and 80 (36%) answered "NO". A total of 29 NO responders went on to have an ablation/maze procedure, of which, 19 (66%) were deemed to be successful. Five of the NO responders stated that their intervention program had been partially successful, but they decided to undergo an ablation or maze procedure anyway. Overall, 45 of the 248 respondents (18%) had undergone an ablation/maze procedure with 25 or 56% being successful.

There were no significant differences in baseline characteristics between YES and NO responders. The division into the two groups is clearly subjective since it is based on the respondents' feeling about the benefits of their chosen protocols. Nevertheless, some interesting differences stand out.

- The difference in percentage of mixed and vagal afibbers (27% vs 45% and 56% vs 38%) between the YES and NO responders was statistically significant (p = 0.03). This difference would indicate that vagal afib is comparatively easier to manage than is mixed afib.

- There was no significant difference in afib burden prior to program implementation when comparing YES responders to NO responders indicating that initial afib burden, as such, is not a determinant of ultimate success in reducing or eliminating afib.

- The most popular intervention program was trigger avoidance engaged in by 88% of all respondents. This was followed by supplementation (84%), therapy with pharmaceutical drugs (79%), dietary changes (55%), and other therapies (55%).

- Avoidance of caffeine had been found useful by 67% of respondents, alcohol avoidance by 56%, and avoidance of aspartame and MSG by 38% and 34% respectively. Altogether, respondents had identified 17 important triggers.

- The most important dietary changes were elimination of wheat, gluten and dairy products, and a switch to the Paleo diet. These changes were significantly more successful among females and vagal afibbers.

- Eighty-five percent of responders had tried supplementation. The most effective supplement was magnesium glycinate, which had been found beneficial by 48% of those who had tried it. Potassium supplementation (including low-sodium V8 juice) had been tried by 79% of all respondents and found beneficial by 43%. Taurine had been tried by 43% and found beneficial by 32%. About half of those supplementing with magnesium also took potassium and taurine.

- The most successful pharmaceutical drug was amiodarone, which had been tried by 10% and found beneficial by 65%. Flecainide (Tambocor) was the most popular antiarrhythmic. It had been tried by 38% of all respondents and been found successful by 60%.

- Breathing exercises and relaxation therapy were the most commonly tried stress reduction measures and had been found successful by 39% and 34% respectively. Yoga had been tried by 19% and found beneficial by 52%.

- Dealing with GERD, digestive problems, and food allergies had benefited 26-30% for those who dealt with these conditions. This clearly indicates that digestive problems are an important component of afib.

- The percentages of YES responders who believed that the various therapies had been beneficial on their own, or in combination with other measures, are given below:

Protocol	Sole Therapy	Combination
Trigger avoidance	36%	50%
Dietary changes	30%	55%
Supplementation	25%	53%
Drug therapy	56%	25%
Other therapies	19%	53%
Disease treatment	35%	44%

- About 50% of respondents had found a way of shortening their episodes. On-demand (pill-in-pocket) flecainide had been found effective by 25%, light exercise by 24%, and resting by 21%. The most effective therapies for women were hydrotherapy, meditation, tranquilizers and resting, while the most effective therapy for men was vigorous exercise. This is not surprising since vigorous exercise will increase adrenergic tone and 80% of respondents who had found vigorous exercise beneficial were male, vagal afibbers.

- A third of respondents had found ways of preventing ectopics with supplementation with the magnesium/potassium/taurine combination being the most popular followed by the consumption of low-sodium V8 juice.

- A comparison between 46 afibbers (Group A) who had managed to completely eliminate their afib episodes over the most recent 6 months and 40 afibbers (Group B) whose condition had worsened or remained constant revealed the following:

  - The median birth weight in Group A was substantially lower than in Group B.
  - There was no indication that members of Group B had tried fewer interventions than had those members in Group A.
  - Group B had achieved no improvement at all through dietary changes, while Group A had achieved significant benefits, especially by changing to the Paleo diet (75%), avoiding dairy (60%), and eliminating wheat and gluten (33%).
  - Group A had achieved very significant benefits from supplementing with magnesium, potassium and taurine, while Group B had seen little or no benefit from supplementing.
  - Amiodarone was the most effective antiarrhythmic, but its use, in 50% of cases, was accompanied by adverse effects, notably thyroid problems. Tranquilizers (Ativan, Xanax, Valium) were found to be quite effective for mixed afibbers. Flecainide had been found effective by 41% of those who had tried it.
  - The treatment of sleep apnea and GERD had benefited 50% and 27% respectively.

Overall, it would appear that Groups A and B and indeed, YES and NO responders, are markedly different in that practically nothing worked for NO responders and those in Group B, while several different protocols worked quite well for YES responders and those in Group A.

It is not apparent what the difference is since there is no indication that NO responders were less diligent in their approach than were YES responders. It is possible that the statistically significant lower birth weight in Group A could contain a clue, but it is certainly not obvious what that clue might be, especially since a higher birth weight is generally associated with better cardiovascular health.

I have discussed the birth weight finding with Pat Chambers, MD and he points out that a higher birth weight such as found in Group B is associated with increased baroreflex sensitivity [2] and that an increased baroreflex sensitivity, in turn, is associated with more difficulty in dealing with sudden changes in autonomic tone that could lead to an afib episode. Thus, it may well be that lone afibbers can be divided into two groups - those (like in Group A) whose main underlying problems are magnesium deficiency, wheat sensitivity, etc. and those (like in Group B) whose main underlying problem is an increased baroreflex sensitivity. Clearly, it would be much easier to correct a magnesium deficiency than an increased baroreflex sensitivity, perhaps explaining why "nothing worked" for Group B. It is also intriguing to speculate that the reason why mixed type afibbers (neither pure adrenergic nor pure vagal) have a more difficult time reducing their afib burden could be that they have increased baroreflex sensitivity. Hopefully, medical researchers will someday cast more light on this finding.

Protocol for Afib Reduction/Elimination

The following 12-step program is based on the findings of this survey, numerous Bulletin Board postings, and with supporting information from my first book *Lone Atrial Fibrillation: Towards a Cure.*

1. Ensure that your condition is indeed **lone** atrial fibrillation (no underlying heart disease) and rule out known causes such as thyroid disorders, hypoglycemia, hyperaldosteronism (Conn's Syndrome) and pheochromocytoma.

2. Ensure that your liver and kidney functions are normal before embarking on an abatement program based on pharmaceutical drugs or supplements. This would involve BUN, creatinine and liver enzyme tests. It is also a good idea to establish your baseline electrolyte concentrations. This can be done through a simple blood test. Although the results are not very indicative of the concentration where it matters, namely in the myocytes (heart muscle cells) they will alert you to serious deficiencies. If the potassium level is below 4.5 mEq/L then supplementation is likely necessary to bring the daily intake up to the recommended 4500 mg/day. Magnesium level is best determined in red blood cells (RBCs) or in scrapings from the mouth (Exatest). NOTE: Probably close to 90% of lone afibbers test low for magnesium when using the Exatest. Finally, it would also be advisable to determine if systemic inflammation is present. A high-sensitivity C-reactive protein (hs-CRP) level above 1.0 mg/L (0.1 mg/dL) may indicate the need for supplementation with an effective anti-inflammatory such as beta-sitosterol or Zyflamend.

3. If not already doing so start keeping a detailed journal of the timing, duration and likely triggers of your afib episodes. This is essential in helping you determine the nature of your afib (adrenergic, mixed or vagal) and in establishing a successful abatement program.

4. Determine what your triggers are and scrupulously avoid them. If you are not yet sure what they are try avoiding caffeine, alcohol, MSG, aspartame, wheat, tyramine-containing foods, sugar and sleeping on your left side and see if that improves your situation.

5. Unless your magnesium and potassium levels are excessive begin supplementing with the magnesium, potassium, taurine combo to see if that is beneficial in your specific case. If your sun exposure is limited supplement with vitamin D as well to ensure optimum absorption of magnesium.

6. Eliminate wheat and gluten-containing grains from your diet. Rice is OK and oats and rye may be as well, but this needs to be determined on an individual basis. Also avoid high glycemic load foods, *trans*-fatty acids and tyramine-containing foods. Avoid large meals and if hypoglycemia is a problem have a light snack mid-morning and mid-afternoon. Ensure adequate hydration; daily water intake, in addition to that supplied by food, should be 1-1.5 liters (32-48 oz.)

7. Determine if you have any disease conditions associated with atrial fibrillation such as sleep apnea, GERD (gastroesophageal reflux disease), hyperthyroidism or hypoglycemia and take appropriate steps to deal with them. Also ensure that your digestive process is functioning properly. Bloating and gas formation in the stomach often cause ectopics and in some cases, atrial fibrillation. If this is a problem supplementation with pancreatic enzymes and betaine hydrochloride may be helpful. If bloating and gas occur close to bedtime an 80 mg simethicone tablet may help (best taken about 45 minutes prior to bedtime).

8. Find a relaxation therapy or other alternative protocol helpful in relieving stress that works for you and practice it daily.

9. If following steps 1-8 does not provide relief switch to a strict paleo diet. This combined with magnesium/potassium/taurine supplementation is probably the most effective step you can take, but it does require a very significant commitment, persistence, self-discipline and full cooperation from your spouse or significant other.

10. Try the on-demand (pill-in-pocket) approach to terminating episodes quickly with flecainide crushed and swallowed with lukewarm water at the start of an episode (200 mg for people weighing less than 70 kg (154 lbs) and 300 mg for people weighing more than 70 kg). In the case of a heart rate exceeding 100 bpm taking a beta-blocker first may be advisable. Propafenone (Rythmol) can also be used for the on-demand approach (450 mg for people weighing less than 70 kg and 600 mg for people weighing over 70 kg).

11. Consider going on an antiarrhythmic drug full time. Flecainide (Tambocor), possibly in combination with a beta-blocker, would appear to be most successful and should generally be tried first (50-100 mg every 12 hours).

12. If steps 1-11 have been faithfully followed and doing so has brought no relief get in line for an ablation or maze procedure with a highly skilled and experienced electrophysiologist or cardiac surgeon.

Why not go directly to an antiarrhythmic or ablation you may ask? Because, there is no guarantee of success and both have the potential for serious adverse effects, while improving your diet, eliminating wheat and supplementing with magnesium only have positive effects.

REFERENCES

1. King, DE, et al. Dietary magnesium and C-reactive protein levels. Journal of the American College of Nutrition, Vol. 24, No. 3, 2005, pp. 166-71
2. Leotta, G, et al. Effects of birth weight on spontaneous baroreflex sensitivity in adult life. Nutrition, Metabolism and Cardiovascular Diseases, Vol. 17, May 2007, pp. 303-10

2008 Ablation/Maze Survey

By Hans R. Larsen [2008]

The 2008 Ablation/Maze Survey produced 323 responses, 162 of which were updates to responses submitted in earlier surveys. Combining the 516 respondents to earlier surveys with the 161 new respondents contributing their experience in 2008 results in a total database of 677 patients having undergone a total of 1045 procedures.

Evaluation of Background Data

Distribution of procedures

Six hundred and seventy-seven afibbers responded to the survey and provided data for a total of 1045 procedures distributed as follows:

RF Ablation Procedures					
	1st	2nd	3rd	Further	Total
Focal ablation	52	26	7	0	85
Pulmonary vein ablation (PVA)	191	71	15	1	278
Segmental PVI	65	37	10	0	112
Circumferential PVI	55	23	5	2	85
Antrum PVI	127	37	13	3	180
Right atrial flutter ablation	50	17	6	0	73
Left atrial flutter ablation	5	6	4	0	15
Ablation for SVT	4	2	2	0	8
Unspecified	62	32	9	13	116
Total RF ablation procedures	611	251	71	19	952
Other Procedures					
Cryoablation	8	4	0	0	12
Maze	20	3	1	2	26
Mini-maze	29	3	6	2	40
AV node ablation + pacemaker	9	3	1	2	15
Total other procedures	66	13	8	6	93
GRAND TOTAL	677	264	79	25	1045
% undergoing procedure	100	39	12	4	-

The majority of procedures (90%) were radiofrequency (RF) ablation procedures. Thirty-nine percent of the 677 respondents underwent a second procedure, 12% a third procedure, and 4% underwent further procedures. The most widely used AF ablation procedure was the generic pulmonary vein ablation (PVA) followed by the pulmonary vein antrum isolation (Natale), the segmental PVI (Haissaguerre), and the circumferential PVI (Pappone).

Demographics

Demographics	Male	Female	Total
Gender distribution, %	78	22	100
Average (median) age, yrs*	58	59	58
Median age at diagnosis, yrs(1)	47	49	48
Age range at diagnosis, yrs(1)	5-74	10-79	5-79
Years since diagnosis(1)	8	8	8
Years since diagnosis (range)	1-45	1-44	1-45
Underlying heart disease, %	9	7	8
LAF confirmed by diagnosis, %	92	90	92
Median age at last proc., yrs(1)	56	56	56
Age range (last proc.), yrs(1)	26-81	26-85	26-85

* At time of completing survey
(1) From 2007 ablation/maze survey

There are no significant differences between males and females as far as demographic variables are concerned.

Afib type and burden

A total of 584 respondents had provided detailed information regarding their type of AF (adrenergic, mixed, vagal) prior to their procedure. The distribution was as follows:

Type of AF	Male	Female	Total
# of respondents	453	131	584
Adrenergic, %	5	4	5
Mixed, %	43	48	44
Vagal, %	25	24	24
Total paroxysmal, %	72	76	73
Persistent, %	10	10	10
Permanent, %	17	15	17
TOTAL, %	100	100	100
NOTE: 93 respondents were uncertain as to which type of afib they had			

The majority of the 2008 respondents (73%) had paroxysmal AF, while 10% had persistent, and 17% had permanent AF. Mixed (random) AF was the most common paroxysmal type for both sexes followed by vagal and adrenergic.

Although not specifically dealt with in this survey, the 2007 survey did provide data concerning the frequency of episodes and the total burden (frequency x duration) experienced among 478 afibbers.

The majority of respondents (79%) experienced episodes at least once a week and 40% were in afib every day (including permanent afibbers). Only 6% of those seeking a cure through ablation or surgical procedures had episodes less frequent than once a month. This indicates that most afibbers only opt for a procedure when the frequency of episodes becomes intolerable or permanent AF becomes a reality.

The median duration of paroxysmal episodes was 9 hours with a wide range of from a few minutes to 120 hours. There was no statistically significant difference in afib burden between paroxysmal afibbers taking antiarrhythmics or blockers and those taking no medications on a continuous basis.

The total average (median) burden over a 3-month period was 208 hours for mixed afibbers, 163 hours for vagal afibbers, and 104 hours for adrenergic.

Radiofrequency LAF Ablations

Demographics
A total of 552 afibbers underwent a RF ablation of the left atrium for the purpose of curing afib as their first procedure. The majority of the 481 respondents who knew their type of afib had the paroxysmal form (74%), 10% had persistent afib, while the remaining 16% were in permanent afib. Among the 352 paroxysmal afibbers who were aware of the initiating circumstances for their episodes, 58% characterized themselves as mixed, 35% were vagal, and 7% were adrenergic.

Twenty-three percent of respondents were female. Six percent of respondents had been diagnosed with heart disease.

Initial procedure results
Only afibbers who had undergone their first RF ablation at least 6 months prior to completing the survey questionnaire were considered in this evaluation in order to avoid making premature conclusions as to success. Thus, 475 afibbers who knew the outcome of their first ablation were included.

Ablation Outcome	# in Group	Complete Success, %	Partial Success, %	Failure, %
Adrenergic	20	44	6	50
Mixed	188	35	6	58
Vagal	99	33	3	64
Paroxysmal – not sure	49	24	7	69
Total paroxysmal	356	33	6	61
Persistent	42	46	8	46
Permanent	70	42	5	53
Not sure	7	29	14	57
GRAND TOTAL	475	34	5	61
Other Possible Variables				
Underlying heart disease	30	20	7	73
Outcome for males	367	36	4	61
Outcome for females	108	28	10	62

The overall rate of complete success (no afib, no antiarrhythmics) for a first RF ablation was 34%. The rate of partial success (no afib, but on antiarrhythmics) was 5%, and the overall failure rate was a disappointing 61%. There were no statistically significant differences in success or failure rates between the three types of paroxysmal AF (adrenergic, mixed and vagal). The failure rate for afibbers with underlying heart disease was somewhat higher than the average; however, this difference was not statistically significant, nor was the difference in complete success between male and female ablatees.

The overall complete success rate (34%) for the initial RF ablation is clearly disappointing. However, as previous surveys have shown, success rates are mostly dependent on the skill and experience of the EP performing the procedure. The possible influence of episode duration and frequency on procedure outcome was evaluated in the 2007 ablation/maze survey. Episode duration, somewhat surprisingly, did not play a statistically significant role in determining the outcome of the first ablation. The risk of failure did, however, increase with increasing episode frequency. Afibbers who experienced episodes every week or more frequently had a 65% risk of failure, while those with less frequent episodes had a failure risk of 49%. This difference is statistically significant (p=0.03) and may indicate that ablation should be considered if episode frequency approaches once a week. However, in assessing the validity of any possible correlation such as this, it should always be kept in mind that the overriding factors in any evaluation of ablation success are the skills and experience of the EP performing the procedure.

Second and third procedure results
Only afibbers who had undergone their 2nd and 3rd afib ablations at least 6 months prior to completing the survey and were certain of the outcome were included in this tabulation in order to avoid making premature conclusions as to success. Results are presented in the table below.

Procedure Outcome	# in Group	Complete Success, %	Partial Success, %	Failure, %
1st procedure	475	34	5	61
2nd procedure	193	34	5	61
3rd procedure	46	35	17	48
Total/average	714	34	6	60

The percentage of complete success of the 2nd and 3rd procedures is not significantly different from that of the first procedure, thus supporting the claim by many EPs that a follow-up procedure is not materially different from the initial procedure. The remainder of this section will thus combine the results for all RF afib ablation procedures for which the outcome is known (after a 6-month wait period) including the 4th, 5th and 6th procedures.

It is of interest to note that the rate of partial success (no afib, but on antiarrhythmic drugs) is substantially higher after the 3rd procedure than after the 1st and 2nd procedures (17% vs. 5%). This difference is statistically highly significant and may indicate that the chance of antiarrhythmics working is greater after multiple ablations.

Procedure Outcome – Left Atrial RF Ablation

Complete Success by Year of Procedure, %					
Procedure	1998-2004 Success	2005 Success	2006 Success	2007-08 Success	1998-2008 Success
Focal ablation	11	30	33	33	19
PV ablation (PVA)	19	37	26	43	28
Segmental PVI	32	43	43	41	40
Circumferential PVI	30	20	18	67	34
Antrum PVI (PVAI)	52	63	63	59	59
Unspecified	11	18	11	38	18
Total/Average	24	39	33	48	34
# of procedures	276	148	140	165	729

The average complete success rate for 729 individual left atrium RF ablation procedures (including 4th, 5th, and 6th) performed during the period 1998-2008 was 34%. Complete success rates have doubled from the average 24% observed for the 1998-2004 period to 48% for the year 2007 and first 4 months of 2008. This remarkable improvement in single procedure success is reflected in an overall average increase in final (complete) success rate from 47% in the period 1998-2004 to 66% in the period 2007-2008.

The most successful procedure is clearly the pulmonary vein antrum isolation procedure (Natale method) with an average single procedure success rate of 59%. The second most successful procedure is the segmental PVI (Haissaguerre method) as practiced in Bordeaux and several other clinics with an average single procedure success rate of 40%. The circumferential PVI (Pappone method) had an overall success rate of 34%, but improved markedly in the last year or so to reach an average complete success rate of 67%. This remarkable improvement could be due to the introduction of more reliable mapping procedures, the increasing experience of the EPs performing the procedure, but could also be due to a preference for selecting paroxysmal afibbers for the procedure. In the period 2007-2008, 95% of patients undergoing the circumferential procedure had the paroxysmal form of AF. In contrast, only 65% of patients undergoing the pulmonary vein antrum isolation procedure had paroxysmal AF. Similarly, only 62% of afibbers treated with the segmental procedure had paroxysmal AF.

The usage pattern of the different procedures in relation to the type of afib ablated is shown below.

Success Rate – Single Procedure, 2005-08							
		Procedure Use, %			Complete Success Rate, %		
Procedure	# in Group	Parox.	Persist.	Perm.	Parox.	Persist.	Perm.
Focal ablation	28	71	7	21	35	100	0
PV ablation (PVA)	129	79	12	9	36	38	18
Segmental PVI	85	74	12	14	40	40	58
Circumferential PVI	50	90	6	4	36	67	0
Antrum PVI (PVAI)	99	65	7	28	69	57	46
Unspecified	51	76	6	18	21	100	0
Total/Average	-	75	9	15	41	51	32
# in group	442	333	41	68	137	21	22

It is clear that the circumferential PVI is primarily used in paroxysmal afib and has an average success rate for this type (36%). The PVAI procedure, on the other hand, has an excellent success rate for both paroxysmal (69%) and permanent (46%) afib, and only 65% of patients undergoing this procedure had paroxysmal afib. The best success rate for permanent afib (58%) was observed for the segmental PVI, no doubt, because 67% of the procedures were carried out by the Bordeaux team of Profs. Haissaguerre and Jais. Similarly, the 46% success rate for single procedure PVAI for permanent afib is, no doubt, due to the fact that 66% of the procedures were carried out by Dr. Natale. The average success rate for persistent afib was surprisingly high at 51%. I have no explanation for this other than the fact that most procedures for persistent afib were carried out at top-ranked institutions.

Adverse events

The 2008 ablation/maze survey did not specifically enquire about adverse events. However, the 2006 survey did and since the incidence of adverse events is an important consideration in deciding on an ablation, I have repeated the results of the 2006 survey.

The tables below show the incidence of adverse events that occurred during or shortly following 358 RF ablation procedures performed during the period 1998-2006. Fifty-nine percent of all procedures were not accompanied by an adverse event, while 41% were associated with one or more events.

Incidence of Adverse Events, %						
	1998-2004			2005-06		
	Compl. Success	Part. Success	Failure	Compl. Success	Part. Success	Failure
None	74	63	55	69	30	48
One or more	26	38	45	31	70	52
Total, %	100	100	100	100	100	100

Incidence of Adverse Events, %				
1998-2006				
	Compl. Success	Part. Success	Failure	Total Events
None	71	50	52	59%
One or more	29	50	48	41%
Total, %	100	100	100	100

It is clear that the risk of adverse events is substantially higher in the case of a failed ablation (48%) than in the case of a successful one (29%). This difference is statistically very significant (p=0.002). About 70% of all adverse events reported were fully resolved at the time the survey was completed.

The following tables show the distribution of events. The percentage of events relates to the number of procedures (not the total number of events). Thus, the sum of adverse events and no adverse events may not always equal 100% since some procedures were accompanied by more than one adverse event.

Type of Adverse Events, %						
	1998-2004			2005-06		
	Compl. Success	Part. Success	Failure	Compl. Success	Part. Success	Failure
None	74	63	55	69	30	48
Hematoma	13	13	19	14	10	21
TIA	2	0	1	0	0	1
Stroke	0	0	2	0	0	0
PV stenosis	2	0	6	0	10	0
Pericarditis	0	0	3	3	10	1
Tamponade	0	0	2	0	0	0
Fistula	2	0	0	0	0	0
Left flutter	2	31	12	8	20	21
Right flutter	2	0	8	3	30	8
Minor events	5	0	3	7	10	1
Life-threat.	0	0	1	0	0	0
Permanent	0	0	2	0	0	0

Type of Adverse Events, %				
1998-2006				
	Compl. Success	Part. Success	Failure	Total Events
None	71	50	52	59%
Hematoma	13	12	20	17%
TIA	1	0	1	0.8%
Stroke	0	0	1	0.6%
PV stenosis	1	4	4	2.5%
Pericarditis	1	4	3	2.1%
Tamponade	0	0	2	0.8%

Type of Adverse Events, %				
1998-2006				
	Compl. Success	Part. Success	Failure	Total Events
Fistula	1	0	0	0.3%
Left atrial flutter	5	27	15	12%
Right atrial flutter	2	12	8	6%
Minor events	6	4	3	4%
Life-threatening.	0	0	1	0.6%
Permanent	0	0	1	0.6%

Over the period 1998-2006 hematoma in the groin and thigh area was the most common adverse effect at 17%.

Fortunately, this adverse event was short-lived and was completely resolved at the time the survey was submitted. The second most common adverse event was the development of post-procedural left atrial tachycardia/flutter. This complication arose in 44 of 358 procedures (12%). The left atrial tachycardia/flutter resolved on its own in about 40% of cases, but 6 (14%) ablatees underwent another ablation to deal with it. Post-procedure right atrial flutter was reported by 22 ablatees (6%) and 8 (36%) subsequently underwent an ablation to eliminate it.

In the remaining 64% the right atrial flutter was temporary and resolved itself prior to completion of the survey. NOTE: One hundred and fourteen (32%) of all ablation procedures included a right atrial flutter ablation as a precautionary measure.

Minor reversible events occurred during 4% of all procedures, pulmonary vein stenosis during 2.5%, and stroke and TIA accounted for 0.6% and 0.8% respectively. Tamponade (piercing of the heart wall) occurred during 3 procedures and thus accounted for 0.8% of events, pericarditis (inflammation of the heart wall) followed 8 procedures (2.1%), and one ablatee experienced a non-fatal fistula (0.3%). One respondent sustained permanent damage to the mitral valve, and another experienced a life-threatening event.

Afib episodes after procedure(s)
Questions about the occurrence of afib episodes after each procedure were not included in the 2008 survey, so the results from the 2007 survey are repeated below.

Continuing AF Episodes				
	# in Group	Complete Success, %	Partial Success, %	Failure, %
None	156	69	33	8
Less than 1 month	83	12	27	21

Continuing AF Episodes				
	# in Group	Complete Success, %	Partial Success, %	Failure, %
One month	21	7	3	3
Two months	30	6	7	7
Three months	21	3	3	5
More than 3 mos.	155	2	27	56
TOTAL	466	100	100	100

Complete success was associated with only an 11% incidence of continuing afib episodes after the first, often unstable month. Failure, on the other hand, was associated with a 68% incidence of continuing episodes after the first month. This difference was extremely significant ($p < 0.0001$). It is also evident that experiencing episodes beyond 3 months post-procedure is a strong indicator of ultimate failure. While only 2% of successfully ablated afibbers experienced episodes beyond 3 months, 56% of those ultimately unsuccessful did. These findings support the observation made by Italian researchers that patients who continue to have episodes beyond the first month post-procedure only have a 10% probability of eventual cure [1].

Recovery time

A question about recovery time was not included in the 2008 ablation/maze survey, so the results from the 2007 survey are repeated below.

Time to Full Recovery					
	# in Group	Complete Success, %	Partial Success, %	Failure, %	Average, %
Less than 1 month	96	28	29	33	31
1-2 months	84	26	25	28	27
2-3 months	54	24	8	14	17
More than 3 mos.	75	21	38	25	24
TOTAL	309	100	100	100	100

About 58% of all ablatees recovered fully in less than 2 months, but 24% took longer than 3 months to return to their pre-ablation level of stamina.

Patient Outcome

Four hundred and sixty-one patients had undergone one or more RF ablation procedures in order to cure their AF, knew the outcome of their final procedure, and had gone at least 6 months since that last procedure. The average (median) observation period after the most recent ablation was 18 months with a range of 6 months to 11 years.

Two hundred and fifty-six of the 461 respondents (56%) were no longer experiencing afib episodes and were no longer taking antiarrhythmic drugs (compete success). Ten percent were also afib-free, but only with the help of antiarrhythmics (partial success), while the remaining 156 (34%) were still experiencing episodes with or without the use of antiarrhythmics. Thus, the overall outcome after an average 1.5 procedures per patient was as follows:

	Objective Judgment	Subjective Judgment
Complete success	56%	64%
Partial success	10%	20%
Failure	34%	16%
TOTAL	100%	100%

The subjectively judged success rate is clearly higher than actually warranted by the actual outcome. It is likely that some afibbers considered their procedure a success even though they still experienced episodes, but generally of lesser frequency and/or shorter duration. Many also were less sensitive to former triggers adding to the feeling of success.

In interpreting the objective judgment numbers, it should be kept in mind that they are applicable to the 11-year period 1998-2008. If only the latest period 2007-2008 is considered, then the percentages become:

	Objective Judgment
Complete success	66%
Partial success	8%
Failure	26%
TOTAL	100%

Trigger avoidance
While 79% of successful ablatees no longer needed to avoid previous triggers, only 23% of those having undergone an unsuccessful procedure were so lucky. Nevertheless, it would seem that any ablation, whether successful or not, does help to reduce trigger sensitivity.

Trigger Avoidance					
	# in Group	Complete Success, %	Partial Success, %	Failure, %	Average, %
No longer necessary	264	79	51	23	57
Still necessary	85	5	16	42	18
Much less sensitive	72	10	18	24	16
Uncertain	39	6	14	11	8
TOTAL	460	100	100	100	100

Changes in heart rate

The 2008 ablation/maze survey did not enquire about post-procedural changes in heart rate. However, the 2007 survey did and produced the following results. Changes in resting heart rate after RF ablation were quite common among paroxysmal and persistent afibbers.

Changes in Heart Rate					
	# in Group	Complete Success, %	Partial Success, %	Failure, %	Average, %
Increase	137	67	56	41	57
No change	67	23	36	33	28
Decrease	36	10	8	26	15
TOTAL	240	100	100	100	100

The most frequent post-procedural change was an increase in heart rate (experienced by 57%). This increase was most common among afibbers who had undergone successful procedure(s) (67%) and least common among those whose procedures had failed to cure the afib (41%). This difference was statistically significant (p=0.04). A decrease in heart rate was fairly rare among successfully ablated afibbers (10%), but more common (26%) among those whose procedure had failed.

The reason for the increase in heart rate after an ablation is that a significant portion of vagal nerve endings is damaged during the RF ablation procedure. Because the vagal nerves imbedded in the myocardium serve as "speed controllers" counteracting the adrenergic influence, a reduction in the number of effective vagal nerves would be expected to lead to an increased heart rate. Thus, it is possible that a more "aggressive" ablation, as indicated by a higher heart rate after the procedure, is more likely to be successful. However, this is speculation on my part and obviously assumes that the "aggression" is directed at the right spots on the atrium walls and pulmonary vein ostia.

It is generally assumed that the increase is temporary; however, this may not always be the case. A mini-survey (2006 survey) of 25 afibbers who had experienced a significant increase (average of 20 bpm) in post-procedure resting heart rate revealed that for 13 out of 25 respondents (52%) the heart rate was still significantly elevated a year or more after the last procedure. From personal experience I know that a substantial increase in heart rate (to 90 bpm or higher) can be very uncomfortable, so it is to be hoped that afib researchers will eventually address this problem.

Post-procedure arrhythmias

One hundred and forty-seven afibbers provided data as to whether they had experienced episodes of ectopics (PACs and PVCs), supraventricular tachycardia (SVT) including inappropriate sinus tachycardia, or flutter beyond 6 months following their final left atrium ablation procedure for the purpose of curing afib. When completing the survey they had five choices in answering the questions:

1. Do you still experience ectopics?
2. Do you still experience tachycardia?
3. Do you still experience flutter?

The five possible answers were:
- Yes
- No
- No, but did experience episodes for some time following the procedure
- No, never did experience episodes after the procedure
- Not sure

The answers were evaluated against the following two variables:

- Success of left atrium ablation procedure
- Previous or concomitant right atrial flutter ablation

	# in Group	Never, %	No, %	Sometimes, %	Yes, %	Unsure, %
Experiencing Post-Procedure Ectopics						
Related to outcome of ablation(1)						
Compl. success	103	2	29	8	50	12
Failure	34	0	21	0	71	9
Related to right atrial flutter ablations(2)						
None previous	74	3	22	7	59	10
Right flutter abl.	73	4	24	7	50	15

(1) Outcome of final RF ablation in left atrium
(2) Right atrial flutter ablation as part of left atrium ablation, or separate procedure preceding final left atrium ablation

It is clear that continuing to experience episodes of ectopic beats (PACs and PVCs) even 6 months following a left atrium ablation procedure is very common with 50% of ablatees having undergone a successful procedure, and 71% of those whose procedure had failed experiencing ectopics. This difference is statistically significant and shows that an increase in ectopic episodes goes hand in hand with a failed procedure. It is also clear that even a successful ablation does not solve the problem of ectopics, but merely prevents them from precipitating afib. The idea has been advanced that the ectopic beats originate in the pulmonary veins, but cannot initiate afib, because the electrical impulse generated by them is unable to cross the barrier (lesions) isolating the veins from the left atrium. I posed this possibility to Prof. Pierre Jais and his reply was, "*In my opinion, you cannot feel ectopics from the isolated veins. There is no atrial contraction associated with the isolated beat*". It is thus likely that the source of the ectopics is the atrium wall itself and that an additional ablation may be required in order to deal with them. However, I should point out that many afibbers have found that supplementation with magnesium, potassium, and taurine significantly reduces ectopics.

There was no indication that having a right atrial flutter ablation prior to or during the left atrium ablation reduced the incidence of ectopics.

	# in Group	Never, %	No, %	Sometimes, %	Yes, %	Unsure, %
Experiencing Post-Procedure Tachycardia						
Related to outcome of ablation(1)						
Compl. success	103	7	70	10	12	2
Failure	34	6	41	3	44	6
Related to right atrial flutter ablations (2)						
None previous	74	4	66	7	19	4
Right flutter abl.	73	9	59	9	22	0

(1) Outcome of final RF ablation in left atrium
(2) Right atrial flutter ablation as part of left atrium ablation, or separate procedure preceding final left atrium ablation

Tachycardia is a less common post-procedural complication than ectopics and unless actually diagnosed may be mistaken for flutter or vice versa. Again, it is clear that a failed left atrium ablation is associated with a substantially higher risk of experiencing post-procedural tachycardia than if the procedure is successful (44% vs. 12%). Having undergone a right atrial flutter ablation as part of or prior to the left atrium ablation did not affect the incidence of post-procedure tachycardia.

	# in Group	Never, %	No, %	Sometimes, %	Yes, %	Unsure, %
Experiencing Post-Procedure Flutter						
Related to outcome of ablation(1)						
Compl. success	103	11	72	5	7	6
Failure	34	0	32	3	41	24
Related to right atrial flutter ablations(2)						
None previous	74	7	62	5	14	12
Right flutter abl.	73	9	62	5	15	8

(1) Outcome of final RF ablation in left atrium
(2) Right atrial flutter ablation as part of left atrium ablation, or separate procedure preceding final left atrium ablation

The incidence of post-procedure flutter is substantially higher in the case of a failed left atrium ablation than in the case of a successful one (41% vs. 7%). Unfortunately, I have no data to enable me to determine whether the flutter originated in the left or right atrium. However, the finding that having undergone a right atrial flutter ablation made no difference to the incidence of post-procedural flutter may indicate that most of the post-procedure flutter was left atrial flutter.

Quality of life

Although the main concern of the medical profession when it comes to lone atrial fibrillation is stroke risk, the overwhelming concern of the patient is quality of life. As all afibbers know, being in permanent afib or awaiting the next episode in a state of anxiety has a devastating effect on ones quality of life and radically changes the life of those nearest and dearest to us.

Considering quality of life improvement rather than strictly success or failure of RF ablation procedures, it becomes clear that even a failed ablation may improve life quality. The average complete success rate found in this survey (after an average 1.5 procedures) is 56%. Adding to this partial success (where afib is kept at bay with antiarrhythmics) brings the percentage of afibbers whose lives have been improved through RF ablation to 66%. Further considering that, according to the 2007 ablation/maze survey, about 70% of ablatees whose procedure failed still reduced their afib burden by at least 50% brings one to the conclusion that RF ablation, whether successful or not, is likely to improve quality of life in close to 90% of those undergoing the procedure. A significant portion of the remaining 10% may however, see a worsening of their condition or may experience a serious adverse event.

Performance Rating – LAF Ablation Procedures

Previous ablation/maze surveys have all arrived at the conclusion that the most important factor in determining the outcome of a RF ablation is the skill and experience of the EP performing it. In order to provide some guidance in regard to the likelihood of undergoing a successful left atrium AF ablation at a particular institution, I have developed a Performance Rating scheme. This rating takes into account the success rates reported by afibbers treated at specific institutions and by specific EPs. The rating is calculated using the following rating scores:

Success score
- Completely successful left atrium ablation Score = 10
- Partially successful left atrium ablation   Score = 5
- Failed ablation (continuing afib episodes) Score = 0

Please note that in this evaluation of 729 single RF left atrium afib ablation procedures, a procedure is not considered a failure unless followed by another RF left atrium afib ablation or continued afib episodes. The subsequent occurrence of left or right atrial flutter or tachycardia is treated here as an adverse event and not as an ablation failure.

It is clear that a performance rating is not very indicative in cases where just one or two procedures have been performed. Thus, performance ratings have only been established for institutions that had reports on 6 or more procedures. The data used to calculate performance ratings [ranked by complete success rate] is presented below [in detail for 15 institutions with a performance rating of 3.0 or higher [Top-ranked] and in summary for the remaining 13 institutions].

Single Procedure Performance Rating						
Rank	Institution	# of Proced.	Rating	Complete Success	Partial Success	Failure, %
1	Cleveland Clinic, OH	83	6.4	61%	6%	33
2	Cleveland Clinic, FL	7	7.1	57%	29%	14
3	California Pacific(1)	55	5.9	56%	5%	38
4	Mayo Clinic, MN	14	5.7	50%	14%	36
5	Freeman Hospital	8	5.0	50%	0%	50
6	Bordeaux, France	73	4.7	47%	1%	52
7	MUSC	11	5.0	45%	9%	45
8	Univ. of Pennsylvania	20	5.0	45%	10%	45
9	Good Samaritan, CA	14	4.3	43%	0%	57
10	Loyola Medical, IL	7	4.3	43%	0%	57
11	Sequoia,Redwood City	11	3.6	36%	0%	64
12	Johns Hopkins	6	5.0	33%	33%	33
13	Aurora/Sinai,	6	4.2	33%	17%	50
14	Univ. of Michigan	13	3.5	31%	8%	62
15	NYU Medical Center	14	3.2	29%	7%	64
	Total top-ranked	342	5.3	50%	6%	44
	Other institutions	387	2.4	21%	5%	74
	All institutions	729	3.7	34%	6%	60

(1) Includes procedures carried out by Drs. Natale and Hao at Marin General

The statistics presented above are indeed sobering. Undergoing a single RF ablation procedure of the left atrium at an institution not included in the top 15 is associated with an average complete success rate of 21%, a partial success rate of 5%, and a failure rate of 74%.

The following electrophysiologists performed the procedures in the top-ranked institutions:

Institution	Electrophysiologists
Cleveland Clinic, OH	Drs. Andrea Natale*, Robert Schweikert**, Walid Saliba, Patrick Tchou, Oussama Wazni
Cleveland Clinic, FL	Dr. Sergio Pinski
California Pacific	Drs. Andrea Natale, Steven Hao
Mayo Clinic, Rochester, MN	Drs. Douglas Packer, Thomas Munger, Paul Friedman, Peter Brady
Freeman, Newcastle, UK	Dr. Stephen Furniss***
Bordeaux, France	Drs. Michel Haissaguerre, Pierre Jais
MUSC	Dr. Marcus Wharton
University of Pennsylvania	Drs. David Callans, Frank Marchlinski, David Lin
Good Samaritan, Los Angeles	Drs. Anil Bhandari, Neala Hunter, David Cannom, Mark Girski
Loyola Medical, Maywood, IL	Drs. David Wilber, Albert Lin
Sequoia, Redwood City, CA	Drs. Rob Patrawala, Roger Winkle
Johns Hopkins	Drs. Hugh Calkins, Ronald Berger
Aurora/Sinai, Milwaukee, WI	Dr. Jasbir Sra
University of Michigan	Drs. Fred Morady, Hakan Oral, Frank Pelosi, Eric Good
NYU Medical Center	Dr. Larry Chinitz

NOTE: 90% of the procedures performed at the Cleveland Clinic, OH were done by Dr. Natale or Dr. Schweikert

* Now at St. David's Medical Center, Austin, TX and California Pacific Medical Center, San Francisco
** Now at Akron General Medical Center, OH
*** Now at Eastbourne General Hospital, East Sussex, UK

The average performance rating for the top-ranked institutions is 5.3 as compared to 2.4 for the remaining institutions (387 single procedures). In evaluating the results for the top-ranked institutions it should be kept in mind that some may have a greater load of "difficult cases" than do others. The following table shows the relative proportion of paroxysmal, persistent, and permanent afibbers treated at the top-ranked institutions.

It is clear that a significant percentage of procedures performed at the Cleveland Clinic in Ohio (31%), Hopital Cardiologique du Haut Leveque in Bordeaux (30%), California Pacific Medical Center in San Francisco (37%), Good Samaritan Hospital in Los Angeles (46%), and Sequoia Hospital in Redwood City, CA (36%) involved patients with permanent or persistent afib. In contrast, the cases treated at Freeman Hospital in Newcastle, UK, the Cleveland Clinic in Weston, FL, Medical University of South Carolina, NYU Medical Center, Johns Hopkins, and the Mayo Clinic in Rochester did not include any permanent or persistent afibbers.

Institution	# of Procedures.	Paroxysmal %	Persistent %	Permanent %
Cleveland Clinic, OH	83	69	7	24
Cleveland Clinic, FL	7	100	0	0
California Pacific*	55	63	2	35
Mayo Clinic, MN	14	100	0	0
Freeman Hospital	8	100	0	0
Bordeaux, France	73	70	15	15
MUSC	11	100	0	0
Univ. of Pennsylvania	20	85	10	5
Good Samaritan, CA	14	54	23	23
Loyola Medical, IL	7	86	0	14
Sequoia, RedwoodCity	11	64	18	18
Johns Hopkins	6	100	0	0
Aurora/Sinai,Milwaukee	6	67	0	33
Univ. of Michigan	13	85	8	8
NYU Medical center	14	100	0	0
Total top-ranked	342	74	8	18
Other institutions	387	80	9	11
All institutions	729	77	9	14

*Includes procedures carried out by Drs. Natale and Hao at Marin General

Final outcome

The ultimate measure of success for the individual patient is, of course, whether or not they are cured of afib irrespective of how many procedures it takes. In other words, the crucial question to an afibber seeking a solution is, "If I go to institution X what are my chances of getting cured?"

This part of the evaluation includes 461 individual patients whose last reported procedures were RF ablations in the left atrium for the purpose of curing AF. All patients reported their afib status 6 months following their last procedure. The patients underwent a total of 729 procedures at 168 different institutions. A substantial number of the 200 repeat ablations were performed at institutions other than the ones doing the original procedure, so as far as this evaluation is concerned, a total of 531 patients were treated. Results of the evaluation are presented in the following table.

Final Performance Rating – Top-Ranked Institutions							
Rank	Institution	# of Proced.	# of Patien	Repeat Rate,%	Compl. Succ.%	Partial Succ.%	Fail. %
1	Cleveland Clinic, OH	83	72	15	72	7	21
2	Bordeaux, France	73	47	55	72	2	26
3	California Pacific	55	46	20	67	7	26
4	Cleveland Clinic, FL	7	6	17	67	33	0
5	Freeman Hospital	8	6	33	67	0	33
6	Mayo Clinic, MN	14	11	27	64	18	18
7	MUSC	11	8	38	63	13	25
8	Good Samaritan	14	10	40	60	0	40

Final Performance Rating – Top-Ranked Institutions							
Rank	Institution	# of Proced.	# of Patien	Repeat Rate, %	Compl. Succ, %	Partial Succ, %	Fail. %
9	Univ. Pennsylvania	20	16	25	56	13	31
10	Loyola	7	6	17	50	0	50
11	Sequoia	11	8	38	50	0	50
12	Aurora/Sinai	6	4	50	50	25	25
13	Johns Hopkins	6	5	20	40	40	20
14	Univ. of Michigan	13	9	44	44	11	44
15	NYU Medical Cen	14	8	63	38	13	50
	Total top-ranked	342	262	30	65	8	27
	Other institutions	387	269	44	32	7	61
	All institutions	729	531	37	48	8	44

NOTES:
- Ranking is by highest % of patients achieving complete elimination of AF without use of antiarrhythmics
- Repeat rate is calculated as # of repeat ablations divided by # of initial procedures performed at the institutions
- First repeat procedure on patients who came to the institution from another one is not counted as a repeat

The average complete success rate for the 15 top-ranked institutions is 65% with a failure rate of 27%. This compares to a complete success rate of 32%, and a failure rate of 61% at other than top-ranked institutions. The average repeat rate is 30% at top-ranked institutions versus 44% at other institutions.

In evaluating the results of the final performance rating it should be kept in mind that they, in order to optimize the statistical power of the survey, reflect the 11-year period 1998-2008. Techniques and outcomes have improved markedly from the period 1998-2004 to the period 2007-2008. For example, the final success rate for the three top-rated RF ablation centers (Cleveland Clinic (Ohio), Hopital Cardiologique du Haut Leveque (Bordeaux), and California Pacific Medical center (San Francisco)) has increased almost 10% to average 82% for the period 2007-2008. A very encouraging trend indeed!

The repeat rate of 55% at Hopital Cardiologique Haut Leveque in Bordeaux is particularly high. This is likely due to the fact that most patients treated in Bordeaux have traveled long distances to get there and probably do not fancy repeating the trip. Thus, the Bordeaux team, at least until recently, used to perform a touch-up procedure as soon as one week following the initial procedure if the patient showed any signs at all that the ablation had not been successful. Over half of the repeat procedures done in Bordeaux were performed within the first month following the initial procedure. Since the first 3 months following an ablation is usually considered a blanking period where irregular heart activity is common without necessarily predicting ultimate failure, it is likely that some of the repeat procedures may not have been necessary, but were done anyway in order to ensure, as far as possible, that the patient returned home cured.

Comparison with other surveys

In 2005 a group of American, British, Italian, and Japanese electrophysiologists published a survey of catheter ablation success rates in 90 centers across the world [Cappato Survey]. The study involved a total of 8745 patients of which 3244 underwent their procedures in a major center [having performed more than 300 procedures] while 2109 patients underwent their procedures in institutions having performed 90 or fewer procedures. [2]

A comparison of the results from the Cappato survey and the afibbers.org 2008 ablation/maze survey is presented below.

Survey	afibbers.org	Cappato
Overall outcome		
Number of patients	531	5353
Complete success	48%	52%
Partial success	8%	24%
Failure	44%	24%
Repeat rate	37%	27%
Outcome – Major centers		
Number of patients	262	3244
Complete success	65%	64%
Partial success	8%	16%
Failure	27%	20%
Repeat rate	30%	
Outcome – Other centers		
Number of patients	269	2109
Complete success	32%	34%
Partial success	7%	33%
Failure	61%	33%
Repeat rate	44%	
Adverse events		
TIA	0.8%	0.7%
Stroke	0.6%	0.3%
PV stenosis	2.5%	1.6%

In 2006 a worldwide survey carried out by Fisher and colleagues at the Montefiore Medical Center in New York reported a complete success rate of 68%, a partial success rate of 8% and a failure rate of 24% for 11,132 patients undergoing pulmonary vein antrum isolation procedures [PVAI–Natale protocol]. The repeat rate was 26%. [3]

Other RF Ablation Procedures

Supraventricular tachycardia

Eight afibbers had undergone an ablation for supraventricular tachycardia (SVT), 4 as their first procedure and 4 following a left atrium ablation procedure. All but one (performed after a left atrium AF ablation) were successful.

Left atrial flutter

Five respondents had received a diagnosis of left atrial flutter as being the likely cause of their afib and underwent an ablation for this condition as their first procedure. Four of the respondents knew the outcome of the procedure and had gone at least 6 months since the procedure. One of the procedures was partially successful (no afib, but still on antiarrhythmics), but the other 3 were not. Two of the three went on to have PVIs, both of which successfully eliminated their afib.

It is estimated that about 10% of afibbers undergoing a PVI develop left atrial flutter or tachycardia following the procedure. If the flutter or tachycardia develops within the first week following the procedure, it is usually transient and requires no treatment. However, it may develop as much as 2-3 months post-procedure and, in this case, treatment is usually required. Treatment may involve re-isolation of the pulmonary veins or the placement of linear ablation lesions to interrupt the flutter circuit.

Ten respondents underwent a left atrial flutter ablation subsequent to a PVI. I have insufficient data to determine the success of these ablations as far as elimination of the flutter is concerned.

Right atrial flutter

Seventy-three respondents had undergone a right atrial flutter ablation either as an initial procedure (50 respondents) or as a follow-up after a PVI, mini-maze or unsuccessful right atrial flutter ablation (23 respondents). In addition, 254 left atrium ablation procedures included a routine right atrial flutter ablation, while 379 did not. The need for a subsequent right atrial flutter ablation was 0.8% in the group having undergone the routine flutter ablation versus 1.8% in the group that did not. This difference was not statistically significant.

Forty-seven of the 50 respondents who underwent a right atrial flutter ablation as their first procedure reported the outcome at least 6 months after their procedure. Five of the procedures were completely successful in eliminating the afib (11%) and 4 (9%) were partially successful (still on antiarrhythmics). Thus, in 80% of cases an initial right atrial flutter ablation failed to eliminate the underlying AF (with or without antiarrhythmics). Somewhat surprisingly, 11% of afibbers underwent a second, and even a third, right atrial flutter ablation in further attempts to cure their afib.

In this regard, it should be mentioned that only 2 of the original 50 initial procedures were carried out at top-ranked RF ablation institutions and both were followed by standard PVI ablations. All told, 56% of initial right atrial flutter ablations were followed by standard RF pulmonary vein ablations.

Atrial flutter and AF are similar in that they both involve abnormal, sustained, rapid contractions of the heart's upper chambers (atria). In atrial flutter the atria contract 220 to 350 times a minute in an orderly rhythm. In AF the rate of contraction may be as high as 500 beats/minute and the rhythm is totally chaotic. The two arrhythmias can both occur as a result of an enlarged atrium or in the aftermath of open-heart surgery, but the mechanism underlying them is quite different. Nevertheless, they can coexist in the same patient and one may convert to the other.

Because the location of the origin of atrial flutter, at least in the common type, is so well known and consistent from patient to patient radio frequency catheter ablation can be used with considerable success to permanently eradicate atrial flutter. Unfortunately, this procedure is unlikely to cure AF, which may often coexist with atrial flutter. There is also some evidence that atrial flutter patients who have a successful right atrial flutter ablation increase their risk of later developing AF by 10-22%. So undergoing RF ablation for atrial flutter may not remove the necessity of dealing with AF.

Because of the close connection between AF and atrial flutter, it was quite common, in the early days of ablation, to perform an atrial flutter ablation in the hope that it would cure the AF. The atrial flutter ablation involves only the right atrium so there is no need to pierce the septum to the left atrium as is done in a PVI.

After the 1998 discovery that 80-90% of paroxysmal episodes originate in the left atrium near the pulmonary veins, the use of the right atrial flutter ablation in an attempt to cure AF became less common, but the procedure is still used as a first attempt in patients with a combination of AF and flutter. It is, of course, also used in patients suffering from right atrial flutter only.

Summary – RF Ablation Procedures

- The 2008 ablation/maze survey included 611 respondents who had undergone a total of 952 RF ablation procedures. The outcome of 729 of these procedures was known (status reported at least 6 months following the procedure).

- The overall objectively-rated complete success rate (no afib, no drugs) for 461 afibbers after an average of 1.5 procedures per patient was 56%, partial success was achieved in 10% of cases, and 34% of all afibbers who underwent one or more RF ablations continued to experience AF episodes.

- The subjective judgment of success by ablatees was somewhat more favourable with 64% feeling that the end result was total success, 20% claiming partial success, and 16% judging their procedures as a failure.

- The objectively rated complete success rate for a single RF ablation procedure was 34% when averaged over the years 1998-2008. For the more recent period 2007-2008, the complete success rate for a single RF ablation procedure averaged 48%. This remarkable improvement in single procedure success is reflected in an overall average increase in final (complete) success rate from 47% in the period 1998-2004 to 66% in the period 2007-2008.

- The complete success rate [after an average of 1.5 procedures] for the 15 top-ranked RF ablation centers was 65% with a failure rate of 27% for the period 1998-2008. This compares to a complete success rate of 32%, and a failure rate of 61% at other than top-ranked institutions. This clearly indicates that the all-important factor in determining the outcome of an RF ablation is the skill and experience of the EP performing it.

- Techniques and outcomes have improved markedly from the period 1998-2004 to the period 2007-2008. For example, the final success rate for the three top-rated RF ablation centers (Cleveland Clinic (Ohio), Hopital Cardiologique du Haut Leveque (Bordeaux), and California Pacific Medical center (San Francisco)) has increased almost 10% to average 82% for the period 2007-2008. A very encouraging trend indeed! The average repeat rate was 30% at top-ranked institutions versus 44% at other institutions.

- The most successful procedure for the period 2005-2008 was the pulmonary vein antrum isolation procedure (Natale method) with a single procedure complete success rate of 62% (paroxysmal, persistent and permanent combined). The segmental PVI (Haissaguerre method) was the second-most successful procedure with an average complete success rate of 42%.

- While 79% of successful ablatees no longer needed to avoid previous triggers, only 23% of those having undergone an unsuccessful ablation were so lucky. Nevertheless, it would seem that any ablation, whether successful or not, does help to reduce trigger sensitivity.

- The incidence of post-procedure ectopics (PACs and PVCs) 6 months or more following the procedure was high at 50% for completely successful ablations and 71% for failed procedures, a difference that is statistically significant. There was no indication that having undergone a right atrial flutter ablation prior to or during the left atrium ablation reduced the incidence of ectopics.

- The incidence of post-procedure tachycardia (SVT and inappropriate sinus tachycardia) was 12% for completely successful and 44% for failed ablations. Having undergone a right atrial flutter ablation as part of or prior to the left atrium ablation did not affect the incidence of post-procedure tachycardia.

- The incidence of post-procedure flutter was 7% for a completely successful ablation and 41% for an unsuccessful one. Having undergone a prior right atrial flutter ablation made no difference to the post-procedure incidence of flutter perhaps indicating that most of the post-procedure flutter was left atrial flutter.

Observations from 2006 Ablation/Maze Survey

- Forty-one percent of 358 RF ablation procedures were accompanied by an adverse event, the most common (17%) being temporary hematoma in the thigh area. Left atrial tachycardia was also a fairly common adverse effect (12%), but resolved by itself in about 50% of cases. Stroke and TIA were rare at 0.6% and 0.8% respectively. About two-thirds of all adverse events were fully resolved at the time the survey was completed. Successful ablations were much less likely to be accompanied by an adverse event than were unsuccessful ones. [From 2006 survey].
- Almost 60% of ablatees recovered fully in less than 2 months, but 24% took longer than 3 months to return to their pre-ablation level of stamina. [From 2006 survey].

Observations from 2007 Ablation/maze survey

- The majority (79%) of respondents experienced AF episodes at least weekly prior to their ablation. [From 2007 survey]
- There was no evidence that age at diagnosis and ablation, gender, years of afib, or type of paroxysmal afib affected the outcome to a significant degree. However, more frequent episodes were associated with a lower success rate. [From 2007 survey]
- A significant majority (69%) of afibbers who had a completely successful ablation experienced no AF episodes at all after the procedure. Only 8% of those "doomed to failure" experienced no episodes at all after their procedure. Only 2% of completely successful ablatees experienced episodes for more than 3 months after the procedure, while 56% of unsuccessful ablatees did so.

Thus, if AF episodes continue beyond 3 months the procedure is almost certainly a failure. On the other hand, if no AF episodes occur during the first month then the procedure is likely to be a success. [From 2007 survey]

- Most (96%) of afibbers who had a completely successful ablation did not continue with warfarin, but 13% of them continued to use natural stroke prevention remedies such as fish oil, nattokinase, vitamin E and ginkgo biloba. Seventeen percent took a daily aspirin for stroke prevention. In contrast, 36% of ablatees with a failed procedure continued on warfarin. [From 2007 survey]

- Even an unsuccessful ablation resulted in a significant reduction in episode frequency in 74% of cases and in 75% of cases was associated with a significant decrease in episode duration. Overall, 70% of unsuccessfully ablated patients experienced a 50% or better decrease in their afib burden. [From 2007 survey]

- Considering a 50% or greater reduction in afib burden (frequency x duration) as an indicator of improvement, it is estimated that close to 90% of RF ablations were ultimately successful in improving quality of life. [From 2007 survey]

- A post-ablation increase in heart rate was a common occurrence. This phenomenon was more prevalent among successful ablatees (67%) than among those whose ablation had failed (41%). This may indicate that a more aggressive approach (increased destruction of vagal nerve endings) is associated with a better outcome. [From 2007 survey]

Conclusion

I have made every effort to ensure that the calculations and conclusions made in this survey are correct. I have observed good internal consistency in the data and am comforted by the fact that the success rates found in this 2008 LAF Ablation/Maze Survey agree reasonably well with those found in published studies. The LAF survey is based on a total of 729 procedures performed on 461 individual patients, not an overly large number, but enough to draw reasonably valid conclusions in general terms. Where the survey results become less "solid" are in the evaluation of the success rates of individual electrophysiologists and institutions. The ratings of the Cleveland Clinic and the Hopital Cardiologique, Bordeaux are probably reasonably indicative since they involve a reasonably large number of patients, but ratings based on just 5 or 6 patients are clearly much less reliable, and it is quite possible that larger samples would produce different results.

Nevertheless, there is still a considerable gap in outcomes between top-ranked institutions and other centers. By far the best chance of success can be had at the top-ranked institutions, particularly one of the top three. That said, it is also clear that most, probably as many as 90%, of RF ablations result in a significant improvement in quality of life whether they are completely successful or not. This also means that 10% of all afibbers embarking on the ablation path can expect no improvement and in a significant proportion, a worsening of afib or a major adverse event.

Procedures Other Than RF Ablation

The procedures used to cure atrial fibrillation can be divided into two groups – catheterization procedures and surgical procedures. Both types involve the creation of lesions on the heart wall (right and/or left atrium) in order to stop the propagation of impulses not involved in conducting the heart beat "signal" from the sino-atrial (SA) node to the atrio-ventricular (AV) node.

Catheterization procedures create the lesions from the inside via an ablation catheter threaded through the femoral vein and are performed by electrophysiologists (EPs). Surgical procedures create the lesions from the outside and access is either through incisions between the ribs or may involve open-heart surgery and the use of a heart/lung machine. Surgical procedures are carried out by cardiothoracic surgeons.

The original surgical procedure, the full maze or Cox procedure, used a cut and sew protocol for creating lesions forming a "maze" that conducted the electrical impulse from the SA to the AV node, while at the same time interrupting any "rogue" circuits. The cut and sew method has now largely been replaced by the use of RF-powered devices, but cryosurgery, microwave application, and high-intensity focused ultrasound (HIFU) have all been tried as well and are preferred by some surgeons.

The so-called mini-maze procedure also involves lesions on the outside of the heart wall, but access to the heart is through incisions between the ribs rather than via open-heart surgery. The mini-maze may involve the creation of the full maze set of lesions, but usually focuses on pulmonary vein isolation. The procedure does not involve the use of a heart/lung machine.

Most of the rogue electrical impulses that create afib originate in the area where the pulmonary veins join the left atrium. Thus, all catheterization procedures aimed at curing afib involve electrical isolation of the pulmonary veins from the left atrium wall. Depending on the origin of the afib, catheterization procedures may also involve ablations of the superior vena cava and coronary sinus (thoracic veins), linear ablation of the left atrial roof, and a standard cavotricuspid isthmus (right flutter) ablation.

Surgical procedures, except for the full maze, also focus on isolating the pulmonary veins, but in addition may involve lesion creation at specific spots located by mapping, removal of the left atrial appendage, and disconnection of the ligaments of Marshall – a potent source of vagal input.

The procedures covered in this part of the survey are cryoablation, AV node ablation + pacemaker installation, the maze procedure, and the so-called "mini-maze" procedure (thoracoscopic epicardial pulmonary vein isolation). The main difference between the full maze and the mini-maze procedure is the method of access to the heart. The maze involves a 6-12 inch long cut through the breastbone, while the mini-maze provides access through two or more 2-inch incisions between the ribs. Another important difference is that the maze procedure requires the use of a heart/lung machine, while the mini-maze does not.

Distribution of procedures

Eighty-seven afibbers had undergone one or more surgical procedures (maze, mini-maze, AV node + pacemaker installation) or cryoablation. The distribution of these procedures is detailed below.

Distribution of Procedures					
Procedures	1st	2nd	3rd	Further	Total
Cryoablation	8	4	0	0	12
Maze	20	3	1	2	26
Mini-maze	29	4	6	2	41
AV node ablation + pacemaker	9	3	1	2	15
Total	66	14	8	6	94
RF ablation*	21	18	10	5	54
Total procedures	87	32	18	11	148

*RF ablations performed before or after cryoablation, maze, mini-maze, or AV node ablation + pacemaker implantation procedure

Sixty-six respondents had undergone a surgical procedure or cryoablation as the initial attempt to cure their afib. Another 21 had theirs following an initial RF ablation – right atrial flutter (2), PVI or focal ablation (19).

Demographics and Afib Type
The general background data for the 87 respondents whose treatments for the purpose of curing atrial fibrillation included one or more cryoablation, maze, mini-maze or AV node ablations is given below.

Demographics and Afib Type			
	Male	Female	Total/Av.
Gender distribution, %	80	20	100
Average (median) age, yrs*	62	61	62
Underlying heart disease, %	22	29	23
LAF confirmed by diagnosis, %	100	100	100

	Male	Female	Total/Av.
Adrenergic, %	1	6	2
Mixed, %	37	50	39
Vagal, %	18	6	15
Uncertain, %	12	6	11
Total paroxysmal, %	68	69	68
Persistent, %	7	19	10
Permanent, %	25	13	23
TOTAL	100	100	100

* At time of completing questionnaire

The only statistically significant difference between this group and the group undergoing RF ablations is the considerably higher incidence of underlying heart disease (23% vs 8%).

The majority of the cryoablation/maze group had paroxysmal afib (68%). Mixed (random) AF was the most common type of paroxysmal afib, followed by vagal and adrenergic. There were no statistically significant differences in afib type between this group and the RF ablation group.

Cryoablation
The cryoablation procedure is similar to the standard RF ablation procedure except that the ablation catheter is cooled by liquid nitrogen or argon rather than electrically heated. The advantage of cryoablation is that it reduces procedure stroke risk and does not create pulmonary vein stenosis even if the ablation is done inside the pulmonary veins.

Eight paroxysmal afibbers with no underlying heart disease (7 male, 1 female) had undergone cryoablation as their first procedure. Three of these procedures were fully successful (no afib, no drugs) giving a first procedure complete success rate of 38%.

Three of the unsuccessful ablatees went on to have other procedures – 2 had another cryoablation of which one was a success, while the third had an unsuccessful PVI procedure. The 2 remaining unsuccessful ablatees went on to have RF ablations, one of which was successful. Two respondents underwent a cryoablation following a failed PVI. One was partially successful (afib controlled with antiarrhythmics).

The outcome (at least 6 months after procedure) was known for 12 cryoablation procedures. Four (33%) were fully successful and one (9%) was partly successful. The average single procedure complete success rate for cryoablation is thus 33%, not significantly different from the average single procedure complete success rate for PVI procedures at 34%. There is insufficient data to say what the final success rate would be after repeated cryoablations.

AV node ablation + pacemaker implantation

Palpitations, elevated heart rate, and other major symptoms of an atrial fibrillation episode are associated with rapid and irregular contractions of the left ventricle rather than with the actual "quivering" of the left atrium. So, although the root cause of AF is found in the left atrium, its symptomatic effects can, to a large extent, be eliminated by isolating the AV node (the ventricular beat controller) from impulses originating in the left atrium and feeding the ventricles their "marching orders" from an implanted pacemaker. AV node ablation + pacemaker installation is a relatively simple procedure and is therefore mostly successful. It does also provide substantial symptom relief allowing afibbers to live a fairly normal life. Nevertheless, the procedure is considered a last resort for the following reasons:

- It does nothing to stop the fibrillation in the atrium and may, in fact, hasten the progression to permanent AF.
- It does not reduce stroke risk as do successful PVIs and maze procedures. Thus, the patient must continue on warfarin for life.
- It makes the patient dependent on the pacemaker. If it or the leads malfunction, or the battery runs out the patient may die.
- It does little to prevent the fatigue and reduced exercise capacity felt by some afibbers during an episode.

Fourteen respondents (36% female) underwent AV node ablation + pacemaker implantation procedures. One had a second procedure to replace a pacemaker lead after 6 years. Of the 14 patients, 29% had underlying heart disease; the median age of the patients was 65 years.

Nine patients underwent the AV node ablation as their first procedure in an attempt to alleviate their afib symptoms (44% had underlying heart disease and 60% had permanent afib). Six patients had no further follow-up, while of the remaining three, one had a pacemaker replacement (6 years after the initial one), one had a PVI (partially successful), and one had a maze procedure (partially successful) with no further follow-up.

Two respondents underwent their AV node ablation following a failed PVI and a failed maze procedure respectively. One respondent had his procedure after 2 failed focal ablations, and one had his as a fifth procedure after 3 PVIs and a mini-maze. Finally, one respondent had his AV node procedure after 3 failed right atrial flutter ablations and 3 failed PVIs.

It is somewhat difficult to evaluate the success of an AV node ablation + pacemaker implantation since it, at best, provides symptomatic relief only. Eighty percent of respondents felt (subjectively) that their procedure had been a success, while the remaining 20% felt that it had been partially successful.

Based on this small sample of 14 respondents, it is clear that AV node ablation + pacemaker installation is usually a successful procedure and provides significant symptomatic relief even though it does not eliminate AF. Nevertheless, it is still the procedure of last resort.

Maze procedure

Twenty-six respondents reported having undergone a full maze procedure – 20 as their initial procedure, 5 after failed PVIs or focal ablations, and 1 after an AV node ablation + pacemaker implantation. The maze group differed significantly from the group of 552 afibbers who underwent catheter ablation. While the percentage of patients in the RF ablation group who had underlying heart disease was only 6%, it was 35% in the maze group. Also, while the percentage of patients having permanent afib was only 15% in the ablation group, it was 33% in the maze group. Both differences were statistically highly significant.

Five of the 26 procedures were cryo-maze. In other words, the maze lesions were applied with a nitrogen-cooled or argon-cooled catheter rather than with RF energy or the cut-and-sew approach. Only 2 of these procedures were successful. One of the unsuccessful patients went on to undergo a pulmonary vein isolation procedure with Dr. Natale, which was a complete success.

Twenty-three patients had gone 6 months or more following their maze procedure and knew the outcome. It is problematical, perhaps even unwise, to pronounce on success rates with only 23 procedures in the sample. Nevertheless, as with catheterization procedures, there would appear to be a definite trend for procedures performed by top-ranked cardiac surgeons to be more successful than those performed by less prominent ones.

Procedural Success				
Surgeon	# of Procedures	Complete Success, %	Partial Success, %	Failure %
Top-ranked	8	88	0	13
Other	15	33	7	60
Total	23	52	4	43

It is, of course, open to argument who is and who is not "top-ranked", but I do believe that the surgeons in the above group (Drs. Niv Ad, Ralph Damiano, Dale Geiss, Marc Gillinov and Patrick McCarthy) would all fall in this category.

The complete success rate for top-ranked surgeons is thus 88%, very close to the oft-quoted 90% success rate for maze procedures. [4,5] However, the complete success rate for other than top-ranked surgeons is only 33%, very close to the 34% found for other than top-ranked EPs performing RF ablation procedures.

Our results, albeit based on a very small sample, lead to the conclusion that, just as in the case of conventional PVIs, the choice of surgeon or EP is the all-important variable with the type of procedure playing a lesser role in the final outcome.

As reported in the 2006 Ablation/Maze Survey, 7 out of 12 (58%) of patients undergoing the maze procedure experienced one or more adverse events, some of them quite serious. Two suffered a transient ischemic attack (TIA, mini-stroke), one reported excessive fluid retention, and one pericarditis. This rate of serious adverse events is higher than experienced in any other procedure.

A comparison of objective and subjective success rates show that the respondents' subjective impression of outcome is identical to the actual (objective evaluation) when it comes to complete success (no afib, no antiarrhythmics). However, it would seem that respondents were more likely to feel that even a failed procedure (still experiencing afib episodes) was at least partially successful.

	Objective Judgment	Subjective Judgment
Complete success	52%	52%
Partial success	4%	26%
Failure	43%	22%
TOTAL	99%	100%

As far as post-procedure problems (trigger avoidance, ectopics, tachycardia, flutter) are concerned, it is clear that a successful maze procedure is far less likely to be accompanied by post-procedure problems than is an unsuccessful one. Although a similar trend was observed for catheter ablations, it is far more pronounced for the full maze procedure.

Post-procedure problems		
Variable*	Complete Success, %	Failure, %
Still need to avoid triggers	15	100
Still experience ectopics	33	100
Still experience tachycardia	17	100
Still experience flutter	0	33

*As observed at least 6 months following procedure

The full maze procedure performed by a top-ranked cardiac surgeon provides the best chance of being cured of afib with one single procedure. However, full maze procedures performed by less skilled surgeons tend to be considerably less successful. This, combined with the potential for significant adverse effects (especially associated with the use of the heart/lung machine), would lead one to the conclusion that it may be "overkill" for a paroxysmal afibber, with no underlying heart disease, to select the full maze over a conventional radiofrequency PVI or mini-maze procedure.

This conclusion is supported by the following quote from an article reporting the results of 130 Cox-maze IV procedures, "It is a weakness of this study that we did not examine pulmonary vein isolation in patients who had lone AF. Further data are needed to evaluate the efficacy of this procedure in this group. However, our historical results with the cut-and-sew procedure (Cox-Maze III) had higher success rates in patients who had AF associated with concomitant cardiac pathology as opposed to those who had lone AF".[4]

Of course, the full maze procedure is obviously preferred if other heart surgery is needed.

Mini-maze procedure
Forty-one respondents (17% female) reported undergoing a mini-maze procedure, 29 as their initial procedure and 12 after one or more failed radiofrequency (RF) PVIs. The 12 patients had undergone a total of 22 PVIs before their mini-maze. Only 3 of the failed PVIs were performed at top-ranked institutions. A total of 8 patients underwent PVIs (7) or AV node ablation + pacemaker implantation (1) following a failed mini-maze. There were no repeat mini-mazes. The incidence of underlying heart disease was significantly higher in the mini-maze group than in the RF ablation group (20% vs. 6%).

The majority of procedures (84%) used RF energy in creating the ablation lesions, 13% used microwave energy, and the remaining 3% (1 procedure) used high-intensity focused ultrasound (HIFU). The HIFU procedure was unsuccessful as were 3 of the microwave procedures.

The final outcome at least 6 months following the procedure was known for 31 procedures. Of these, 13 were carried out by 4 top-ranked cardiac surgeons.

- Dr. Randall Wolf, University of Cincinnati Hospital - 8 procedures
- Dr. Michael Mack, Medical City, Dallas, TX - 3 procedures
- Dr. James Cox*, Ohio State University Hospital - 1 procedure
- Dr. Adam Saltman**, University of Massachusetts - 1 procedure

* Now medical director at ATS Medical Inc, Minneapolis, MN
** Now at Maimonides Medical Center, Brooklyn, NY

RF-powered catheters or clamps were used for lesion creation in all procedures.

Outcome of mini-maze procedures				
Surgeon	# of Procedures	Complete Success, %	Partial Success, %	Failure %
Top-ranked	13	62	8	31
Other	18	50	6	44
Total	31	55	6	39

The average complete success rate for top-ranked cardiothoracic surgeons is 62%. This is very close to the initial procedure complete success rate of 61% experienced at the Cleveland Clinic, but significantly better than the average 50% single procedure complete success rate obtained at the 15 top-ranked RF ablation institutions. Considering both top-ranked and other institutions, the 55% average complete success rate for the mini-maze is clearly superior to the average single procedure success rate of 34% for RF ablation.

The standard RF ablation can, of course, be repeated, whereas I have not seen any example of full maze and mini-maze patients being given the option of undergoing a second procedure if the initial one fails. The complete success rate after an average of 1.5 RF ablation procedures is 65% for the 15 top-ranked centers and is now 82% at the 3 top-ranked centers – Cleveland Clinic, OH, Hopital Cardiologique du Haut Leveque, Bordeaux, and California Pacific Medical Center, San Francisco. The overall mini-maze success rate of 50% with other than top-ranked surgeons is, however, superior to the "other institutions" RF ablation complete success rate of 32% after repeat ablations.

A mini-maze procedure performed by a top-ranked cardiac surgeon provides the second-best chance (after the full maze procedure) of being cured of afib with one single procedure, although the Cleveland Clinic single procedure success rate of 61% is very close. It is also likely that even a mini-maze performed by a less than top-ranked surgeon will have a substantially better outcome than a standard RF ablation performed by a less than top-ranked EP.

The incidence of adverse events (as per the 2006 survey) tended to be slightly higher than for RF ablations and involved pneumonia (9%), tamponade (4%), serious hemorrhage (4%), and subcutaneous nerve pain (4%). As far as post-procedure problems (trigger avoidance, ectopics, tachycardia and flutter) are concerned, it is clear (see Table 28) that a successful mini-maze procedure is far less likely to be accompanied by post-procedure problems than is an unsuccessful one. A similar trend has also been observed for the maze procedure and RF ablations.

Incidence of adverse events		
Variable*	Complete Success, %	Failure, %
Still need to avoid triggers	6	63
Still experience ectopics	25	100
Still experience tachycardia	10	40
Still experience flutter	10	75

*As observed at least 6 months following procedure

Published studies on effectiveness
Several studies have been published regarding the efficacy of the mini-maze procedure with complete success rates (no afib, no antiarrhythmics) varying between 58% and 91%.

- A group of cardiothoracic surgeons (including Dr. Randall Wolf) reported on the success of 27 mini-mazes performed in 2003-2004. The complete success rate (no afib, no antiarrhythmics) after 3 months was 65%, which compares well with the 62% observed in this survey for top-ranked surgeons. The average hospital stay was 3.3 days and the average procedure time was about 3 hours. [6]

- Cardiothoracic surgeons at the Ohio State University treated 32 patients with persistent or permanent afib with laparoscopic full maze procedures and observed a complete success rate of 88%. [7]

- A group of American and Japanese cardiothoracic surgeons treated 20 patients (80% paroxysmal, 20% persistent) with the mini-maze procedure and observed a complete success rate of 85% after 6 months. No major adverse events were reported. [8]

- An American team based in Florida treated 100 lone afibbers (64% paroxysmal, 11% persistent, 25% permanent) with a mini-maze procedure using microwave energy for lesion creation. [9]. The complete success rate after 6 months was only 31% and adverse effects were serious (3 patients died following the procedure, 2 patients experienced a TIA (mini-stroke), and 2 had a stroke). These results confirm the survey findings of a 25% success rate with microwave energy (based on a sample of only 4 patients).

- A team at the Nebraska Heart Hospital treated 22 paroxysmal afibbers with a mini-maze procedure and observed a complete success rate of 91% after an average follow-up of 18 months. [10]

Summary – Non RF Ablation Procedures

A total of 94 procedures, other than the conventional RF ablation (PVI), were performed in attempts to eliminate AF. The following observations were made:

- The outcome (at least 6 months after procedure) was known for 12 cryoablation procedures. Four (33%) were fully successful and one (9%) was partly successful. The average single procedure complete success rate of cryoablation is thus 33%, not significantly different from the average single procedure complete success rate of PVI procedures at 34%. There is insufficient data to say what the final success rate would be after repeated cryoablations.

- It is not possible, based on a small sample, to evaluate the success rate of an AV node + pacemaker implantation since it, at best, provides symptomatic relief only. Eighty percent of respondents felt (subjectively) that their procedure had been a success, while the remaining 20% felt that it has been partially successful. Thus, based on a small sample of 14 respondents it would appear that AV node ablation + pacemaker installation is usually a successful procedure and provides significant symptomatic relief even though it does not eliminate the fibrillation of the atria. Nevertheless, it is still the procedure of last resort.

- The full maze procedure performed by a top-ranked cardiac surgeon provides the best chance of being cured of afib with one single procedure (complete success rate of 88%). However, full maze procedures performed by less skilled surgeons tend to be considerably less successful. This, combined with the potential for significant adverse events (especially associated with the use of the heart/lung machine), would lead one to the conclusion that it may be "overkill" for a paroxysmal afibbers, with no underlying heart disease, to select the full maze over a conventional RF ablation or mini-maze procedure.

- A mini-maze procedure performed by a top-ranked cardiac surgeon provides the second-best chance of being cured of afib with one single procedure. It is also likely that even a mini-maze performed by a less than top-ranked surgeon will have a substantially better outcome than a single standard RF ablation performed by a less than top-ranked EP. However, the risk of adverse effects accompanying the mini-maze procedure is somewhat higher than for RF ablations.

REFERENCES

1. Bertaglia, E, et al. Predictive value of early atrial tachyarrhythmias recurrence after circumferential anatomical pulmonary vein ablation. PACE, Vol. 28, May 2005, pp. 366-71
2. Cappato, R, et al. Worldwide survey on the methods, efficacy, and safety of catheter ablation for human atrial fibrillation. Circulation, Vol. 111, March 8, 2005, pp. 1100-05
3. Fisher, JD, et al. Atrial fibrillation: Reaching the mainstream. PACE, Vol. 29, May 2006, pp. 523-37
4. Melby, SJ, et al. A new era in the surgical treatment of atrial fibrillation: The impact of ablation technology and lesion set on procedural efficacy. Annals of Surgery, Vol. 244, No. 4, October 2006, pp. 583-92
5. Khargi, K, et al. Surgical treatment of atrial fibrillation: A systematic review. European Journal of Cardiothorac. Surgery, Vol. 27, No. 2, February 2005, pp. 258-65
6. Wolf, RK, et al. Video-assisted bilateral pulmonary vein isolation and left atrial appendage exclusion for atrial fibrillation. Journal of Thoracic and Cardiovascular Surgery, Vol. 130, September 2005, pp. 797-802

7. Sirak, J, et al. Toward a definitive, totally thoracoscopic procedure for atrial fibrillation. Ann Thorac Surg, Vol. 86, No. 6, December 2008, pp. 1960-64

8. Matsutani, N, et al. Minimally invasive cardiothoracic surgery for atrial fibrillation. Circ J, Vol. 72, March 2008, pp. 434-36

9. Pruitt, JC, et al. Minimally invasive surgical ablation of atrial fibrillation: the thoracoscopic box lesion approach. J Interv Card Electrophysiol, Vol. 20, No. 3, December 2007, pp. 83-87

10. Wudel, JH, et al. Video-assisted epicardial ablation and left atrial appendage exclusion for atrial fibrillation. Ann Thorac Surg, Vol. 85, January 2008, pp. 34-38

2013 Ablation/Maze Survey

By Hans R. Larsen [2013]

Summary

The 2013 ablation survey involved 54 respondents who had, at least 8 years ago, undergone a total of 76 catheter ablation procedures for the purpose of curing afib.

There were no significant differences in demographics between the respondents to the 2013 survey and those participating in the 2008 survey (677 respondents having undergone 1045 procedures). Thus, the 2013 survey respondents would appear to be a representative sample of the general lone atrial fibrillation population.

Prior to their initial ablation procedure 85% of respondents experienced episodes at least once a week and 42% were in afib every day (including permanent afibbers). The majority of respondents (90%) experienced episodes lasting more than 1 hour and 39% had episodes lasting 24 hours or longer (including permanent afibbers). Only 7% of those seeking a cure through catheter ablation experienced episodes less frequent than once a month. This indicates that most afibbers only opt for a procedure when the frequency of episodes becomes intolerable or permanent AF becomes a reality.

The average paroxysmal afibber spent about 7% of their time in afib as compared to a permanent afibber who, of course, spent 100% of their time in afib. There was a trend (p=0.056) for female afibbers to spend more time (14% on average) in afib than did male afibbers (7%).

The overall mean severity score was 3.9 indicating that afibbers only opt for an ablation or surgical procedure when episodes become very symptomatic. More women (90%) than men (64%) reported a severity score of 4 or 5, but this difference was not statistically significant.

Paroxysmal, female afibbers had a statistically significant higher *Impact on Quality of Life* (IQoL) score than paroxysmal, male afibbers (54 vs. 13); this is not surprising as paroxysmal female afibbers on average spent more time in afib (14%) than did male paroxysmal afibbers (7%) and also had more severe episodes. The difference in IQoL between permanent afibbers (score of 350) and paroxysmal afibbers (average score of 14) was also statistically extremely significant (p<0.0001).

All but one of the 76 procedures reported in this survey (99%) were radiofrequency (RF) catheter ablations. Of the 54 patients undergoing RF ablation as their final or initial procedure, 32 (59%) underwent only one procedure, while 22 patients (41%) underwent 2 procedures for the purpose of curing AF.

The most widely reported ablation procedure was the pulmonary vein antrum isolation procedure (Natale protocol) at 31% of all RF ablations. The second most widely reported procedure was the segmental pulmonary vein isolation procedure (Haissaguerre protocol) at 20%.

The most successful procedures were the pulmonary vein antrum isolation (Natale protocol) and the segmental pulmonary vein isolation (Haissaguerre protocol) with success rates of 76% and 56% for the initial procedures. The poorest performers were the circumferential pulmonary vein isolation procedure (Pappone protocol), at 29%, focal ablation at 17% and generic pulmonary vein ablation at 22%. The overall success rate for initial RF ablations was 44%.

It is clear that having an initially successful final ablation is of prime importance in determining the long-term success of the procedure. The average (mean) complete success rate (no afib, no antiarrhythmics) at the end of year 8 was 86% for those whose last procedure was initially successful versus 42% for those who had not experienced an afib-free index period or who had been on antiarrhythmics during the index period. Corresponding complete success rates for year 10 were 91% and 17% respectively based on a small sample of only 15 respondents.

Of the 40 respondents who were afib-free (without the use of antiarrhythmics) in year 4 only 2 (5%) reverted to having afib episodes by year 8. One more afibber (9% of the 11 for whom data was available in year 10) reverted to having afib in year 10 indicating that status at year 4 is a good indicator of long-term prognosis.

Forty-three per cent of afibbers still experiencing afib believed that their episodes were always, or most of the time, associated with the same triggers that initiated episodes prior to the initial ablation/maze procedure for the purpose of curing afib. Only 8% were quite certain that their episodes were not associated with pre-procedure triggers, while 32% were not certain whether or not they were. Thus, it would seem prudent for afibbers who have experienced an episode following their last procedure to avoid, as much as possible, the triggers that initiated their episodes prior to undergoing the initial ablation or maze procedure.

At year 4 the afib burden and percent time spent in afib were reduced by an average (median) of 98% over the pre-ablation burden among paroxysmal afibbers whose ablation had not been successful. This was reflected in a 97% reduction in impact on quality of life. The reduction in afib burden and percent

248

time spent in afib were also reduced in year 8 as compared to pre-ablation values; however, the reduction (80%) was no longer statistically significant, but the reduction in impact on quality of life (88%) remained statistically significant. These findings may indicate that, while an unsuccessful ablation still results in a significantly lower afib burden and improved quality of life in paroxysmal afibbers at the 4 year mark, the beneficial effects of the ablation may begin to wear off at the 8 year mark.

Only 3 permanent afibbers had provided data for pre-ablation and year 8. Average reductions in afib burden and percent time spent in afib were close to 100% and reduction in impact on quality of life was 99%.

It is clear that afibbers whose latest ablation had been a complete success experienced fewer episodes of other arrhythmias (mostly ectopics) than did those who were still experiencing afib episodes (failures) or were keeping episodes at bay with antiarrhythmics (partial success). On average (over the 8-year evaluation period) 34% of afibbers having undergone a completely successful ablation experienced other arrhythmias as compared to 71% (p=0.003) among those with a partially successful ablation, and 63% (p=0.05) among afibbers with a failed ablation. The presence of other arrhythmias was still common among even successful afibbers and very common among those controlling their episodes with antiarrhythmics. The reason for this is unclear, but it may be that ectopics experienced by successful afibbers are mainly PVCs, the frequency of which would not be affected even by a successful ablation procedure. As for the high level of other arrhythmias experienced by afibbers taking antiarrhythmics, it is possible that they are related to the inherent pro-arrhythmic effect of most antiarrhythmics.

The two most important, statistically significant, factors associated with being afib-free in year 8 were not having afib episodes during the **index period** and having, as the final or only ablation, a pulmonary vein antrum isolation procedure (Natale protocol). There was a trend for having undergone the final or only procedure at a top-ranked institution to be associated with a favourable 8-year outcome, as was having been on antiarrhythmics prior to the initial procedure and not having needed antiarrhythmics during the index period.

The most important factors associated with an afib-free **index period** were:

- Having undergone the final or only ablation procedure at a top-ranked institution;
- Having, as the final or only ablation, a pulmonary vein antrum isolation procedure (Natale protocol) or a segmental pulmonary isolation procedure (Haissaguerre protocol);
- Being male;
- Not experiencing atrial fibrillation or atrial flutter during the blanking period;
- Not experiencing atrial flutter during the index period;

- Not needing beta- or calcium channel blockers during the blanking and index periods.

Survey Details

The 2008 ablation/maze survey evaluated the short- to medium-term success rates for a total of 1045 catheter ablation, maze, and mini-maze procedures involving 677 patients. The results of the survey provided a good basis for judging the likely outcome of the various procedures aimed at curing atrial fibrillation. However, the question uppermost in the mind of any afibber having undergone or contemplating a catheter ablation, maze or mini-maze procedure is "How long will a successful procedure keep me in normal sinus rhythm?" – In other words, "How long will it last?"

In the survey questionnaire the term "initially successful" is defined as not being on antiarrhythmic drugs and not having experienced any AF episodes during the last 6 months of the 12-month period following the latest procedure for the purpose of curing AF (**Index Period**). The first 6 months following the procedure is considered a "blanking period" and AF episodes and episodes of other arrhythmias do not "count" during this period.

Demographics

	2013	2008
# of participants	54	677
% male	81	78
% female	19	22
Average age at first episode, yrs	50	48
Age range at first episode, yrs	19-67	5-79
Years since diagnosis[1]	17	8
Years since diagnosis (range)[1]	8-28	1-45
Underlying heart disease, %	9	8
Enlarged left atrium, %	22	
Aver. age at last procedure, yrs	57	56
Age range at last procedure, yrs	22-72	26-85
Years to last procedure[2]	7	
Years to last procedure (range)[2]	0-20	

[1] Years [average] elapsed since first episode and completion of survey
[2] Average (median) # of years from initial diagnosis to final procedure

There are no significant differences in demographics between the respondents to the 2013 ablation/maze survey and those participating in the 2008 survey except that the 2013 respondents experienced their first afib episode 9 years earlier than did the 2008 respondents. Thus, conclusions reached in the 2013 survey should be applicable to the lone AF population in general.

Afib type

A total of 51 respondents in the 2013 survey and 584 in the 2008 survey had provided detailed information regarding their type of AF prior to their initial procedure for the purpose of curing AF. The distribution is as follows:

Type of AF	2013 Survey	2008 Survey
# of respondents	51	584
Adrenergic, %	2	5
Mixed, %	51	44
Vagal, %	23	24
Total paroxysmal, %	76	73
Persistent, %	2	10
Permanent, %	22	17
TOTAL	100	100

Again, there are no major differences in the afib type of respondents to the 2013 survey when compared to the 2008 survey.

Episode frequency

The distribution of episode frequency prior to the initial ablation procedure is presented below for the 51 afibbers participating in the 2013 survey:

Episode Frequency	Episodes/6 months	Respondents, %
Permanent (24/7)	182	20
Daily	182	22
Twice weekly	52	26
Weekly	26	17
Twice a month	12	4
Monthly	6	4
Every 2 months	3	7
TOTAL	-	100

The majority of respondents (85%) experienced episodes at least once a week and 42% were in afib every day (including permanent afibbers). Only 7% of those seeking a cure through catheter ablation procedures experienced episodes less frequent than once a month. This indicates that most afibbers only opt for a procedure when the frequency of episodes becomes intolerable or permanent AF becomes a reality.

Episode duration

The distribution of episode duration prior to the initial ablation procedure is presented in the following table:

Episode Duration	Aver. Duration, hrs	Respondents, %
Less than 30 min	0.25	2
Between 30 min and 1 hour	0.75	7

Episode Duration	Aver. Duration, hrs	Respondents, %
Between 1 and 3 hours	2	19
Between 3 and 10 hours	6	15
Between 10 and 24 hours	17	15
Between 24 and 48 hours	36	4
More than 48 hours, but self-converted	48	11
More than 7 days or required cardioversion	168	2
Permanent (24/7)	24	20
Not sure	-	5
TOTAL	-	100

The majority of respondents (90%) experienced episodes lasting more than 1 hour and 37% had episodes lasting 24 hours or longer (including permanent afibbers).

Afib burden

By multiplying the number of episodes with their average duration for each respondent it is possible to obtain an estimate of the afib burden experienced over a 6-month period for various types of AF. Results are presented below:

Afib Burden		
Average AF Burden/6 mos.	Burden, hrs.	Time Spent in AF, %
Paroxysmal male afibbers	156	4
Paroxysmal female afibbers	624	14
Vagal afibbers	260	6
Mixed afibbers	312	7
Adrenergic afibbers	144	3
Paroxysmal afibbers	312	7
Permanent afibbers	4368	100

Over a 6-month period the average paroxysmal afibber spent 7% of their time in afib (range 0.1 – 71%). There was no statistically significant difference in afib burden between the different types of paroxysmal afib nor was the difference between male and female afibbers statistically significant ($p=0.056$), although there was a trend for female paroxysmal afibbers to carry a heavier burden.

Episode severity [On a scale from 1 to 5]

1. Barely noticeable
2. Mildly symptomatic
3. Symptomatic, but tolerable
4. Very symptomatic, but tolerable
5. Debilitating

% Respondents with Indicated Score						
Severity Score (1-5)	1	2	3	4	5	Mean Score
Male afibbers	2	7	27	37	27	3.8
Female afibbers	-	-	10	40	50	4.4
Vagal afibbers	-	8	31	15	46	4.0
Mixed afibbers	-	-	19	58	23	4.0
Adrenergic afibbers	-	-	100	-	-	3.0
Paroxysmal afibbers	-	2	26	40	31	4.0
Persistent afibbers	-	-	-	-	100	5.0
Permanent afibbers	9	18	18	36	18	3.4
Overall	2	6	24	39	30	3.9

The overall mean severity score was 3.9 indicating that afibbers only opt for an ablation or surgical procedure when episodes become very symptomatic. More women (90%) than men (64%) reported a severity score of 4 or 5, but this difference was not statistically significant.

Quality of life

It may be possible to get some idea of the *impact on quality of life (IQoL)* of afib by calculating an *IQoL* score using the percent afib burden and the severity score. For a permanent afibber with disabling afib the impact on quality of life score would thus be 500 (severity score x % spent in afib), while for a person with no afib the *IQoL* score would be zero. The average (median) *IQoL* score for the entire group of respondents was 40. *IQoL* scores for various categories of afib, calculated using this definition, are shown below.

Respondents	IQoL Score
Paroxysmal male afibbers	13
Paroxysmal female afibbers	54
Vagal afibbers	40
Mixed afibbers	18
Adrenergic afibbers	10
Paroxysmal afibbers	14
Permanent afibbers	350

Paroxysmal female afibbers had a statistically significant higher *IQoL* score (poorer quality of life) than paroxysmal male afibbers (54 vs. 13); this is not surprising as paroxysmal female afibbers, on average, spent more time in afib (14%) than did male paroxysmal afibbers (4%) and also had more severe episodes. The difference in *IQoL* between permanent afibbers (score of 350) and paroxysmal afibbers (score of 14) was also statistically extremely significant ($p < 0.0001$). This is perhaps not surprising since experiencing very symptomatic afib for 24 hours a day every day must have a very detrimental impact on quality of life. On the other hand, paroxysmal afibbers suffer from the constant dread of not knowing when the next episode will happen. So overall, a paroxysmal afibber with debilitating episodes may be just as bad off psychologically as a permanent afibber with symptomatic but tolerable episodes. This whole area of the impact of afib on quality of life could certainly benefit from more research.

Procedure Outcomes

Fifty-four afibbers provided data for a total of 76 RF catheter ablation procedures. In addition to these 76 "free-standing" procedures, 31 patients also underwent a right atrial flutter ablation as part of their initial or final procedure for the purpose of curing afib. Adding these 31 procedures to the 8 performed separately means that 39 patients underwent a right atrial flutter ablation as part of their treatment to become free of arrhythmia.

Of the 54 patients undergoing RF ablation, 32 (59%) underwent only one procedure, while 22 patients (41%) underwent 2 or more procedures for the purpose of curing AF.

The most widely reported ablation procedure was the pulmonary vein antrum isolation procedure (Natale protocol) at 31% of all RF ablations. The second most widely reported procedure was the segmental pulmonary vein ablation (Haissaguerre protocol) at 20%.

Distribution of Procedures				
Number of Procedures	Initial	Final	Total	% of Total
Focal ablation	6	6	12	16
Pulmonary vein ablation (PVA)	8	1	9	12
Segmental PVI	9	6	15	20
Circumferential PVI	7	1	8	11
Antrum PVI	17	7	24	31
Unspecified	6	1	7	9
Cryoablation	1	0	1	1
Total ablation procedures	54	22	76	100
Adjuvant right flutter ablation[1]	20	11	31	-

[1] Right atrial flutter ablation carried out as part of main procedure

The success rates for the different types of procedures are shown below. Complete success is defined as being afib-free without the use of antiarrhythmics at the end of the first year following the initial procedure (ignoring the outcome of any follow-up procedures that may have been done within the first year). The most successful procedures were the pulmonary vein antrum isolation (Natale protocol) and the segmental pulmonary vein isolation (Haissaguerre protocol) with success rates of 76% and 56% for the initial procedures. The poorest performers were the circumferential pulmonary vein isolation procedure (Pappone protocol) at 29%, focal ablation at 17% and generic pulmonary vein ablation at 22%. The overall success rate for initial RF ablations was 44%.

Complete Success Rate, Initial Procedure		
Procedure	# in Group	Success, %*
Focal ablation	6	17
Pulmonary vein ablation (PVA)	8	22
Segmental PVI	9	56
Circumferential PVI	7	29
Antrum PVI	17	76
Unspecified	6	17
Cryoablation	1	0
Total catheter ablation procedures	54	44

* Defined as being AF-free without use of antiarrhythmics 1 year
   from date of initial ablation

The outcome of the final procedure (which was the initial procedure in 59% of cases) for various categories of afib and respondent characteristics is presented below.

Outcome of Final Procedure				
Type of Afib	# in Group	Complete Success, %	Partial Success, %	Failure, %
Adrenergic	1	100	0	0
Mixed	26	77	19	4
Vagal	12	75	8	17
Paroxysmal – not sure	3	67	33	0
Total paroxysmal	42	76	17	7
Persistent	1	0	0	100
Permanent*	11	91	0	9
Overall success	54	78	13	9

* 78% of procedures done by Pr. Haissaguerre or Dr. Natale

The goal of the 2013 ablation survey was to determine the "longevity" of procedures which had been initially successful, defined as being afib-free without the use of antiarrhythmics, during the index period following the final (or only) procedure for the purpose of curing AF. Index period, in turn, is defined as the last 6 months of the 12-month period following completion of the final procedure. In the 2013 survey, 42 respondents met this rather strict definition, while the remaining 12 did not – they were either experiencing afib episodes or using antiarrhythmics during the index period. Nevertheless, all 54 respondents were included in the evaluation of procedure outcome in order to determine the importance of an afib-free index period for the long-term prognosis.

All 54 respondents provided data until the end of the 8th year following their final procedure – 33 provided data for year 9, 17 provided data for year 10, and 3 provided data for year 11 after their latest ablation.

The outcomes, by year, for all ablations as well as for initially successful (no afib, no antiarrhythmics during index period) and initially unsuccessful (afib episodes or use of antiarrhythmics during index period) catheter ablations are presented below.

Overall Procedure Outcome						
	Yr 1	Yr 4	Yr 8	Yr 9	Yr 10	Yr 11
Paroxysmal						
# of respondents[1]	42	42	42	27	15	2
Complete success, %	76	57	63	59	67	50
Partial success, %	7	4	4	7	7	0
Failure, %	17	22	16	33	27	50
Persistent & Permanent						
# of respondents[1]	12	12	12	6	2	1
Compl. success, %[2]	83	85	64	67	50	0
Partial success, %	0	0	0	0	0	50
Failure, %	17	8	21	33	50	0
Total						
# of respondents[1]	54	54	54	33	17	3
Complete success, %	78	74	76	61	65	33
Partial success, %	6	4	4	6	6	33
Failure, %	17	22	20	33	29	33

[1] # of respondents who reported their afib status and use of antiarrhythmics for indicated period
[2] 78% of procedures done by Pr. Haissaguerre or Dr. Natale

Outcome for Initially Successful Ablation Procedures[1]						
	Yr 1	Yr 4	Yr 8	Yr 9	Yr 10	Yr 11
Paroxysmal						
# of respondents[2]	32	32	32	19	10	2
Complete success, %	100	81	88	79	90	50
Partial success, %	0	0	0	0	0	0
Failure, %	0	19	13	21	10	50
Persistent & Permanent						
# of respondents[2]	10	10	10	5	1	0
Compl. success, %[3]	100	100	80	80	100	
Partial success, %	0	0	0	0	0	
Failure, %	0	0	20	20	0	
Total						
# of respondents[2]	42	42	42	24	11	2
Complete success, %	100	86	86	79	91	50
Partial success, %	0	0	0	0	0	0
Failure, %	0	14	14	21	9	50

Initially Unsuccessful Ablation Procedure[1]						
	Yr 1	Yr 4	Yr 8	Yr 9	Yr 10	Yr 11
Paroxysmal						
# of respondents[2]	10	10	10	8	5	0
Compl. success, %	0	30	40	13	20	
Partial success, %	30	20	20	25	20	
Failure, %	70	50	40	63	60	
Persistent & Permanent						
# of respondents[2]	2	2	2	1	1	0
Compl. success, %	0	50	50	0	0	
Partial success, %	0	0	0	0	0	
Failure, %	100	50	50	100	100	
Total						
# of respondents[2]	12	12	12	9	6	0
Compl. success, %	0	33	42	11	17	
Partial success, %	25	17	17	22	17	
Failure, %	75	50	42	67	67	

It is clear that having an initially successful final ablation is of prime importance
in determining the long-term success of the procedure. The average (median)
complete success rate (no afib, no antiarrhythmics) at the end of year 8 was
86% for those whose last procedure was initially successful versus 42% for
those who had not experienced an afib-free index period or who had been on
antiarrhythmics during the index period. This difference is statistically
significant (p=0.01).

It will no doubt be of interest to many afibbers that, of the 40 respondents who
were afib-free (without the use of antiarrhythmics) in year 4, only 2 (5%)
reverted to having afib episodes by year 8. One more afibber (9% of the 11
afibbers for whom data was available in year 10) reverted to having afib in year
10, indicating that status at year 4 is a good indicator of long-term prognosis.

Change in afib burden

Prior to the initial catheter ablation, all respondents experienced symptomatic paroxysmal AF episodes or were in permanent (24/7) AF. At the end of the 4th year following the last catheter ablation 6 paroxysmal afibbers who were not on antiarrhythmics provided data allowing a comparison between pre-ablation afib burden and year 4 afib burden. Their afib burden and percent time spent in afib were reduced by an average (median) of 98% (p=0.03). This was reflected in a 97% reduction in impact on quality of life (p=0.04).

The reduction in afib burden and percent time spent in afib were also reduced in year 8 as compared to pre-ablation values; however, the reduction (80%) was no longer statistically significant (p=0.06) but the reduction in impact on quality of life (88%) remained statistically significant (p=0.05). NOTE: It is of course likely that the differences would be statistically significant if a larger sample size had been available.

These findings may indicate that, while an unsuccessful ablation still results in a significantly lower afib burden and improved quality of life in paroxysmal afibbers at the 4 year mark, the beneficial effects of the ablation may begin to wear off at the 8 year mark.

Only 3 permanent afibbers had provided data for pre-ablation and year 8. Average reductions in afib burden and percent time spent in afib were close to 100% (p<0.0001) and reduction in impact on quality of life was 99% (p=0.0004).

Change in AF Burden – Year 4				
6 paroxysmal afibbers[1]	Pre-ablation	Year 4	Reduction, %	P-value[2]
Episode frequency – median	52	13	75	0.03
Episode duration, hrs – median	21	4	81	0.1
Episode burden, hrs – median	806	11	99	0.03
Time spent in AF, % - median	19	0.3	98	0.03
Severity score (1-5) – mean	4	3	25	0.05
Impact on QoL[3] – mean	102	3	97	0.04

[1] All values are averages for 6-month periods (182 days) and apply to catheter ablation only
[2] Statistical significance (two-tailed p-value) of difference between median pre-procedure values and values for year 4
[3] Impact on Quality of Life is calculated as severity score multiplied with % time spent in AF. A score of zero corresponds to no AF, while a score of 500 corresponds to being in debilitating permanent (24/7) AF. NOTE: No data available for permanent afibbers in year 4

258

Change in AF Burden – Year 8				
6 paroxysmal afibbers[1]	Pre-ablation	Year 8	Reduction, %	P-value[2]
Episode frequency – median	52	36	31	0.4
Episode duration, hrs – median	21	6	71	0.3
Episode burden, hrs – median	806	158	80	0.06
Time spent in AF, % - median	19	3.6	81	0.06
Severity score (1-5) – mean	4	3	25	0.02
Impact on QoL[3] – mean	102	12	88	0.05
3 permanent afibbers[1]				
Episode frequency – median	182	1	99	<0.0001
Episode duration, hrs – median	24	18	25	0.8
Episode burden, hrs – median	4368	18	100	<0.0001
Time spent in AF, % - median	100	0.4	100	<0.0001
Severity score (1-5) – mean	3.6	4.3	(19)	0.4
Impact on QoL[3] – mean	366	3.3	99	0.0004

[1] All values are averages for 6-month periods (182 days) and apply to catheter ablation only. Pre-ablation burden is for burden prior to 1st ablation for AF

[2] Statistical significance (two-tailed p-value) of difference between median pre-procedure values and values for year 8

[3] Impact on Quality of Life is calculated as severity score multiplied with % time spent in AF. A score of zero corresponds to no AF, while a score of 500 corresponds to being in debilitating permanent (24/7) AF

Change in triggers

A previous LAF survey involving 198 afibbers uncovered a number of triggers involved in initiating afib episodes. The most common were:

- Caffeine
- Alcohol
- Physical overexertion
- Heavy evening meals
- Aspartame
- Sleeping on left side
- Emotional stress
- Dehydration
- Monosodium glutamate (MSG)
- High glycemic index foods
- Cold drinks
- Tyramine-containing foods

Since these triggers can all be avoided it would be of interest to see if afib episodes occurring after the final ablation/maze procedure are associated with pre-procedure triggers. NOTE: The following data is from a previous survey.

Triggers – Same Trigger as Before Final Procedure					
	Year 2, %	Yrs 3-4, %	Yrs 5-6, %	Yrs 7-10, %	Average, %
Yes	29	36	37	20	33
Yes, most of the time	10	4	16	10	10
Yes, sometimes	19	16	21	10	18
Not certain	29	36	21	40	32
No	14	8	5	0	8
# of respondents[1]	21	25	19	10	-

[1] # of respondents answering question concerning triggers

It is apparent that 43% of afibbers still experiencing afib believe that their episodes were always, or most of the time, associated with the same triggers that initiated episodes prior to the initial ablation/maze procedure for the purpose of curing AF. Only 8% were quite certain that their episodes were not associated with pre-procedure triggers, while 32% were not certain whether or not they were.

Thus, it would seem prudent for afibbers who have experienced an episode following their last procedure to avoid, as much as possible, the triggers that initiated their episodes prior to undergoing the initial ablation or maze procedure.

Other arrhythmias

The incidence of other arrhythmias (atrial flutter, tachycardia and ectopics) following the final procedure is tabulated in Table 14 below.

Other Arrhythmias[1]				
	Index Period	Year 4	Year 8	Average
Complete success[2]	36%	40%	27%	34%
Partial success[3]	67%	50%	100%	71%
Failure[4]	67%	67%	55%	63%
Total respondents	54	54	54	-

[1] Respondents whose latest procedure was a catheter ablation done at least 8 years ago
[2] No AF episodes and no use of antiarrhythmics during indicated period
[3] No AF episodes, but using antiarrhythmics during indicated period
[4] Experiencing AF episodes with or without the use of antiarrhythmics

It is clear that afibbers whose latest ablation had been a complete success experienced fewer episodes of other arrhythmias than did those who were still experiencing afib episodes (failures) or were keeping episodes at bay with antiarrhythmics (partial success). On average (over the 8 year evaluation period) 34% of afibbers having undergone a completely successful ablation experienced other arrhythmias as compared to 71% (p=0.003) among those with a partially successful ablation and 63% (p=0.05) among afibbers with a failed ablation. The presence of other arrhythmias (mostly ectopics) was still common among even successful afibbers and very common among those controlling their episodes with antiarrhythmics. The reason for this is unclear, but it may be that ectopics experienced by successful afibbers are mainly PVCs, the frequency of which would not be affected even by a successful ablation procedure. As for the high level of other arrhythmias (mostly ectopics) experienced by afibbers taking antiarrhythmics, it is possible that they are related to the inherent pro-arrhythmic effect of most antiarrhythmics.

Factors affecting year 8 outcome

The factors that may affect long-term outcome of catheter ablations were evaluated for 54 respondents who knew their afib status at the end of year 8. The respondents were divided into two groups – group 1 consisted of 41 afibbers who had not used antiarrhythmics and who had not experienced any episodes during year 8 (complete success: 100%); group 2 consisted of 13 afibbers who either experienced episodes during year 8 (failure: 85%), or had remained free of episodes through the use of antiarrhythmics (partial success: 15%).

Table 15 compares a number of factors that could potentially explain the significant outcome differences between the two groups. In considering this analysis it should be kept in mind that differences that are found to be statistically non-significant (NS or p>0.05) may well prove to be significant in studies involving a larger number of participants.

Comparative Data at Year 8			
	Group 1 Success	Group 2 Failure	Significance of Difference
Number of participants	41	13	-
Demographics			
Percent male	83	77	NS
Percent female	17	23	NS
Average (mean) age at 1st episode, years	51	48	NS
Underlying heart disease, %	7	15	NS
Enlarged left atrium, %	22	23	NS
AF burden prior to 1st procedure[1]			
Episode frequency (# in 6-month period)	52	52	NS
Episode duration (median), hours	6	6	NS
AF burden (hrs spent in AF in 6 months)	156	432	NS
AF burden (% time spent in AF in 6 months)	4	10	NS
AF severity (mean – scale of 1 to 5)	3.7	4.1	NS
Impact on QoL (mean range 0-500)	74	49	NS

Arrhythmias during blanking period			
No arrhythmias, %	22	0	NS
Atrial fibrillation, %	20	38	NS
Atrial flutter, %	7	38	p=0.005
Tachycardia, %	10	38	p=0.02
Ectopics (PACs and PVCs), %	34	46	NS
Arrhythmias during index period			
No arrhythmias, %	65	17	p=0.003
Atrial fibrillation, %	10	42	p=0.01
Atrial flutter, %	0	33	p=<0.0001
Tachycardia, %	5	33	p=0.006
Ectopics (PACs and PVCs), %	23	33	NS
Timing of procedures			
Average (mean) age at 1st procedure	57	56	NS
Years from 1st episode to initial procedure	6	7	NS
Average (mean) age at last procedure	58	56	NS
Years from 1st procedure to last procedure	7	8	NS
Average number of procedures	1.4	1.5	NS
Months (average) between procedures	19	14	NS
Type of last or only procedure			
Circumferential PVI, %	12	0	NS
Pulmonary vein antrum isolation, %	49	15	p=0.03
Segmental PVI, %	22	15	NS
Generic PVA, %	5	31	p=0.009
Focal ablation, %	10	31	p=0.07
Other catheter ablation procedures, %	2	8	NS
Right atrial flutter ablation, %[2]	53	62	NS
Procedures done at top institutions, %[3]	73	46	p=0.07
Medications prior to initial procedure			
Antiarrhythmics, %	71	15	p=0.08
Beta or calcium channel blockers, %	26	0	NS
Medications during blanking period			
Antiarrhythmics, %	0	0	NS
Beta or calcium channel blockers, %	23	27	NS
Medications during index period			
Antiarrhythmics, %	7	27	p=0.06
Beta or calcium channel blockers, %	16	27	NS
Supplementation			
With the "essential trio", %[4]	47	27	NS

[1] Paroxysmal afibbers only
[2] Right atrial flutter ablation done as part of AF ablation
[3] % of procedures done at top 15 institutions as determined in
2008 Ablation/Maze Survey
[4] Supplementation with one or more of the "essential trio"
components (magnesium, potassium, and taurine) during the 1st year
following last procedure.

There are no statistically significant differences in general background variables between the two groups. Afib burden and severity prior to the initial procedure are also not significantly different between the two groups indicating that the long-term outcome of an ablation is independent of how bad the afib status was prior to the initial procedure.

The difference in the frequency of arrhythmias observed during the index period is however, not surprisingly, statistically extremely significant, again confirming that the absence of afib episodes during the index period is of crucial importance in predicting a favourable long-term outcome. It is also evident that experiencing atrial flutter or tachycardia during the index period heralds a poor 8-year outcome as does experiencing these arrhythmias during the blanking period.

Age at time of procedures and duration of afib prior to procedures did not affect year 8 outcome and the number of procedures and the time span between them did not affect long-term outcome either.

The type of ablation procedure did, however, affect year 8 outcome. Forty-nine per cent of afibbers in group 1 had undergone a pulmonary vein antrum isolation (PVAI) procedure while only 15% had done so in group 2. This difference was statistically significant (p=0.03). In contrast, 31% of members of group 2 had undergone a "generic" pulmonary vein ablation (PVA) while only 5% of members of group 1 had done so. This difference again was statistically significant (p=0.009). Focal ablations were also associated with a poorer long term outcome. There was a trend (p=0.07) for ablations done at top-ranked institutions to have a better long-term outcome with 73% of group 1 members having undergone their ablation at such an institution as compared to only 46% of group 2 having done so. This observation is strongly supportive of the results of previous ablation surveys, which have all concluded that the all-important factor in short-term (1 year) success is the experience and expertise of the EPs performing the procedures.

Finally, there was a trend for long-term outcome being better among afibbers who had been on antiarrhythmics prior to their initial procedure (p=0.08) while afibbers who had needed antiarrhythmics during the index period tended to have a poorer year 8 outcome (p=0.06).

Clearly, a very important factor in predicting the long-term (8 year) outcome of a catheter ablation is the absence of arrhythmias (atrial fibrillation, flutter and tachycardia) during the index period (last 6 months of the 12-month period following the final procedure for the purpose of curing AF). The factors that significantly influence afib occurrence during the index period are listed below.

Comparative Data for Index Period			
	Group 1 Success	Group 2 Failure	Significance of Difference
Number of participants	42	12	-
Demographics			
Percent female	12	42	0.02
Arrhythmias during blanking period			
Atrial fibrillation, %	17	46	0.02
Atrial flutter, %	10	31	0.04
Arrhythmias during index period			
Atrial flutter, %	2	25	0.008
Type of last or only procedure			
Segmental or antrum PVI procedure, %	74	17	0.0002
Procedure done at top institutions, %[1]	76	33	0.005
Medications during blanking period			
Beta or calcium channel blockers, %	19	50	0.03
Medications during index period			
Beta or calcium channel blockers, %	10	50	0.001

[1] Procedures done at top 15 institutions as determined in the 2008 Ablation/Maze Survey

It is again clear that the skill and expertise of the EPs doing the procedures are the key factors in determining whether or not the index period will be free of afib episodes. Seventy-six per cent of successful procedures (group 1: no afib and no antiarrhythmics during index period) were done at top-ranked institutions and 74% involved either a PVAI or a segmental PVI. In contrast, only 33% of failed procedures (group 2: afib episodes or use of antiarrhythmics during index period) were done at top-ranked institutions and only 17% involved a PVAI or segmental PVI procedure. Both of these differences are statistically extremely significant (p=0.005 and p=0.0002).

Female afibbers were more likely to be found in group 2 (42%) than in group 1 (12%) and this difference was statistically significant (p=0.02). Experiencing atrial fibrillation or atrial flutter during the blanking period was also associated with a greater chance of not experiencing an afib-free index period, as was experiencing atrial flutter during the index period itself (p=0.008). Finally, needing beta-blockers or calcium channel blockers during the blanking period and the index period was also associated with a significantly reduced chance of being afib-free during the index period.

Case Histories
From The AFIB Report
April 2008 – April 2009

The following case histories describe the protocols used by six afibbers to either completely eliminate their afib or reduce their afib burden by at least 95%.

56-year-old woman with vagal afib

Demographics and Afib Burden

Years of AF	10 years
Underlying heart disease?	No
# of episodes prior to protocol*	48
Afib burden prior to protocol*	192 hours
# of episodes after protocol*	2
Afib burden after protocol*	2 hours
Time on protocol	6 months
Trigger avoidance?	Yes, but much less so

*over a 6-month period

Main Components of Protocol

Trigger avoidance	MSG, aspartame, other excitatory food additives, caffeine, high glycemic foods, heavy evening meals, dehydration
Diet changes	Elimination of wheat and adopted Zone diet
Supplementation	Magnesium, potassium, taurine, coenzyme Q10
Drug therapy	None
Stress management	Relaxation therapy, breathing exercises
Approaches to shorten episodes	Light exercise, hydrotherapy (ice baths, icy water on hands, hot/cold showers)
Approaches to reduce ectopics	Supplementation with magnesium, potassium, taurine, and low-sodium V8 juice

Background and Details

I was having increased episodes with the use of Toprol XL which my doctor prescribed. I had taken the drug for 2 years. I began suffering with PACs and ectopics every day as well. During that time I was faithfully avoiding every trigger I could. My situation only got worse. The first thing I did was to purchase Hans' book. I determined, with the help of his book, the web site, and the people participating on the Bulletin Board, that I was probably vagal and needed to eliminate the beta-blocker. I stopped the beta-blocker (slowly) at the same time I began experimenting with adding supplements. I experimented with dosages of magnesium to determine my bowel tolerance.

I had always taken calcium and fish oil. I stopped those because my research indicated that they could be counter-productive. All the while I had changed my diet and continued to exercise, but not with the vengeance I used to. I eat breakfast now; I never used to. I eliminated bread and have increased my veggies. I'm not a fruit eater, but admittedly I have always had a lousy diet. I avoid triggers, watch my diet, exercise, drink lots of water and take my supplements. My biggest trigger is a large meal, especially in the evening. I try to walk or stay active at night after a meal. All this with my EP's blessing. He has given me Toprol for pill-in-the-pocket usage, but I have yet to use them. I am an avid golfer and will play in the heat of the day. I am very careful to avoid becoming dehydrated all the time, but especially when I am out golfing. I carry my own bag and walk, so I'm loaded down with water. All of these supplements are taken after food: one 500-mg magnesium in the morning and one in the evening, one 500-mg taurine in the morning and one in the evening. All of these are in the morning only - 1 multi, 500 mg Vit C, 100 mg of potassium, 150 mg CoQ10, 325 mg aspirin (doctor's continued wish, although I have only age and afib as risk factors) I know some of these doses (taurine, Vit C, magnesium) are low, but they are currently working. Perhaps I can increase them if things change.

I started out purchasing my supplements at the corner drug store out of frustration. Once my current supply is gone, I fully intend to use the services in Hans' supplement store. My education has included the need to be careful with supplements and I need to purchase the best forms of the products I take. I have yet to avoid an activity or an opportunity because of afib. Once, I played a round of golf while in afib. It did affect my putting! I think a positive attitude will go a long way in meeting this condition head on. Lastly, I'm very lucky because my condition is mild compared to many. I know from reading postings that some people suffer far more than I do. For that, I am grateful, but I have compassion for those who are not as fortunate.

Demographics and Afib Burden

Years of AF	25 years
Underlying heart disease?	No
# of episodes prior to protocol*	Permanent
Afib burden prior to protocol*	2160 hrs.
# of episodes after protocol*	3
Afib burden after protocol*	6 hours
Time on protocol	7.5 years
Trigger avoidance?	No

*over a 6-month period

Main Components of Protocol

Trigger avoidance	MSG, aspartame, alcohol, caffeine, high glycemic index foods, dehydration
Diet changes	Changed to Paleo diet
Supplementation	None
Drug therapy	None
Stress management	None
Approaches to shorten episodes	Not applicable
Approaches to reduce ectopics	Paleo diet

Background and Details

I first experienced AF at 22 years of age. It came out of the blue after the birth of my first son. Unfortunately, sometimes when it happened I would pass out. Witnesses said I convulsed, so the diagnosis came as epilepsy. I was put on anticonvulsants which never worked. In the beginning my AF was maybe twice or three times a week. Always at rest. It was short-lived, well the really fast racing part was short lived – maybe 2 to 4 hours (in the end it could go on for days, then became permanent). Every so often I would visit my GP and complain, but was told it was just palpitations and I was being over anxious. So decided they must be panic attacks and gave up on doctors.

Nine years later I was finally diagnosed with atrial fibrillation and was put on digoxin which I stayed on for 10 years. In 2000 I finally saw a new cardiologist who said that I should never have been put on digoxin. I was then put on Rythmol (propafenone) and when this did not work sotalol, flecainide, and atenolol followed.

All these drugs had terrible side effects, so in December 2001 I stopped taking all medications. In October of 2000 I had started a program of trigger elimination (notably MSG and food additives) and had also adopted the paleo diet. In hindsight my diet had been very refined which led to leaky gut (with no digestive symptoms) so that my body was very low on all nutrients. The paleo diet cut out the problem foods, helped heal the gut, didn't feed bad bacteria and allowed good bacteria to flourish, thus allowing absorptions of all the major nutrients. Excitatory neurotransmitters such as MSG, aspartame, etc. played havoc since there were not enough minerals, vitamins, etc to make inhibitory neurotransmitters, hormones, etc. and the liver was under undue stress and unable to break down and eliminate toxins. Starchy foods such as grains and potatoes played havoc with blood sugar levels as there were no glycogen stores in the liver or muscle to fall back on.

This was verified by hair tissue analysis which showed that I was still low on all minerals except vitamin K which was very high (and had an inverse ratio with Na – very low), meaning that K is not readily available for use in the body. The lack of available K meant it was difficult for insulin to be delivered into cell walls for storage, and also couldn't polarize nerve impulses. As mineral levels increased the problems subsided. Obviously, the whole scenario is a lot more complex than discussed above; however, it is my opinion that my AF was a culmination of long-term malnutrition that could not be sorted out by taking supplements since they could not be metabolized, and the underlying reasons had to be dealt with first.

Since then I have played around with my diet, as after curing my AF, I became aware of reactive hypoglycemia. Happily, I have overcome this, but of course, I have to stick to my paleo diet. I prefer it this way since I have regained my health. I have cured more than just AF – don't suffer from fibromyalgia, headaches, tremors, seizures, and fainting. The only thing I have not solved is low blood pressure, but I can live with that!

52-year-old man with vagal afib

Demographics and Afib Burden

Years of AF	4 years
Underlying heart disease?	No
# of episodes prior to protocol*	7
Afib burden prior to protocol*	49 hours
# of episodes after protocol*	0
Afib burden after protocol*	0 hours.
Time on protocol	43 months
Trigger avoidance?	No

*over a 6-month period

268

Main Components of Protocol

Trigger avoidance	None
Diet changes	None
Supplementation	Magnesium, potassium, taurine
Drug therapy	Pill-in-pocket flecainide
Stress management	None
Approaches to shorten episodes	Pill-in-pocket flecainide
Approaches to reduce ectopics	Magnesium, potassium, taurine

Background and Details

I am a vagal afibber and a life-long exerciser. I am sufficiently fit to compete annually in a 13-mile race up Pike's Peak (14,100', 4,300m elevation, 7850' elevation gain). In the summer of 2004 several days after a long training day on a 14'er, I woke up with a rapid, irregular heart beat and was subsequently diagnosed with lone atrial fibrillation. During the next 2 months I experienced 5 more classically vagal episodes starting around 3 AM. These either converted on their own or converted with exercise after about 7 hours. The next episode, however, lasted 2.5 months, but I was eventually able to convert it by taking 300 mg of flecainide (conversion took 20 hours).

Early on, I found the LAF Bulletin Board and purchased Hans' first book. I looked at low potassium (hypokalemia) as a potential issue. Prior to afib, I'd had two annual blood tests with serum potassium levels at the low end of normal - 3.5 mmol/l. The day of my first episode, my level was 3.2 in the ER. Five days later it was 4.2 in the doctor's office.

My conclusion was that I had intermittent hypokalemia. I set out to design a supplement program that would keep my serum K above 4.2. This program includes 3 grams of potassium as citrate, 0.8 grams magnesium as glycinate and 4 grams of taurine per day. All doses are divided and taken morning and evening around meal time. I proposed to my EP that I use on-demand flecainide as a back-up in case the supplements failed. He agreed.

After ending the 2.5-month episode, I started supplements. Here are the subsequent episodes:

1. 1 month – 3 AM episode, converted 20 hours after taking 300 mg flecainide
2. 4.5 months – midnight episode, converted 20 minutes after taking 300 mg flecainide
3. 5.5 months – 3 AM episode, converted 20 minutes after taking 300 mg flecainide
4. 2.5 years – 11 PM episode, in vagal period after sexual climax. Converted 50 minutes after taking 300 mg flecainide.

Notes – prior to episodes 2 & 3, I'd run out of taurine and not bothered to replace it. Episode 4 occurred, 3 days after ceasing all supplements. This was evidence that all three supplements are essential for me. Episode 2 was a bit unusual, as I'd snow-shoed for 4 hours through heavy snow with a 75-pound pack and then spent 6 hours of hard work constructing a snow cave. It came on after I'd gone to bed. Normally I would crush the flecainide in warm water, however all I had was partially frozen water bottle. I chewed the flecainide tablets and washed them down with near freezing water – still effective.

When I started the supplement program, I also started a monitoring program with a Polar S810 heart rate monitor and a FreezeFramer heart rate monitor. Using them I was able to count PAC and PVC rates/hour. PAC's typically run 0-2/hr and PVC's 0-20/hr. My monitoring concept is that an increase in ectopic rates will foreshadow afib. The results could also be used to "tweak" the supplement program.

For anyone copying this program, I recommend BUN and creatinine tests to make sure your kidneys are OK. Also start slowly with the supplements and gradually increase dosages.

A couple of other, perhaps unrelated notes. When I was out of rhythm for 2.5 months, I gained 20 lbs (9.1 kg). I decided a good approach to losing weight would be to keep my blood sugar low and level. I purchased the most accurate home glucometer I could find – Bayer Ascencia Contour. I sampled my blood sugar 45 minutes (usually maximum spike) after eating and would modify my meals such that I'd keep this spike to around 100 or 110 mg/dL (6.1 mmol/l) or less. This allowed me to drop the excess weight in around 2 months. This did not have any bearing on my success at keeping afib in remission, I only include it for general information.

The reason I stopped all supplements prior to episode 4 is that I thought I might be allergic to the fillers in the pills. I subsequently underwent an Elisa IgE/IgG test and determined that I was allergic to wheat, dairy, eggs, soy, almonds, grapes ... These were the source of my allergy, not the pills.

I have had a regular meditation habit for many years (before and after I ended up with afib). I have not seen any effect on afib by meditation.

In summary, I'm very happy with my program. I am still very active, exercising on the excessive side of moderate. However I no longer train for endurance activities and try to keep my heart rate under 130 BPM during daily exercise (in fact, a lot of my exercise is in the 100 to 110 BPM range). However, I have done long hard days of exercise with high HR without adverse effect. I just try not to make it too regular a habit and limit them to FUN activities – not training. I do pay attention to my early morning resting HR. If it is elevated by 10 BPM or more, it is a sign that: 1) I've overdone it the day before, or 2) I'm coming down with some illness. In either case, I take it very easy.

65-year-old woman with vagal afib

Demographics and Afib Burden

Years of AF	7 years
Underlying heart disease?	No
# of episodes prior to protocol*	4-5
Afib burden prior to protocol*	4 hours
# of episodes after protocol*	0
Afib burden after protocol*	0 hours.
Time on protocol	58 months
Trigger avoidance?	No

*over a 6-month period

Main Components of Protocol

Trigger avoidance	MSG, caffeine, high glycemic index foods, dehydration, emotional stress
Diet changes	Eliminated gluten and wheat, sharply reduced intake of dairy products, switched to Paleo diet
Supplementation	Magnesium, potassium, taurine and low-sodium V8 juice
Drug therapy	Lisinopril (Zestril) 10 mg/day
Stress management	Avoid stressful relationships
Approaches to shorten episodes	None
Approaches to reduce ectopics	Potassium and low-sodium V8 juice

Background and Details

My first brush with afib was in late '99 while working a stressful job. I was 57 years old, seriously overweight, had that year gone through a lot of stressful life changes, was eating poorly [whatever I could pick up in the convenience store I worked in], it was hot weather and I had no air conditioning, and I was surviving on coffee. I had a couple of short episodes that went away before I could get to a doctor, and of course when I did get to the doctor he found nothing wrong. Then I had one that did not go away, and ended up in the hospital for 3 days. I changed jobs after that, and worked more normal hours, dropped the

271

coffee and ate better [more vegetables, less junk], and had no more afib until August 2000, when I was hospitalized again with another "just-won't-go-away" episode. This again was associated with caffeine [green tea this time, dozens of cups of it, trying to stay awake at work] and hot weather, compounded by lack of sleep. After that I dropped caffeine altogether, and got an air conditioner.

For the next several years I had short episodes occasionally, but they always went away by themselves, and in any case, I was getting turned off by hospital emergency rooms. I had learned a little about using computers by that time, and was researching better nutrition. I retired and moved back to Maine, and eventually got my own computer, and found Hans' site. Here I found there were a lot of people taking various drugs, and none of these drugs seemed to be curing their afib. They were still getting afib attacks, trading drug advice, going on different drugs, and still getting afib. Some of them were talking about, and some even resorting to, heart surgery. I couldn't blame them for doing this, because their afib had started small and gradually increased until it ruled their lives. I was afraid mine would do that too.

Worse yet, by no means all of those ablation patients had gotten rid of their afib either. Two of them had had near-death experiences, and I was pretty sure that the reason there were not more stories like that was because most ablations that went bad had resulted in death, and of course, we are not very likely to hear from those people. And then there were 2 people posting who claimed to have gotten rid of their afib by diet and supplements. These were Fran and Erling.

Well, I thought, if these 2 people so different from one another can do that, maybe I can too. Food choices are something I can control. So I changed to a mostly paleo diet, and sent away for some Carlson's magnesium glycinate. At first I still did get some short, mild afib episodes, but then I began seeing posts about low sodium V8 juice, 850 mg potassium per 8 oz. glass. I was having trouble consuming enough vegetables and fruits to get in 3-5 grams K a day, and this seemed like just what I needed, and sure enough it was. The taurine I added later when I began to experience loose bowels from my usual dosage of magnesium glycinate.

The Paleo diet
The paleo diet is based on the premise that the human body thrives best on the diet of our hunter/gatherer forebears of 10,000 years ago, ie. before the introduction of agriculture. The proponents of the diet point out that the human genomic make-up is very slow to change and has not had a chance to adjust to the very major changes in diet that have occurred since the Stone Age. The hunter/gatherers of the Stone Age consumed a diet based on fish and meat from wild animals, vegetables, berries, fruits and nuts. Grains and dairy

products were not available. The paleo diet thus emphasizes the above food sources and excludes dairy products, grains, starchy vegetables, sugar and legumes, and of course, chemical food additives. The paleo diet is described in detail in the book "The Paleo Diet" by Loren Cordain, PhD and at www.paleodiet.com

Concerning those few short, mild episodes, I think a lot of what paleo did for me was eliminated postprandial hypoglycemia. A paleo diet pretty much prohibits high glycemic load foods. Jackie and others had called my attention to the fact that a lot of my afib symptoms were the same symptoms as those of reactive hypoglycemia - shaky, lightheadedness, cold sweat, panic - and sure enough, the minor episodes I got soon after converting to paleo lacked just those features. I wasn't sorry to see them go.

Also, I need to mention that those last episodes, mild though they were, appeared right after use of a seasoning containing MSG. I had never had an afib episode that I could tie to MSG before, but then I had never been without it for any period of time before either. For all I really know, they could have all had to do with MSG, in combination with stress, hypoglycemia, dehydration, electrolyte deficiency, caffeine, and any of the other myriad stressors of modern life.

Any paleo diet purist will point out that I ingest a lot of stuff that isn't paleo. The V8 certainly isn't, and neither are the supplements I take. I do eat a little cheese, too, though not the plasticized processed cheese. I cannot afford organic food, so I make do with what I can find in the local supermarket, cheapest first. I go out to eat sometimes, and on those occasions I commit excesses like baked potato and gravy, or bread on sandwiches. I cheat outrageously sometimes, too, particularly with chocolate baked goods.

Speaking of bread, gravy, and bakery goodies, if I hadn't gone to paleo I would also never have realized that I have a bad reaction to wheat. Since taking up the paleo diet my antacid consumption has gone way down, except when I eat anything with wheat in it. That will have me eating antacids for a good 12 hours and sometimes more.

Another good thing about the paleo diet is that I fit the classic profile for insulin resistance - fat, high blood pressure, relatively inactive, cholesterol a bit on the high side - and the paleo diet is good for insulin resistance. I hope to avoid type 2 diabetes this way, or at least to slow it down.

For those concerned about whether my afib is "really cured", I do not think I can expect to be cured of needing proper nutrition, any more than cars are cured of needing gasoline. I don't think I am going to ever again be just like I was in my 20's either. To use the same metaphor, old cars are never again just like they were when new.

I think afib is one of the long latency deficiency diseases, and that is why, in most people, it does not appear until a relatively 'older' age, and why it appears in the context of stress so often. I am still old, fat, and lame in the knees, but I don't have afib anymore. If I can do this, you can too.

47-year-old man with mixed afib

Demographics and Afib Burden

Years of AF	12 years
Underlying heart disease?	No
# of episodes prior to protocol*	45
Afib burden prior to protocol*	630 hours
# of episodes after protocol*	3
Afib burden after protocol*	30 hours.
Time on protocol	28 months
Trigger avoidance?	Yes

*over a 6-month period

Main Components of Protocol

Trigger avoidance	MSG, caffeine, high glycemic index foods, stress, heavy evening meals, physical overexertion, alcohol, mercury (tuna)
Diet changes	Zone diet and 4-5 small meals throughout day
Supplementation	Magnesium, potassium, taurine, fish oil, coenzyme Q10
Drug therapy	Beta-blocker + flecainide
Stress management	Regular exercise
Approaches to shorten episodes	On demand beta-blocker + flecainide
Approaches to reduce ectopics	Beta-blocker

Background and Details

I started off with the recommendations on Hans' website and publications. Largely a change in lifestyle with emphasis on taking things a bit easier, avoiding large meals (especially at bedtime) and taking the above supplements, including large doses of fish oil (3 500-mg enteric-coated fish oil capsules and one large fish oil gel cap daily). I also had some benefits from eliminating all tuna (mercury issue) and limiting swordfish to about once/month. Anecdotally,

I believe this helped. Also, I believe MSG was a trigger and tried to avoid this. Later, I discovered that a diet with lots of protein and complex carbs (similar to zone diet) was helpful.

Typically I have a hearty breakfast with eggs and some type of low-fat meat (Canadian bacon or turkey sausage or bacon) and some kind of fresh fruit. Just before (late afternoon) exercise, yogurt mixed with more fruit. After exercise a protein shake mixed with a banana and some nuts.

Then I try to have a healthy Zone diet type dinner in the evening (meat about the size of a deck of cards and a vegetable). I try to have no bread whatsoever. I also drink about 3 liters of water daily and steer clear of all refined sugar products.

The above protocol was helpful, but I was still having persistent attacks which inhibited my ability to exercise in the day (adrenergic attack) or would wake me up in the middle of the night (vagal). Generally, once the attack went from persistent arrhythmia to full afib, they would go on all night and convert sometime between late morning and early afternoon. Some attacks lasted almost 24 hours. I worked through a cardiologist, who put me on a few beta-blockers and we finally settled on Toprol - 4 x 25 mg/day. I experimented with the timing of taking the pills and try to take a pill around 11:00, 2:00, 5:00 and 8:00. This helped with the daytime attacks but still not satisfactory. Also would "bite" one or two metoprolol during daytime attacks and this seemed to help me convert back within a couple of hours. Unfortunately, the night time attacks were no better. Metoprolol would not help with evening attacks, and may have made some worse. Many sleepless nights were spent listening to the "frog in my chest trying to get out".

I strongly considered ablation, but wanted to give procedure development more time so I opted for flecainide. Flecainide proved to be the final "plank" needed for my program. This worked in two ways. The dosage (3 x 50 mg/day) strongly curtailed the frequency of the attacks. Secondly, if I do get an episode, I have taken up to five additional pills (about three is sufficient most of the time) and will convert in 2-4 hours) - I don't believe I have had a single monster 20-24 hr attack since. Added benefit at this point was "normal sinus rhythm promotes more normal rhythm" - it felt like, over time, the attacks become fewer and fewer, which I think is due to some restoration of "normal" heart circuitry.

So to summarize my (largely successful but not perfect) program (in order of perceived effectiveness/benefit is): - 150 mg flecainide - timed to take most in the evening to address vagal attacks; additional "bite down" flecainide to convert if full afib attack occurs; 100 mg Toprol - timed to keep adrenergic attacks (and PACs) to a minimum; additional "bite down" of 25-50 mg of metoprolol if attacks are adrenergic (daytime); strong magnesium and potassium supplementation; avoidance of heavy meals or heavy drinking to avoid vagal attacks; avoidance of severe mental or emotional stress and over-working; avoidance of mercury and MSG; heavy doses of fish oil; sitting up or standing during the onset of a vagal attack (i.e. lots of PACs or persistent arrhythmia); sitting down during onset of adrenergic attack; Zone-type diet; exercise (weight training) and cardio exercise (possible since I started taking flecainide); listening to your own body - sense when you are more susceptible and be proactive. And finally, take responsibility for your own "cure" - our current medical establishment will only do so much.

60-year-old woman with vagal afib

Demographics and Afib Burden

Years of AF	6 years
Underlying heart disease?	No
# of episodes prior to protocol*	25
Afib burden prior to protocol*	1000 hours
# of episodes after protocol*	0
Afib burden after protocol*	0 hours.
Time on protocol	33 months
Trigger avoidance?	Yes

*over a 6-month period

Main Components of Protocol

Trigger avoidance	MSG, aspartame, caffeine, high glycemic index foods, heavy evening meals, alcohol, dehydration, sleeping on left side
Diet changes	Eliminated gluten and wheat, modified Paleo diet
Supplementation	Magnesium, taurine
Drug therapy	None
Stress management	Breathing exercises, yoga
Approaches to shorten episodes	None
Approaches to reduce ectopics	Magnesium and taurine

Background and Details

I began supplementing with magnesium and taurine almost 2 years ago. I was already supplementing with omega-3 oil, Multibionta, coenzyme Q10, vitamin E, etc., but did not notice any difference until the taurine was added. I now supplement with 4 grams a day. I adopted a modified paleo diet and after

276

having tests for allergies gave up eating wheat and gluten products as I reacted badly to them during the tests. This has resulted in no afib at all for 33 months. Once my cardiologist took me off warfarin, I had an immediate improvement to what remained of my GERD problem. This had already been helped by the supplements. Within a month of stopping the warfarin, the GERD disappeared completely and has not returned. My dietary regimen is very strict and absolute avoidance of triggers is a must, but it continues to be worth the effort.

Details of Content

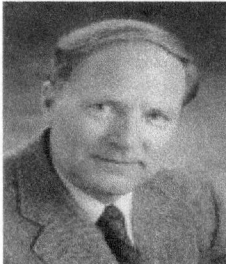

Hans Larsen is a Professional Engineer and holds a Master's degree in chemical engineering from the Technical University of Denmark. He developed a lifelong interest in biochemistry and nutrition through his early studies with Professor Henrik Dam, the Nobel Prize-winning discoverer of vitamin K.

After having been diagnosed with atrial fibrillation and doing extensive research in the field of lone atrial fibrillation and stroke prevention Hans published *Lone Atrial Fibrillation: Towards a Cure* in December 2002. [A revised edition was published in November 2015] followed by *Thrombosis and Stroke Prevention* – a layman's guide to the causes and prevention of ischemic stroke published in 2007. [A third edition of this very popular book was published in April 2018].

Hans' latest book, *The LAF Surveys – What we learned about the causes and treatment of lone atrial fibrillation*, was published in April 2020.

www.ingramcontent.com/pod-product-compliance
Lightning Source LLC
Chambersburg PA
CBHW081459200326
41518CB00015B/2313